# INTERVENTIONAL CARDIOLOGY CLINICS

www.interventional.theclinics.com

*Editor-in-Chief*

MATTHEW J. PRICE

# Interventional Heart Failure

July 2017 • Volume 6 • Number 3

*Editor*

SRIHARI S. NAIDU

**ELSEVIER**

1600 John F. Kennedy Boulevard • Suite 1800 • Philadelphia, Pennsylvania, 19103-2899

http://www.theclinics.com

INTERVENTIONAL CARDIOLOGY CLINICS Volume 6, Number 3
July 2017 ISSN 2211-7458, ISBN-13: 978-0-323-53136-8

Editor: Lauren Boyle
Developmental Editor: Donald Mumford

*Interventional Cardiology Clinics* (ISSN 2211-7458) is published quarterly by Elsevier Inc., 360 Park Avenue South, New York, NY 10010-1710. Months of issue are January, April, July, and October. Subscription prices are USD 195 per year for US individuals, USD 449 for US institutions, USD 100 per year for US students, USD 195 per year for Canadian individuals, USD 536 for Canadian institutions, USD 150 per year for Canadian students, USD 295 per year for international individuals, USD 536 for international institutions, and USD 150 per year for international students. To receive student/resident rate, orders must be accompanied by name of affiliated institution, date of term, and the *signature* of program/residency coordinator on institution letterhead. Orders will be billed at individual rate until proof of status is received. Foreign air speed delivery is included in all *Clinics* subscription prices. All prices are subject to change without notice. **POSTMASTER:** Send address changes to *Interventional Cardiology Clinics*, Elsevier Health Sciences Division, Subscription Customer Service, 3251 Riverport Lane, Maryland Heights, MO 63043. **Customer Service: Telephone: 1-800-654-2452** (U.S. and Canada); **1-314-447-8871** (outside U.S. and Canada). **Fax: 1-314-447-8029. E-mail: journalscustomerservice-usa@elsevier.com (for print support); journalsonlinesupport-usa@elsevier.com (for online support).**

*Reprints.* For copies of 100 or more of articles in this publication, please contact the Commercial Reprints Department, Elsevier Inc., 360 Park Avenue South, New York, NY 10010-1710. Tel.: 212-633-3874; Fax: 212-633-3820; E-mail: reprints@elsevier.com.

# CONTRIBUTORS

**EDITOR-IN-CHIEF**

**MATTHEW J. PRICE, MD**
Director, Cardiac Catheterization Laboratory,
Division of Cardiovascular Diseases, Scripps
Clinic, Assistant Professor, Scripps
Translational Science Institute, La Jolla,
California

**EDITOR**

**SRIHARI S. NAIDU, MD, FACC, FAHA,
FSCAI**
Director, Hypertrophic Cardiomyopathy
Program, Interventional Cardiologist,
Westchester Medical Center, Associate
Professor of Medicine, New York Medical
College, Valhalla, New York

**AUTHORS**

**ANITA W. ASGAR, MD, MSc**
Assistant Professor, Department of Medicine,
Montreal Heart Institute, Universite de
Montreal, Montreal, Quebec, Canada

**GANESH ATHAPPAN, MD**
Valve Science Center, Minneapolis Heart
Institute Foundation; Center for Valve and
Structural Heart Disease, Minneapolis Heart
Institute, Abbott Northwestern Hospital,
Minneapolis, Minnesota

**SUKHDEEP BASRA, MD, MPH**
Department of Cardiology, The Heart Hospital
Baylor Plano, Plano, Texas

**DANIEL BURKHOFF, MD, PhD**
Division of Cardiology, Columbia University,
Cardiovascular Research Foundation, New
York, New York

**CARLOS D. DAVILA, MD**
Interventional Heart Failure Fellow; The Acute
Mechanical Support Working Group, The
Cardiovascular Center, Tufts Medical Center,
Boston, Massachusetts

**V. VIVIAN DIMAS, MD**
Division of Cardiology, Associate Professor,
Department of Pediatrics, University of Texas
Southwestern Medical Center, Children's
Health System of Texas, Dallas, Texas

**SIMON DIXON, MBchB**
Chair, Department of Cardiovascular
Medicine, William Beaumont Hospital, Royal
Oak, Michigan

**MICHAEL ESKANDER, MD**
Cardiology Fellow, Division of Cardiology,
Department of Internal Medicine, University of
California, Irvine Health, Orange, California

**DMITRIY N. FELDMAN, MD**
Associate Professor of Medicine, Division of
Cardiology, Interventional Cardiology and
Endovascular Laboratory, Weill Cornell
Medical College, New York Presbyterian
Hospital, New York, New York

**ARIEL FURER, MD**
Internal Medicine T, Tel-Aviv Sourasky Medical
Center, Tel Aviv, Israel

**JAMES A. GOLDSTEIN, MD**
Director, Cardiovascular Research and
Education, Department of Cardiovascular
Medicine, William Beaumont Hospital, Royal
Oak, Michigan

**GEORGE S. HANZEL, MD**
Director, Cardiac Catheterization Laboratory,
Department of Cardiovascular Medicine,
William Beaumont Hospital, Royal Oak,
Michigan

PRAKASH HARIKRISHNAN, MD
Division of Cardiology, Westchester Medical
Center, New York Medical College, Valhalla,
New York

ZIYAD M. HIJAZI, MD, MPH, FACC,
MSCAI, FAHA
Director, Sidra Cardiac Program; Chair,
Department of Pediatrics, Sidra Medical and
Research Center, Professor of Pediatrics, Weill
Cornell Medicine, Doha, Qatar

RAVI S. HIRA, MD
Division of Cardiology, University of
Washington, School of Medicine, Seattle,
Washington

SEI IWAI, MD, FACC, FHRS
Professor of Clinical Medicine, Director of
Cardiac Electrophysiology, Division of
Cardiology, Westchester Medical Center, New
York Medical College, Valhalla, New York

JASON T. JACOBSON, MD, FACC, FHRS
Associate Professor of Cinical Medicine,
Division of Cardiology, Westchester Medical
Center, New York Medical College, Valhalla,
New York

MARWAN F. JUMEAN, MD
Assistant Professor of Medicine, Interventional
Cardiology and Advanced Heart Failure
Programs; Center for Advanced Heart Failure,
University of Texas Health Medical School,
Houston, Texas

NAVIN K. KAPUR, MD
Associate Professor of Medicine,
Interventional Cardiology and Advanced
Heart Failure Programs; Director, The Acute
Mechanical Support Working Group, The
Cardiovascular Center, Tufts Medical Center,
Boston, Massachusetts

MORTON J. KERN, MD, MSCAI, FACC,
FAHA
Chief, Department of Medicine, VA Long Beach,
Long Beach, California; Professor of Medicine,
Department of Internal Medicine, University of
California, Irvine Health, Orange, California

LUKE K. KIM, MD
Division of Cardiology, Interventional
Cardiology and Endovascular Laboratory,
Weill Cornell Medical College, New York
Presbyterian Hospital, New York, New York

SANDEEP K. KRISHNAN, MD
Division of Cardiology, University of
Washington, School of Medicine, Seattle,
Washington

JUSTINE LACHMANN, MD, FACS
Director, Heart Failure Service, Winthrop
Cardiology Associates, PC, NYU-Winthrop
Hospital, Mineola, New York

JOHN M. LASALA, MD, PhD
Professor of Medicine; Director, Structural
Heart Disease, Cardiovascular Division,
Washington University, St Louis, Missouri

WILLIAM L. LOMBARDI, MD
Division of Cardiology, University of
Washington, School of Medicine, Seattle,
Washington

JOSHUA McKAY, MD
Department of Cardiology, Methodist
DeBakey Heart and Vascular Center, Houston
Methodist Hospital, Houston, Texas

SHERIF F. NAGUEH, MD
Department of Cardiology, Methodist
DeBakey Heart and Vascular Center, Houston
Methodist Hospital, Houston, Texas

ALAN W. NUGENT, MBBS
Associate Professor of Pediatrics, Division
of Cardiology, Department of Pediatrics,
University of Texas Southwestern Medical
Center, Children's Health System of Texas,
Dallas, Texas

AMOLE OJO, MD
Division of Cardiology, Westchester Medical
Center, New York Medical College, Valhalla,
New York

MICHELE PIGHI, MD
Department of Medicine, Montreal Heart
Institute, Universite de Montreal, Montreal,
Quebec, Canada

ROBERT F. RILEY, MD, MS
Division of Cardiology, University of
Washington, School of Medicine, Seattle,
Washington

DAVID SILBER, DO
Cardiovascular Fellow, Winthrop Cardiology
Associates, PC, NYU-Winthrop Hospital,
Mineola, New York

NISHTHA SODHI, MD
Interventional and Structural Cardiology
Fellow, Cardiovascular Division, Washington
University, St Louis, Missouri

PAUL SORAJJA, MD
Director, Center for Valve and Structural Heart
Disease, Minneapolis Heart Institute, Abbott
Northwestern Hospital, Valve Science Center,
Minneapolis Heart Institute Foundation,
Minneapolis, Minnesota

HUSSAM S. SURADI, MD, FACC, FSCAI
Director, Structural Heart & Valve Center,
Interventional Cardiology; St. Mary Medical
Center, Hobart, Indiana; Department of
Cardiology, Community Hospital, Munster,
Indiana; Assistant Professor of Internal
Medicine & Pediatrics, Rush Center for
Structural Heart Disease, Rush University
Medical Center, Chicago, Illinois

RAJESH V. SWAMINATHAN, MD
Division of Cardiology, Duke University
Medical Center, Duke Clinical Research
Institute, Durham, North Carolina

MOLLY SZERLIP, MD, FSCAI, FACC
Medical Director of the Inpatient and
Outpatient Valve Program, Department of
Cardiology, The Heart Hospital Baylor Plano,
Plano, Texas

SOHAIB TARIQ, MD
Division of Cardiology, Westchester Medical
Center, New York Medical College, Valhalla,
New York

SURENDRANATH R. VEERAM REDDY, MD
Associate Professor of Pediatrics, Division of
Cardiology, Department of Pediatrics,
University of Texas Southwestern Medical
Center, Children's Health System of Texas,
Dallas, Texas

JEFFREY WESSLER, MD
Division of Cardiology, Columbia University,
New York, New York

THOMAS M. ZELLERS, MD
Professor of Pediatrics, Division of Cardiology,
Department of Pediatrics, University
of Texas Southwestern Medical Center,
Children's Health System of Texas, Dallas,
Texas

MING ZHONG, MD
Division of Cardiology, Interventional
Cardiology and Endovascular Laboratory,
Weill Cornell Medical College, New York
Presbyterian Hospital, New York,
New York

# CONTENTS

## SECTION I - Hemodynamics of Heart Failure Disease States

Heart failure is a clinical diagnosis that is supported by various laboratory, imaging, and invasive hemodynamic measures. There is no single diagnostic test. A variety of structural and/or functional myocardial abnormalities can lead to the inability of the heart to fill or eject blood. Despite ejection fraction being the most commonly assessed measure of systolic function in clinical practice, it is a poor measure of contractility because it is susceptible to loading conditions and chamber size. Invasive hemodynamic assessment remains of great importance in the evaluation of patients with myocardial disease or hypertrophic cardiomyopathy.

Pericardial diseases can be classified broadly as 3 entities: acute pericarditis, cardiac tamponade, and constrictive pericarditis. These disorders can be diagnosed and managed with noninvasive studies following a comprehensive history and physical examination, without the need for cardiac catheterization in most patients. Despite the advances in noninvasive cardiac imaging, there are limitations to their diagnostic accuracy. The invasive hemodynamic study offers the advantage of simultaneous, direct pressure measurement across multiple chambers, with direct examination of blood flow. Herein, the authors review the techniques for obtaining and interpreting invasive hemodynamic data in patients with suspected pericardial disease.

In the current era, diagnosis and follow-up of valvular heart disease is performed noninvasively using echocardiography. In some cases, the results of echocardiographic evaluation are inconclusive or discrepant with the patient's clinical symptoms. In such cases, a well-planned and executed cardiac catheterization is invaluable to clarify the clinical dilemma and assist in planning further management. This article reviews the indications, technique, and interpretation of cardiac catheterization in the setting of valvular stenosis and regurgitation.

Pulmonary hypertension (PH) falls into 5 groups, as defined by the World Health Organization. Swan-Ganz catheters determine precapillary versus post-capillary PH. The hemodynamic values of PH at rest and with vasodilatory challenge categorize the etiology of PH and guide treatment. RV maladaptations to increased pulmonary vascular resistance (PVR) and the chronicity of the right ventricle's (RV) response to increased PH and/or increased PVR can be understood with pressure-volume (PV) loops constructed with use of conductance catheters. These PV loops demonstrate the RV's ability to increase stroke volume in acutely and chronically increased PVR.

Adults with congenital heart disease are a growing population with increasingly more complex disease, in large part due to improvements in delivery of care to the pediatric population. Cardiac catheterization is an integral component of diagnosis and management in these patients. Careful attention to detail and a thorough understanding of intracardiac hemodynamics are critical to performing complete diagnostic evaluations. This article outlines the most commonly encountered lesions with guidelines for invasive assessment to help guide further therapy.

Cardiogenic shock (CS) represents an advanced state of morbidity along the pathophysiologic pathway of end-organ hypoperfusion caused by reduced cardiac output and blood pressure. Acute coronary syndromes remain the most common cause of CS. The spectrum of hypoperfusion states caused by low cardiac output ranges from pre-CS to refractory CS and can be characterized by an array of hemodynamic parameters. This review provides the foundation for a hemodynamic understanding of CS including the use of hemodynamic monitoring for diagnosis and treatment, the cardiac and vascular determinants of CS, and a hemodynamic approach to risk stratification and management of CS.

## SECTION II - Interventional Treatments to Improve/Reverse Heart Failure

Valvular heart diseases such as aortic stenosis and mitral regurgitation are often associated with heart failure, which in turn increases patients' Surgical Thoracic Society (STS) score. A high STS score means the patient is high risk for surgical aortic valve replacement and mitral valve repair/replacement. Transcatheter aortic valve replacement and percutaneous mitral valve repair offer a minimally invasive alternative for the treatment of valvular heart disease in patients with severe heart failure. We aim to review the current evidence on the safety, efficacy, and outcomes of these devices in patients with severe heart failure.

An array of interventional therapeutics is available in the modern era, with uses depending on acute or chronic situations. This article focuses on support in acute decompensated heart failure and cardiogenic shock, including intra-aortic balloon pumps, continuous aortic flow augmentation, and extra-corporeal membrane oxygenation.

This review explores the usefulness of multivessel revascularization with percutaneous coronary intervention in patients with multivessel obstructive coronary artery disease (CAD) presenting with and without cardiogenic shock. We also evaluate the literature regarding complete versus incomplete revascularization for patients with cardiogenic shock, acute coronary syndromes, and stable coronary artery disease.

Cardiac resynchronization therapy (CRT) has emerged as a valued nonpharmacologic therapy in patients with heart failure, reduced ejection fraction (EF), and ventricular dyssynchrony manifest as left bundle branch block. The mechanisms of benefit include remodeling of the left ventricle leading to decreased dimensions and increased EF, as well as a decrease in the severity of mitral regurgitation. This article reviews the rationale, effects, and indications for CRT, and discusses the patient characteristics that predict response and considerations for nonresponders.

Congenital heart disease (CHD) is the most common birth defect, occurring in approximately 0.8% to 1.0% of neonates. Advances in medical and surgical therapies for children with CHD have resulted in a growing population of patients reaching adulthood, with survival rates exceeding 85%. Many of these patients, especially if managed inappropriately, face the prospect of future complications including heart failure and premature death. For adults with uncorrected or previously palliated CHD, percutaneous therapies have become the primary treatment for many forms of CHD. In this article, we discuss the role of transcatheter interventions in the treatment of adults with CHD.

Hypertrophic cardiomyopathy is a commonly encountered inheritable cardiac disorder with variable phenotypic expression. Although most patients will have no or mild symptoms, 10% will develop heart failure symptoms refractory to medical management. This article discusses the mechanisms through which hypertrophic cardiomyopathy induces heart failure and how alcohol septal ablation can reverse each of these mechanisms to lead to clinical improvement.

> Sympathetic overactivation of renal afferent and efferent nerves have been implicated in the development and maintenance of several cardiovascular disease states, including resistant hypertension and heart failure with both reduced and preserved systolic function. With the development of minimally invasive catheter-based techniques, percutaneous renal denervation has become a safe and effective method of attenuating sympathetic overactivation. Percutaneous renal denervation, therefore, has the potential to modify and treat hypertension and congestive heart failure. Although future randomized controlled studies are needed to definitively prove its efficacy, renal denervation has the potential to change the way we view and treat cardiovascular disease.

## SECTION III - Interventional Heart Failure

> Technological advances have promoted challenges to prioritizing and combining therapies for heart failure. The concept of prioritization implies distinct but inextricably linked considerations. They may be viewed from pathophysiologic, clinical, and procedural perspectives, encompassing analysis of hemodynamic status, anatomic considerations, and technical challenges. It is essential to consider factors, including conduction disease, renal and pulmonary function, hematological derangements, and so forth. These considerations allow determination of clinical goals, which determine prioritization and interventional strategies. These considerations then facilitate goal setting for medical and interventional therapies as definitive/destination, preservation/salvage, stepwise, bridge, or palliation.

> Cardiogenic shock remains one of the most common causes of in-hospital death. Recent data have identified an overall increase in patient complexity, with cardiogenic shock in the setting of acute myocardial infarction. The use of percutaneous acute mechanical circulatory support (AMCS) has steadily grown in the past decade. Guidelines and consensus statements addressing proper patient selection, timing of AMCS implantation, device choice, and postimplantation protocol are appearing. The emerging role of interventional heart failure specialists within the heart team includes integration and understanding of advanced hemodynamic and cathether-based therapies, with the goal of improving outcomes.

# INTERVENTIONAL HEART FAILURE

## THE CLINICS ARE NOW AVAILABLE ONLINE!

Access your subscription at:
**www.theclinics.com**

# PREFACE

## Operationalizing Interventional Heart Failure: Adding Substance to the Concept

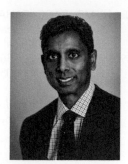

**Srihari S. Naidu, MD, FACC, FAHA, FSCAI**
*Editor*

Although not a new concept, interventional heart failure (IHF) has gained significant ground in recent years due to the explosion of advanced interventional procedures, predominantly in structural heart disease and multivessel revascularization, combined with the growing epidemic of heart failure. Indeed, heart failure is a major economic and societal burden throughout the world, continues to increase in incidence and prevalence, and has become as a result the target of major cost containment strategies for hospitals, insurance companies, and government.

My own interest in IHF evolved from an initial attraction to treating heart failure patients during medical school, when I worked with Drs Alan Gass, Billie Fyfe, John Fallon, and Steven Lansman as part of the heart failure and transplantation team at Mount Sinai Medical Center in New York. It was during my cardiology training at the University of Pennsylvania, however, that I decided to pursue interventional cardiology as a career instead. My early days as an interventional cardiologist found me gravitating toward heart failure nonetheless, including writings and interest in the utilization of novel percutaneous ventricular assist devices in particular. Combined with my interest in another form of heart failure, hypertrophic cardiomyopathy, it soon became clear that heart failure would remain central to my career. In explaining why the combination of interventional cardiology and heart failure

made sense, I launched the Society for Cardiovascular Angiography and Interventions Interventional Heart Failure Working Group, a consortium of interventional cardiology and heart failure experts.

Fundamentally, IHF encompasses spending the requisite time to elaborate on a patient's unique underlying pathophysiology leading to cardiac dysfunction, which is often multifactorial, by focusing on advanced hemodynamics. Following this, we are then able to logically and systematically target and prioritize therapies that have the most impact clinically, in order, from most impactful and lowest risk to the least impactful or most risk. Ultimately, meaningful recovery of function is the goal, with end-stage therapies such as permanent implantable assist devices or heart transplantation reserved for those in whom recovery is not possible.

This issue of *Interventional Cardiology Clinics*, the first of its kind on the topic, presents these concepts sequentially, starting with advanced hemodynamic concepts around various relevant disease states, progressing to a discussion of the effects of invasive therapies on the heart failure state, both anatomically and physiologically, and then culminating in practical approaches to combining therapies and launching training programs on the topic.

It is our hope that this issue provides a valuable resource for the local hospital-based launch of

Intervent Cardiol Clin 6 (2017) xiii–xiv
http://dx.doi.org/10.1016/j.iccl.2017.04.001
2211-7458/17/© 2017 Published by Elsevier Inc.

comprehensive IHF programs, with physician champions in interventional cardiology, heart failure, electrophysiology, and advanced imaging. In addition to cardiologists, trainees and staff should find the information invaluable as they begin to form a logical approach to the care of these complex patients. As programs mature, year-long training programs in IHF may be added, templates for which exist at select programs across the country and are included in this issue.

At my own institution, Westchester Medical Center, we pride ourselves on advanced and complex care of the heart failure and critical care patient, including advanced hemodynamic assessment and interventional approaches when possible, resorting to fully implantable assist devices or heart trans-

plantation in those who fail to recover sufficient function. Multidisciplinary discussions are commonplace and help move the needle on comprehensive and rapid care. That is the goal locally, regionally, and nationally, a goal that it is hoped one day will reduce the burden of heart failure.

Sincerely,

Srihari S. Naidu, MD, FACC, FAHA, FSCAI
Westchester Medical Center
New York Medical College
19 Bradhurst Avenue, Suite 3850
Hawthorne, NY 10532, USA

*E-mail address:*
srihari.naidu@wmchealth.org

# SECTION I - Hemodynamics of Heart Failure Disease States

# Invasive Hemodynamics of Myocardial Disease
## Systolic and Diastolic Dysfunction (and Hypertrophic Obstructive Cardiomyopathy)

Michael Eskander, MD[a],
Morton J. Kern, MD, MSCAI, FACC, FAHA[a,b,*]

**KEYWORDS**

- Hemodynamics • Congestive heart failure • Hypertrophic cardiomyopathy • Ischemia
- Infarction

**KEY POINTS**

- Heart failure is a clinical diagnosis that is supported by various laboratory, imaging, and invasive hemodynamic measures. There is no single diagnostic test.
- A variety of structural and/or functional myocardial abnormalities can lead to the inability of the heart to fill or eject blood.
- Invasive hemodynamic assessment remains of great importance in the evaluation of patients with myocardial disease or hypertrophic cardiomyopathy.
- Several different hemodynamic measures are available to aid in diagnosing systolic and diastolic dysfunction.
- A deep understanding of pressure-volume loops and hemodynamic tracings is necessary in order to appreciate variation in pathology of myocardial disease.

## INTRODUCTION

Invasive assessment of cardiovascular function provides greater insight into the mechanisms of disease not only in classic heart failure due to dilated cardiomyopathy and cardiogenic shock but also in disorders, such as heart failure with preserved ejection fraction (HFpEF), and may explain how patients who have different forms of heart failure respond to various therapies. From the cardiac catheterization laboratory data, hemodynamic pressure waveforms, in addition to echocardiographic information, provide data on left and right heart function, systemic and pulmonary arterial resistances, and cardiac-vascular coupling relationships. These data form therapeutic parameters, such as cardiac preload, afterload, and global left ventricular (LV) function to guide and gauge the efficacy of both medical and mechanical interventions.

## ASSESSMENT OF CARDIAC CONTRACTILITY

The major manifestation of the diseased myocardium is the failure to produce normal contraction

Disclosure Statement: Dr M.J. Kern is a consultant to St. Jude Medical, Philips-Volcano Inc, ACIST Medical, Opsens Medical, and Merit Medical. Dr M. Eskander has nothing to disclose.
[a] Division of Cardiology, Department of Internal Medicine, University of California, Irvine Health, 101 The City Drive South, Suite 400, Orange, CA 92868, USA; [b] Department of Medicine, VA Long Beach, Building 1, Room 417, 5901 East 7th Street, Long Beach, CA 90822, USA
* Corresponding author. Department of Medicine, VA Long Beach, Building 1, Room 417, 5901 East 7th Street, Long Beach, CA 90822.
E-mail address: mortonkern2007@gmail.com

Intervent Cardiol Clin 6 (2017) 297–307
http://dx.doi.org/10.1016/j.iccl.2017.03.001
2211-7458/17/Published by Elsevier Inc.

and in some cases normal relaxation. Systolic contractile effort can be characterized by both global and regional myocardial function as measured by the extent of muscle shortening or thickening producing ejection of blood.[1,2] The ejection of blood from the ventricle can be quantitated by global ejection fraction (EF), segmental LV wall motion, or cardiac output or cardiac work. Contractile ejection is highly sensitive to afterload and really is an expression of ventricular ejection into the arterial resistance, a phenomenon known as vasculo-ventricular coupling. EF is also affected by heart size. Because the denominator of LVEF is end-diastolic volume (EDV), the EF value is more a parameter of remodeling than of contractility. Unfortunately, for simplicity, EF is used as a more binary labeling of myocardial diseases into those with normal versus reduced EF. In reality, the causes and presentation of patients with heart failure is much more complex.

## THE PRESSURE-VOLUME LOOP AND LEFT VENTRICULAR FUNCTION

Parameters of cardiac function can be derived from relations between cardiac pressure and volume. Pressure-volume (PV) loops can be obtained invasively to assess peak systolic and end-diastolic pressures, stroke work, maximal rate of pressure increase during isovolumetric contraction (dP/dtmax), maximal ventricular power (PWR_{max}), elastance, efficiency, and other unique parameters (Fig. 1). By examining the PV loop, myocardial function can be viewed over a range of preload volumes to determine load-independent, cardiac-specific measures.[3]

LV hemodynamics can be represented by a PV loop, which plots the changes of these variables over a cardiac cycle.[4–6] Each PV loop represents one cardiac cycle (see Fig. 1). Beginning at end-diastole (point a), LV volume has received the atrial contribution and is maximal. Isovolumetric contraction (a to b) increases LV pressure with no change in volume. At the end of isovolumetric contraction, LV pressure exceeds aortic pressure, the aortic valve opens, and blood is ejected from the LV into the aorta (point b). Over the systolic ejection phase, LV volume decreases; as ventricular repolarization occurs, LV ejection ceases and relaxation begins. When LV pressure decreases to less than the aortic pressure, the aortic valve closes, a point also known as the end-systolic PV point (ESPV) (point c). Isovolumetric relaxation occurs until LV pressure decreases to less than the atrial pressure, opening the mitral valve (point d).

The stroke volume (SV) is represented by the width of the PV loop, the difference between end-systolic volume (ESV) and EDV. The area within the loop represents stroke work. Load-independent LV contractility, also known as Emax, is defined as the maximal slope of the ESPV points under various loading conditions, the line of these points is the ESPV relationship (ESPVR). Effective arterial elastance (Ea), a measure of LV afterload, is defined as the ratio of end-systolic pressure to SV. Under steady-state conditions, optimal LV contractile efficiency occurs when the ratio of Ea:Emax approaches 1.

## CONTRACTILITY, MYOCARDIAL WORK, AND CARDIAC POWER OUTPUT

Contractility is an intrinsic property of cardiac tissue that determines strength of contraction in response to ventricular load and reflects the level of activation, formation, and cycling of actin and myosin cross-bridges. At a constant preload and afterload, increased contractility results in increased extent and velocity of shortening (Fig. 2A). Contractility is affected by the adrenergic state, drugs, and myocyte injury or loss. Although an increase in heart rate leads to an increase in contractility in normal myocardium (positive force-frequency relationship), this relationship is blunted or even negative in failing myocardium. The most commonly used surrogate variables of contractility, such as EF and peak rate of increase of ventricular pressure (+dP/dt), are load dependent. The use of the end-systolic PV relationship to determine end-systolic elastance (Ees) has been suggested as a load-independent method of assessing myocardial contractility (Fig. 2B–D).

dP/dt_{max} can be assessed using a high-fidelity micromanometer and is used widely as a measure of contractility. dP/dt_{max}, however, depends on cardiac filling (ie, is preload dependent) and heart rate; it may not always reflect contractile function that develops after cardiac ejection is initiated.[2] The relationship between end-systolic pressure and volume from a variety of variably loaded cardiac contractions yields the ESPVR.[7] This slope provides the Ees. The Ees may then provide further information regarding contractile function and chamber stiffness.

The relationship between stroke work and preload, measured from multiple beats under different loading conditions, generates a Sarnoff curve; its slope, often termed *preload recruitable stroke work*, provides a contractile index

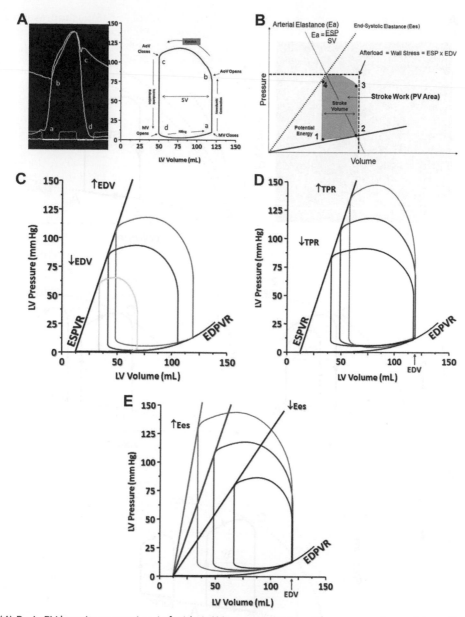

**Fig. 1.** (*A*) Basic PV loop interpretation. Left side is LV pressure tracing with corresponding points on the PV loop (*right side*). Each PV loop represents one cardiac cycle. Beginning at the end of isovolumic relaxation (point a, point 1 on [*B*]), LV volume increases during diastole (a-b). At end-diastole (point b), LV volume is maximal and isovolumic contraction (phase b-c) begins. At the peak of isovolumetric contraction, LV pressure exceeds aortic pressure and blood begins to eject from the LV into the aorta (point c). During this systolic ejection phase, LV volume decreases until aortic pressure exceeds LV pressure and the aortic valve closes, which is known as the end-systolic pressure-volume point (ESPV) (point c). Stroke volume (SV) is represented by the width of the PV loop as the difference between end-systolic and end-diastolic volumes (a-b). (*B*) Load-independent contractility also known as elastance at end-systole (Ees), is defined as the maximal slope of the ESPV point under various loading conditions, known as the ESPV relationship (ESPVR). Effective arterial elastance (Ea) is defined as the ratio of end-systolic pressure (ESP) and SV. Under steady-state conditions, optimal LV pump efficiency occurs when the ratio of Ea:Emax approaches one. Arterial elastance is a component of afterload, which is defined as the resistance to LV ejection throughout systole and can be represented as the product of end-systolic pressure (ESP) and EDV. (*C*). Changes in the PV loops induced by loading (volume), (*D*) total peripheral resistance (TPR), and (*E*) contractility (Ees slope). AoV, aortic valve; MV, mitral valve.

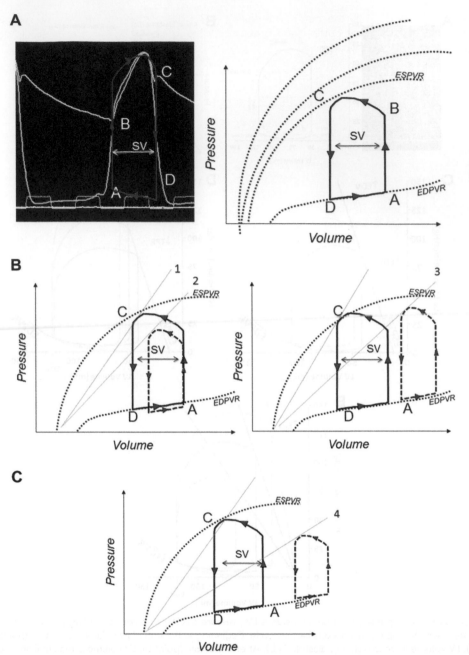

Fig. 2. (A) Hemodynamic conditions associated with myocardial infarction and treatment. Left, hemodynamic tracing describing the PV loop. Right side, A-B-C is ejection to end systole; C-D is isovolumetric relaxation, and D-A is diastolic filling. The ESPV relationship is altered by the contractility represented by the changing Frank-Starling curves. The slope of the ESPVR represents the relationship between SV (and cardiac output) and LV end-diastolic pressure (EDP) or LVEDV. (B) Left, resting conditions are represented by slope 1 and solid-lined PV loops. Increased LVEDP or LVEDV is associated with increased SV. Acute cardiac injury reduces the Frank-Starling curve (slope 2) and end-systole elastance (Ees; *dashed line*) and increases EDV and pressure (*right side*). Chronic systolic heart failure is associated with a reduced Frank-Starling curve (slope 3) and Ees. Patients with compensated systolic heart failure may demonstrate preserved SV (width of the PV loop), increased LVEDV, and normal or mildly increased LVEDP. Increased LVEDP or LVEDV is associated with small increases in SV. (C) Decompensated systolic heart failure or cardiogenic shock is associated with reduced Ees and a flat Frank-Starling curve (slope 4). In this condition, increased LVEDP or LVEDV are not associated with increased SV.

(see Fig. 2B–D). PWR$_{max}$ is the peak instantaneous product of ventricular outflow and pressure and is also quite preload dependent.

## DIASTOLE

Active and passive processes determine diastolic function and contribute to relaxation and chamber filling. Central to cardiac catheterization is the left heart filling pressure, either pulmonary artery occlusion (wedge) pressure or LV end-diastolic pressure (EDP). Fig. 3 shows LV and right ventricular (RV) simultaneous recorded pressure tracings demonstrating different degrees of LV diastolic dysfunction often associated with heart failure.

Aortic valve closure marks the onset of ventricular diastole, whereby relaxation is quantified invasively by the rate of pressure decay, typically expressed by a time constant ($\tau$) that is estimated using several mathematical fits.[8] Even this seemingly straightforward assessment has technical pitfalls. These model fits, usually mono-exponential decays (ie, Pressure = Pressure$_\infty$ + Pressure$_o$e$^{-t/\tau}$ or the same equation without Pressure$_\infty$), may or may not describe adequately the actual decrease in pressure. When used in a setting where they do not fit properly, such as in dilated heart failure, they can lead to erroneous conclusions. This delay in relaxation is common. It frequently accompanies normal aging, but it becomes even more

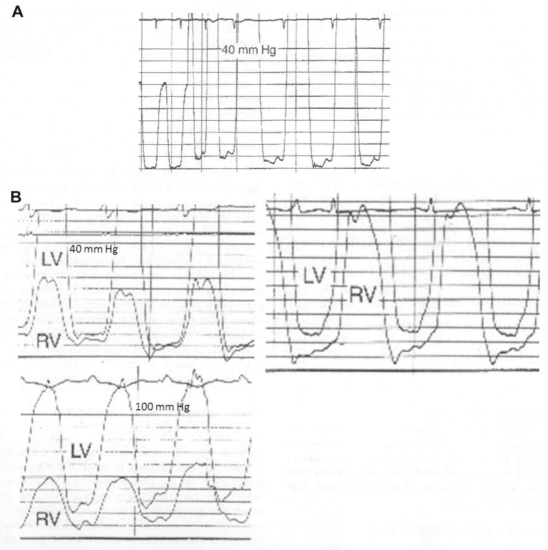

Fig. 3. (A, B) Simultaneously recorded RV and LV pressure tracings demonstrating different degrees of LV diastolic dysfunction often associated with heart failure.

prominent in cardiac failure and with hypertrophy. It has multiple determinants starting with dissociation of the cross-bridge, calcium-handling, and elasticity-restoring forces resulting from the recoil of compressed macromolecules, such as titin.[9] It clearly can affect early filling and pressures, particularly at faster heart rates. Analysis requires invasive high-fidelity micromanometer recordings, although it may be approximated by the time between aortic valve closure and mitral valve opening or inferred from mitral Doppler flow patterns.[10]

Similar to isovolumetric relaxation, passive diastolic chamber stiffness is rarely measured directly in standard clinical practice. LV diastolic PV relationship is curvilinear; thus, compliance is most often expressed by a mono-exponential stiffness coefficient. A more accurate approach is to assess multiple PV loops over a loading range (varying preload) and to connect points at late diastole from these cycles. The apparent chamber stiffness derived from single versus multiple loops can vary substantially, as shown particularly in patients who have genetic hypertrophic cardiomyopathy; in these patients, the use of a single loop markedly underestimated LV stiffness.[11]

## PRELOAD

Preload is related to the amount of blood volume returned to the right side of the heart and transmitted to the LV during diastole. Preload is the EDV at the beginning of systole. The EDV is directly related to the degree of stretch of the myocardial sarcomeres. Atrial pressure is also a surrogate for preload (see **Fig. 1**C).

## AFTERLOAD

LV afterload is LV wall stress over the ejection period and is usually presented as the LV end systole pressure/volume relationship slope. Afterload often referred to as total peripheral resistance (see **Fig. 1**D) represents the degree of resistance the left ventricle must contract against to eject blood.

Afterload is represented by the ventricular pressure at the end of systole (ESP). Ejection stops because the ventricular pressure developed by the myocardial contraction is less than the arterial pressure. Contractility and ESP determine the ESV.

## RIGHT HEART DYSFUNCTION

Right heart dysfunction with or without pulmonary hypertension is increasingly common in patients who have heart failure, regardless of LVEF. The right heart dysfunction potently affects the decline in exercise capacity and clinical outcome.[12] Pulmonary hypertension is defined as a mean pulmonary arterial pressure greater than 25 mm Hg at rest (30 mm Hg with exercise), whereas pulmonary arterial hypertension (ie, pulmonary vascular disease) further requires an elevated pulmonary vascular resistance while maintaining a normal pulmonary capillary wedge pressure.[13] The presence of pulmonary vascular resistance and the ability to reduce it with vasodilators are used commonly for treatment with certain vasodilators and even to establish eligibility for cardiac transplantation. Pulmonary vaso-reactivity testing is conducted with drugs like nitric oxide donators or milrinone and, more recently, the phosphodiesterase 5 inhibitor sildenafil and the natriuretic peptide nesiritide.[14] Although pulmonary artery pressures can be estimated by echo-Doppler methods, invasive assessment is required for definitive diagnosis and to guide treatment decisions.[10]

RV function assessment remains fairly rudimentary as compared with LV assessment. As with the LV, RV pressures are not determined exclusively by the ventricle or vasculature but rather result from the dynamic interaction of the two. The RV PV loop is normally triangular, reflecting the lower resistive load and relatively higher compliance of the pulmonary vascular circuit. It becomes more rectangular (like the LV) in patients who have pulmonary hypertension. Assessment of RV diastolic stiffness is quite rare in the literature and is affected greatly by pericardial restraint and biventricular remodeling. RV vascular impedance consists of mean pulmonary resistance, the proximal stiffness of pulmonary conduit arteries, vascular-ventricular impedance, distal vascular compliance, and reflected waves. There is now renewed interest in how these properties of impedance can impose late-systolic loads on the RV,[12] impacting RV remodeling, relaxation delay, and inefficiency.

## HEART FAILURE WITH PRESERVED EJECTION FRACTION

Invasive hemodynamic assessment of patients presenting with dyspnea in which the diagnosis is not clear can be clinically useful. This assessment may be particularly helpful in cases in which the picture is not so clear, because diastolic dysfunction seen on echo-Doppler imaging is commonly seen and natriuretic peptide levels may be mildly elevated even in the absence of true heart failure.

Filling pressures that are normal at rest but increase with supine exercise at low workload may suggest a cardiac cause of patients' dyspnea. Pulmonary artery pressures may also increase in proportion to the increase in pulmonary wedge, indicating that patients' symptoms probably are caused primarily by HFpEF. Other patients may show filling pressures and cardiac output that are normal both at rest and at maximal workload, arguing against a diagnosis of HFpEF. Finally, others develop pulmonary arterial hypertension with exercise in the absence of an increase in left heart filling pressures, identifying a more isolated lesion at the level of the pulmonary vasculature. In practice, individual patients may embody any of these conditions or, more commonly, present with some combination of all 3; future research is required to understand how best to treat patients who have each type of response.

## HEMODYNAMIC PRESSURE WAVEFORM EXAMPLES OF MYOCARDIAL DYSFUNCTION

### Pulsus Alternans

One common manifestation of the severely impaired LV is a consistent pattern of alternating systolic aortic and LV pressures. **Fig. 4** shows a reduced pressure every other beat of approximately 20 mm Hg. Interestingly, the LV waveform on the weak beats is different by its reduced peak and time to peak pressure as well as a subtle alteration of the rapid phase of relaxation. A similar alteration in peak systolic pressure is also noted on every other beat in the RV and pulmonary artery tracings (**Fig. 5**). Pulmonary and LV diastolic pressures are significantly elevated, consistent with biventricular dysfunction. The time to peak systolic pressure is also prolonged in the weaker beats of right-sided pressures, consistent with the hypothesized mechanism of alternating diminished contractility. RV pulsus alternans may occur independently, concordantly, or discordantly with LV alternans.[15,16]

Pulsus alternans is thought to be primarily due to decreased myocardial contractility on alternate beats, with relatively less effect produced by changes in preload, afterload, or diastolic relaxation.[4,6,17] Weber and colleagues[18] induced pulsus alternans in the canine heart when anaerobic metabolism was reached by increasing the filling volume, heart rate, and contractility and by decreasing coronary perfusion.[18] When the

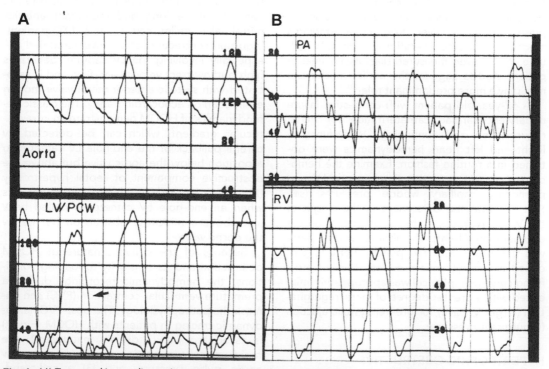

**Fig. 4.** (*A*) Top panel is systolic aortic pressure with simultaneous LV pressure tracing demonstrating approximately 20 mm Hg blood pressure difference in an alternating pattern. Arrow pointing to LV pressure tracing with relative decreased systolic peak. (*B*) Top panel shows pulmonary artery (PA) systolic tracing with simultaneous RV pressure tracing alternating blood pressure of approximately 20 mm Hg. PCW, pulmonary capillary wedge.

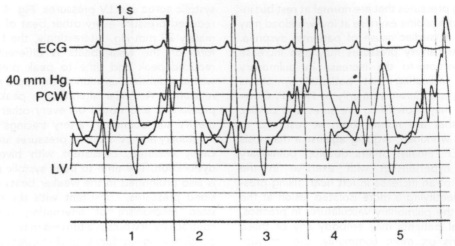

Fig. 5. Simultaneous hemodynamic pressure tracings of the LV and pulmonary capillary wedge (PCW). ECG, electrocardiogram.

aerobic limit of the myocardium was exceeded, myocardial performance declined with resultant pulsus alternans. Decreased contractility is attributed to deletion of the number of myocardial cells contracting on alternate beats. This reduction in the contractile cell population is thought to be caused by intracellular calcium cycling involving the sarcoplasmic reticulum leading to localized electrical mechanical dissociation.[19] Another postulated mechanism for the alternations in pulse pressure evolved from Frank Starling's mechanism due to alterations in diastolic volume.[5,6] However, measured diastolic volumes in patient studies suggest the earlier mechanism may play a more predominant role.[20]

A 62-year-old patient with congestive failure underwent cardiac catheterization for mitral regurgitation and continuing LV dysfunction. Right and left heart hemodynamics were obtained in a routine fashion. Examine the hemodynamic tracings of the simultaneous LV and pulmonary capillary wedge pressures (see Fig. 5). Note the differences in the height of the V and A waves during sinus rhythm on the odd numbered beats. The alternation of V waves was consistent with the pulsus alternans produced in the systemic pressure. The left atrial filling curve (compliance) was appropriately influenced with a greater degree of mitral regurgitation (larger V wave) for greater systolic ejection (regurgitant pressure).

## HYPERTROPHIC OBSTRUCTIVE CARDIOMYOPATHY

Hypertrophic obstructive cardiomyopathy (HOCM) is characterized by an intraventricular

LV outflow (LVOT) gradient. Because of the dynamic nature of the obstruction related to contractile forces and loading conditions, the gradient may be variable even over a brief measurement period. It may be absent at rest and only demonstrated during physiologic maneuvers (eg, Valsalva). HOCM is also associated with significant diastolic dysfunction. The hypertrophy of the interventricular septum, often in concert with a long and redundant anterior mitral valve leaflet, causes the LVOT gradient. Vigorous contraction of the hypertrophied LV, especially involving the LV septum, generates high outflow tract velocity and flow and is associated with systolic anterior mitral valve motion easily seen on echocardiography. The classic hemodynamics of HOCM demonstrate an intraventricular gradient, which can be detected by careful pullback of the end-hole LV catheter to a position below the aortic valve but above the obstructive component of septal hypertrophy (Fig. 6). A large LV-aortic gradient disappears when an end-hole LV catheter is pulled back just above a midcavity obstruction but below the aortic valve.

Because of the dynamic nature of HOCM obstruction and its sensitivity to loading conditions, the hemodynamic recordings during a premature ventricular contraction (PVC) can unmask the pathophysiology. The post-PVC hemodynamic tracing in patients with HOCM (Fig. 7) is associated with 3 distinct features: (1) the rapid upstroke of aortic pressure, (2) a narrow aortic pulse pressure, and (3) a spike-and-dome configuration of early vigorous LV ejection followed by delay in ejection of the remaining LV volume, with the resulting outflow gradient.

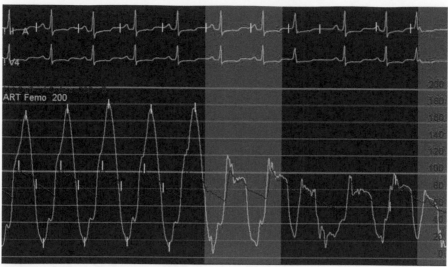

**Fig. 6.** LV catheter pullback from distal LV (*left side*) to subaortic position (*right side*). Note the reduction in LV pressure gradient while still recording LV pressure.

Another method to demonstrate the severity of LVOT obstruction in patients with HOCM is to perform a Valsalva maneuver. At the beginning of Valsalva strain phase, there is an increase in LVEDP and reduced arterial pulse pressure. The LVOT gradient begins to appear and is most pronounced during the plateau phase and may be dramatic during a PVC in this setting (**Fig. 8**).

Both aortic stenosis (AS) and HOCM are associated with systolic outflow obstruction with systolic murmurs. AS can be easily differentiated from HOCM by examining the response to a PVC. A comparison of the post PVC hemodynamic responses between HOCM and AS is shown on **Fig. 8**. In aortic stenosis, the post-PVC hemodynamic tracings show a larger pulse pressure, a consistently slow aortic upstroke of fixed valve obstruction, and no change in the aortic waveform, all in contrast to the HOCM hemodynamics, which show a reduced pulse pressure, brisk aortic pressure upstroke (parallel to LV pressure), and deformation of the aortic waveform with a spike and dome of rapid early ejection with secondary outflow obstruction.

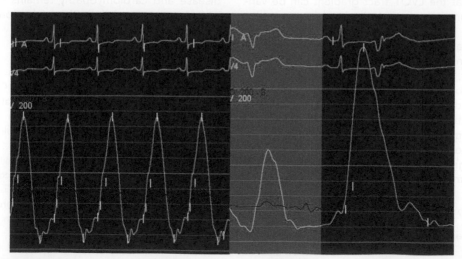

**Fig. 7.** LV (*blue*) and aortic (*red*) pressure tracings in patient with hypertrophic obstructive cardiomyopathy. Note the vertical upstroke of aortic pressure with a delay in mid systole (spike and dome) and the post-PVC reduction of the pulse pressure (the Brockenbrough-Braunwald-Morrow sign).

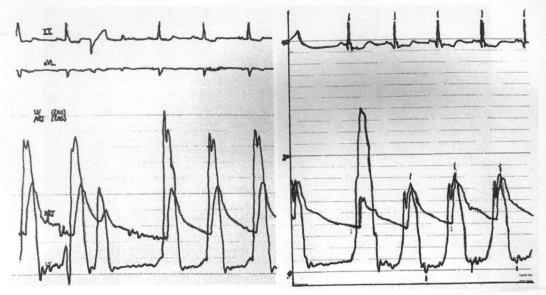

Fig. 8. Comparison of post-PVC hemodynamics of aortic stenosis (AS) (*left*) and HOCM (*right*). The post-PVC beat in the patient with AS shows a large LV-Ao gradient, wider pulse pressure, and persistently delayed upstroke of aortic pressure. The post-PVC pressure in patient with HOCM shows a large LV gradient, but the aortic pulse pressure is narrow; despite a very rapid and preserve aortic upstroke, there is a change in the pulse wave form with a sharp early spike and late plateau (dome) characteristic of hypercontractile ejection and impaired ventricular relaxation. II, aVL, correspond to electrographic (ECG) leads; ART, arterial line transducing aortic pressure.

Individuals with HOCM range from asymptomatic to having severe symptoms, generally correlating with the degree of obstruction that is exquisitely dependent on loading conditions.[21,22] The hemodynamics of the outflow gradient can be obtained through a retrograde approach with an LV catheter, which has side holes only at the distal portion or via a transseptal, antegrade approach.[21] It is important to note that the LVOT tract gradient can be variable during the catheterization laboratory procedure demonstrating significant changes during a single measurement period. If a measurement of less than 30 mm Hg is obtained during rest, Valsalva maneuver or induction of PVCs should be performed in order to ascertain worsening dynamic gradient. Treatment of this obstruction can result in significant reduction of symptoms. Invasive hemodynamic measurement in these patients requires close attention to detail given the potential consequences of errors in measurement.

## SUMMARY

Heart failure is a clinical diagnosis that is supported by various laboratory, imaging, and invasive hemodynamic measures. There is no single diagnostic test. A variety of structural and/or functional myocardial abnormalities can lead to the inability of the heart to fill or eject blood. Despite EF being the most commonly assessed measure of systolic function in clinical practice, it is a poor measure of contractility because it is sensitive to loading conditions and chamber size. The examination of PV loops and factors that influence cardiac output will assist in guiding and gauging therapies. Invasive hemodynamic assessment of valvular disease and cardiomyopathy remains of great importance, especially in the evaluation of patients and selection of therapies.

## REFERENCES

1. Kass DA, Maughan WL, Guo ZM, et al. Comparative influence of load versus inotropic states on indexes of ventricular contractility: experimental and theoretical analysis based on pressure-volume relationships. Circulation 1987;76(6):1422–36.
2. Nagayama T, Takimoto E, Sadayappan S, et al. Control of in vivo left ventricular [correction] contraction/relaxation kinetics by myosin binding protein C: protein kinase A phosphorylation dependent and independent regulation. Circulation 2007;116(21):2399–408.
3. Baicu CF, Zile MR, Aurigemma GP, et al. Left ventricular systolic performance, function, and contractility in patients with diastolic heart failure. Circulation 2005;111(18):2306–12.

4. Borlaug BA, Kass DA. Invasive hemodynamic assessment in heart failure. Cardiol Clin 2011;29: 269–80.

5. Lewis BS, Lewis N, Gotsman MS. Effect of postural changes on pulsus alternans. An echocardiographic study. Chest 1979;75:634–6.

6. McGaughey MD, Maughan WL, Sunagawa K, et al. Alternating contractility in pulsus alternans studied in the isolated canine heart. Circulation 1985;71: 357–62.

7. Suga H, Sagawa K. Instantaneous pressure-volume relationships and their ratio in the excised, supported canine left ventricle. Circ Res 1974;35(1): 117–26.

8. Senzaki H, Fetics B, Chen CH, et al. Comparison of ventricular pressure relaxation assessments in human heart failure: quantitative influence on load and drug sensitivity analysis. J Am Coll Cardiol 1999;34(5):1529–36.

9. Borlaug BA, Kass DA. Mechanisms of diastolic dysfunction in heart failure. Trends Cardiovasc Med 2006;16(8):273–9.

10. Oh JK, Hatle L, Tajik AJ, et al. Diastolic heart failure can be diagnosed by comprehensive two-dimensional and Doppler echocardiography. J Am Coll Cardiol 2006;47(3):500–6.

11. Pak PH, Maughan L, Baughman KL, et al. Marked discordance between dynamic and passive diastolic pressure-volume relations in idiopathic hypertrophic cardiomyopathy. Circulation 1996;94(1):52–60.

12. Haddad F, Doyle R, Murphy DJ, et al. Right ventricular function in cardiovascular disease, part II: pathophysiology, clinical importance, and management of right ventricular failure. Circulation 2008;117(13): 1717–31.

13. McGoon M, Gutterman D, Steen V, et al, American College of Chest Physicians. Screening, early detection, and diagnosis of pulmonary arterial hypertension: ACCP evidence-based clinical practice guidelines. Chest 2004;126(1 Suppl):14S–34S.

14. Alaeddini J, Uber PA, Park MH, et al. Efficacy and safety of sildenafil in the evaluation of pulmonary hypertension in severe heart failure. Am J Cardiol 2004;94(11):1475–7.

15. Kussmaul WG 3rd, Altschuler JA, Matthai WH, et al. Right ventricular-vascular interaction in congestive heart failure. Importance of low-frequency impedance. Circulation 1993;88(3):1010–5.

16. Desser KB, Benchimol A. Phasic left ventricular blood velocity alternans in man. Am J Cardiol 1975;36:309–14.

17. Miller WP, Liedtke AJ, Nellis SH. End systolic pressure diameter relationships during pulsus alternans in intact pig hearts. Am J Physiol 1985;250: H606–11.

18. Weber KT, Janicki JS, Sundram B. Myocardial energetics: experimental and clinical studies to address its determinants and aerobic limit. Basic Res Cardiol 1989;84:237–46.

19. Lab MJ, Lee JA. Changes in intracellular calcium during mechanical alternans in isolated ferret ventricular muscle. Circ Res 1990;66:585–95.

20. Bashore TM, Walker S, Van Fossen D, et al. Pulsus alternans induced by inferior vena caval occlusion in man. Cathet Cardiovasc Diagn 1988;14:24–32.

21. Wigle ED, Sasson Z, Henderson MA, et al. Hypertrophic cardiomyopathy: the importance of the site and the extent of hypertrophy: a review. Prog Cardiovasc Dis 1985;28:1–83.

22. Wigle ED, Rakowski H. Evidence for true obstruction to left ventricular outflow in obstructive hypertrophic cardiomyopathy (muscular or hypertrophic subaortic stenosis). Z Kardiol 1987;76(Suppl 3): 61–8.

# Invasive Hemodynamics of Pericardial Disease

Ganesh Athappan, MD[a,b], Paul Sorajja, MD[a,b,*]

---

## KEYWORDS

- Pericardial disease • Invasive • Hemodynamics

---

## KEY POINTS

- Early rapid ventricular filling (ie, dip-and-plateau pattern) can be seen in patients with constrictive pericarditis, restrictive cardiomyopathy, or any volume-overload state that results in pericardial restraint. Underdamping of fluid-filled catheters may mimic this pattern of ventricular filling.
- Both traditional and dynamic respiratory criteria should be used to distinguish constrictive pericarditis from restrictive cardiomyopathy. Dynamic respiratory criteria for constrictive pericarditis are (1) discordance of the right and left ventricular systolic pressures due to enhanced ventricular interdependence and (2) dissociation of intrathoracic and intracavitary pressures.
- The hemodynamic hallmarks of cardiac tamponade are pulsus paradoxus and loss of the y descent in the atrial waveform. Blunting of early ventricular filling also may occur.

---

Pericardial diseases can be classified broadly as 3 entities: acute pericarditis, cardiac tamponade, and constrictive pericarditis. Of these entities, hemodynamic perturbations occur in tamponade and constriction, whereas acute pericarditis rarely has such consequences. With modern imaging modalities, these disorders can be diagnosed and managed with noninvasive studies following a comprehensive history and physical examination, without the need for cardiac catheterization in most patients.

Nevertheless, despite the advances in noninvasive cardiac imaging, there are limitations to their diagnostic accuracy. The invasive hemodynamic study offers the advantage of simultaneous, direct pressure measurement across multiple chambers, with direct examination of blood flow. These distinctions are important as pathologic conditions that cannot be accurately diagnosed with current noninvasive methods frequently is complex. Herein, the authors review the techniques for obtaining and interpreting invasive hemodynamic data in patients with suspected pericardial disease.

## Approach to Patients

The hemodynamic assessment of these clinical entities should be individualized. Proper planning of the procedure requires a comprehensive differential diagnosis of patients' problems, complete knowledge of the known data, the clinically relevant information that is required from the hemodynamic study, as well as the potential data needed in the event a diagnosis constrictive pericarditis (eg, preoperative coronary angiography) is made. Vascular access sites and the approach to gathering data should be delineated fully before proceeding.

Although all patients should be fasting for the catheterization procedure, intravenous fluids should be administered to patients who have a long waiting period following their last oral intake to prevent measurements from

---

[a] Valve Science Center, Minneapolis Heart Institute Foundation, 800 East 28th Street, Minneapolis, MN 55407, USA; [b] Center for Valve and Structural Heart Disease, Minneapolis Heart Institute, Abbott Northwestern Hospital, 800 East 28th Street, Minneapolis, MN 55407, USA
* Corresponding author. Center for Valve and Structural Heart Disease, Minneapolis Heart Institute, Abbott Northwestern Hospital, 800 East 28th Street, Minneapolis, MN 55407.
E-mail address: paul.sorajja@allina.com

2211-7458/17/© 2017 Elsevier Inc. All rights reserved.

being taken during a low-output, low-volume state. Patients can be lightly sedated but should be awake to simulate the hemodynamic milieu of their outpatient state. No parenteral oxygen should be administered before the procedure to allow measurements of oxygen saturations at steady state for calculation of cardiac output. Temporary pacing should be used in patients with irregular heart rates (eg, atrial fibrillation) to maintain consistent ventricular intervals to improve diagnostic interpretation of the hemodynamic data in these patients. If possible, continuous recording of hemodynamic pressures should be performed to allow retrospective review of these pressures throughout the study.

The accurate measurement of cardiac pressures with fluid-filled catheters requires the use of rigid, large-bore catheters with minimization of the tubing length between the catheter and pressure transducer. Fluid-filled catheters can reliably measure absolute and mean cardiac pressures. However, for analysis of pressure waveforms in patients who may have restriction or constriction, high-fidelity micromanometer-tip catheters (Millar Instruments, Houston, TX) facilitate instantaneous recordings and should be used. These catheters help overcome underdamping, which can mimic early rapid ventricular filling. An alternative method is to use a PressureWire (St. Jude Medical, Fridley, MN), which is relatively higher in fidelity than fluid-filled catheters. In either method, the high-fidelity catheters are calibrated to fluid-filled pressures at baseline and calibration is repeated following any catheter repositioning. A rigid coronary guide catheter for left ventricular pressures and a balloon wedge catheter (Arrow International, Teleflex Medical, Wayne, PA) for right-sided pressures both can be used to accommodate high-fidelity catheters. An appropriate size of these catheters should be chosen to allow calibration to fluid pressures with the micromanometers in place.

## CONSTRICTIVE PERICARDITIS
### Pathophysiology
When right heart failure is out of proportion to the degree of left ventricular dysfunction, constrictive pericarditis should be suspected. The differential diagnosis of right heart failure includes restrictive cardiomyopathy, left to right intracardiac shunting (eg, atrial septal defect), tricuspid regurgitation, pulmonary embolism, right ventricular (RV) infarction, and pulmonary hypertension. Many of these causes can be readily diagnosed with modern noninvasive diagnostic imaging. A common clinical scenario is the inability to distinguish restrictive cardiomyopathy and constrictive pericarditis. These entities have distinct treatments; physicians, therefore, must be able to differentiate the two clinical entities.[1,2]

Constrictive pericarditis is the result of pericardial healing with fibrosis and possibly calcification, following a pericardial insult that leads to loss of elasticity of the pericardial sac. Potential causes are chest radiation, prior cardiac surgery, trauma, and systemic diseases that affect the pericardium (eg, connective tissue disease, tuberculosis, malignancy). Clinical subtypes of constrictive pericarditis include transient constrictive pericarditis, chronic constrictive pericarditis, and effusive constrictive pericarditis. Transient pericarditis is a subform of constrictive pericarditis identified by a reversible pattern of constriction following medical therapy or spontaneous resolution.[3]

The loss of pericardial elasticity leads to impairment in ventricular filling in mid and late diastole, thereby limiting increases in ventricular volume after the end of the early filling period. The end-diastolic pressures become equalized or nearly equalized in all 4 cardiac chambers with the total cardiac volume fixed by the noncompliant pericardium. Because the ventricular septum is not involved, the ventricular septum bulges toward the left during inspiration and returns toward the right during expiration, leading to marked enhancement of ventricular interdependence. This ventricular interaction leads to reciprocal changes in filling and emptying of the right and left ventricles. The rigid, noncompliant pericardium also prevents the complete transmission of intrathoracic pressure to the intracardiac chambers, resulting in dissociation of thoracic and cardiac pressures.

Restrictive cardiomyopathy is a primary myocardial disease characterized by a nondilated rigid ventricle that restricts ventricular filling, leading to hemodynamic changes that can mimic constrictive pericarditis but have distinct differences. Restrictive cardiomyopathy may be primary or secondary due to infiltrative (eg, amyloid), noninfiltrative (eg, hypereosinophilia), and storage disorders (eg, glycogen storage disorders). Mediastinal radiation has also been associated with restrictive cardiomyopathy.

Patients with restrictive cardiomyopathy have severe diastolic dysfunction with high filling pressures in all 4 cardiac chambers. Equalization of pressures is not common, though can be observed. In contrast to constriction, ventricular interdependence is not a prominent feature. Traditional hemodynamic criteria to differentiate restriction from constriction include pulmonary hypertension, left ventricular end-diastolic pressure that exceeds the RV end-diastolic pressure by more than 5 mm Hg, and RV end-diastolic pressure that is less than one-third of the peak systolic pressure.[4] However, these traditional hemodynamic criteria are not as helpful as the determination of exaggerated ventricular dependence for differentiating these two conditions.[5,6]

## Invasive Hemodynamic Assessment

For invasive hemodynamic studies of patients with suspected constrictive pericarditis, the operator should perform right and left heart catheterization with simultaneous assessment of absolute pressures across multiple chambers. The invasive assessment should focus on determining the presence of both enhancement of ventricular interdependence and dissociation of the intrathoracic and intracardiac pressures, while excluding other potential causes of right heart failure. An accurate measurement of cardiac output by either the thermodilution or Fick method should be routinely performed as a part of the invasive hemodynamic assessment in suspected constrictive pericarditis.

On right heart catheterization, rapid fluid administration (ie, >1 L saline bolus) should be performed when the right atrial (RA) pressure is low (ie, <15 mm Hg). In patients with constrictive pericarditis, rapid early ventricular filling results in a prominent y descent. The x decent, which is due to atrial relaxation and downward displacement of the tricuspid valve with isovolumetric contraction, is not affected in constrictive pericarditis. The combination of a prominent y descent and preserved x descent results in a W or M pattern on the RA tracing (**Fig. 1**). It is important to note that a prominent y descent can be seen in patients with many causes of right-sided heart failure (eg, severe tricuspid regurgitation, restrictive cardiomyopathy, RV infarction, and massive pulmonary embolism). An increase in RA pressure during inspiration (ie, Kussmaul sign) is also frequently present but is also not specific for constrictive pericarditis.

The pressure tracings in the RV and left ventricle in constrictive pericarditis characteristically show a dip-and-plateau or a square-root pattern. Rapid, unimpeded early ventricular filling causes the early sharp increase in the diastolic pressure. An abrupt cessation of

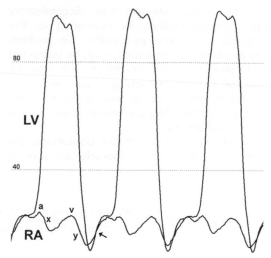

Fig. 1. Ventricular filling pressures in constrictive pericarditis. In the RA tracing, there are rapid x and y descents. The y descent of the RA pressure tracing corresponds to the early rapid filling phase of the ventricular pressure tracing, which demonstrates the typical dip-and-plateau pattern (*arrow*). These hemodynamic tracings were taken using high-fidelity micromanometer catheters from a patient with constrictive pericarditis. LV, left ventricle; RA, right atrium.

ventricular filling in mid and late diastole occurs once the limit for cardiac volume set by the scarred pericardium is achieved. The height of the rapid filling wave is usually greater than 7 mm Hg in constrictive pericarditis. The RV end-diastolic pressure is often elevated, and has been described as commonly being more than one-third of the RV systolic pressure. Pulmonary hypertension is uncommon in patients with constrictive pericarditis. Equalization of diastolic pressures in all four cardiac chambers with inspiration (ie, within 5 mm Hg) is frequently present, but is not specific. Disease states with volume overload, such as decompensated heart failure, acute mitral regurgitation, severe tricuspid regurgitation, and RV infarction that cause relative pericardial restraint can also have diastolic pressure equalization.

Accurate assessment of constrictive pericarditis entails the use of not only single chamber pressure measurements, but also simultaneous left and right heart examinations with dynamic respiration. In patients with low cardiac output and low or normal intracardiac pressures, it is important to perform a fluid challenge (>1 L saline bolus over 6–8 minutes), which can unmask the hemodynamic findings of constrictive pericarditis.[7]

Dissociation of intrathoracic and intracardiac pressures and exaggerated ventricular interdependence are two most discriminatory hemodynamic findings for evaluating for the possible constrictive pericarditis. To perform the assessments, the patient must be instructed to inspire and expire deeply (systolic pressure drop of >10 mm Hg) and gradually, with each of these respiratory phases extended over several diastolic filling periods (at least 5) in the absence of ectopy.

In patients with constrictive pericarditis, the inspiratory decrease in thoracic pressure is increased systemic venous return). These alterations manifest as reciprocal changes in peak systolic pressure, stroke volume, and pulse pressure in both ventricles during respiration.

A quantitative determination of evaluating ventricular interdependence can be performed with measurement of the *systolic area index*. This method examines the ratio of the areas (millimeters of mercury × second) under the RV and left ventricular systolic pressures during inspiration versus expiration (**Figs. 4** and **5**).[5]

$$\text{Systolic area index} = \frac{\text{RV area during inspiration/LV area during inspiration}}{\text{RV area during expiration/LV area during expiration}}$$

transmitted to the pulmonary wedge pressure, but not to the ventricles that are shielded from the respiratory pressure changes by the pericardial scar. By lowering pulmonary wedge and left atrial pressure, inspiration leads to a decrease in the diastolic pressure gradient for ventricular filling (**Fig. 2**). Conversely, during expiration, there is a relatively increase in the pressure gradient for ventricular filling. These findings are described as dissociation of the intrathoracic and intra-cavitary pressures.

Enhancement of ventricular interdependence leads to *discordant* changes in right and left ventricular pressures during respiration that is more exclusive to constrictive pericarditis (**Fig. 3**). This discordance is due to reciprocal changes in ventricular filling mediated by the ventricular septum due to the finite cardiac volume in patients with constrictive pericarditis (not by

In a study of 100 patients, including 59 who had surgically proven constriction, a systolic area index ratio of greater than 1.1 had 97% sensitivity and 100% predictive accuracy for identifying patients with constrictive pericarditis.

Patients with severe tricuspid regurgitation can share hemodynamic findings with those who have constrictive pericarditis.[8] Careful analysis during inspiration can help to differentiate the two disorders. During inspiration, patients with severe tricuspid regurgitation have widening of left ventricular and RV diastolic pressures and accentuation of the height and slope of RV early rapid filling wave (**Fig. 6**). These findings occur more commonly in patients with tricuspid regurgitation because flow into the RV is not limited by a rigid pericardium that is present in constrictive

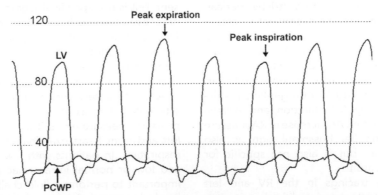

**Fig. 2.** Dissociation of intracavitary and intrathoracic pressures in constrictive pericarditis. In patients with constrictive pericarditis, inspiration leads to a decrease in ventricular filling by decreasing intrathoracic pressure relative to ventricular diastolic pressure. Conversely, during expiration, positive intrathoracic pressure leads to an increase in ventricular filling. These respiratory effects can be seen by examining the changes in the pressure gradient between the pulmonary capillary wedge pressure (PCWP) and ventricular early diastolic pressure (*gray*).

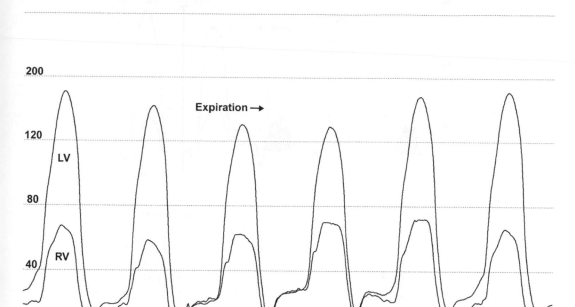

**Fig. 3.** Enhancement of ventricular interdependence in constriction. In patients with constrictive pericarditis, the total ventricular volume is fixed by the noncompliant pericardium. Thus, reciprocal respiratory changes in the filling of each ventricle occur. These changes are described as discordance in pulse pressure, systolic pressure, or stroke volume between the RV and left ventricle (LV) during respiration.

pericarditis. Thus, patients with tricuspid regurgitation have significant enhancement of RV diastolic filling during inspiration with a marked increase in RV diastolic pressures and rapid flow waves.

In patients with restrictive cardiomyopathy, there is neither significant dissociation of intrathoracic and intracavitary pressures nor enhancement of ventricular interdependence. In these patients, respiration affects the pulmonary wedge and left ventricular diastolic pressures equally or nearly equally; thus, the diastolic ventricular filling gradient remains minimally changed with both expiration and inspiration. Because there is not significant enhancement of ventricular interdependence, the left ventricular and RV pressures also move *concordantly* throughout the respiratory cycle (Fig. 7).

## CARDIAC TAMPONADE

Cardiac tamponade occurs when intrapericardial pressure exceeds intracardiac pressure, resulting in compression of cardiac chambers and impairment of ventricular filling throughout the diastolic period. Virtually any disorder that causes pericardial effusion can result in cardiac tamponade. The most common cause is malignancy, with breast and lung cancer being the most frequent. Other important causes are complications of invasive cardiac procedures, idiopathic or viral pericarditis, aortic dissection with disruption of the aortic valve annulus, tuberculosis, uremia, and pericarditis or ventricular wall rupture from myocardial infarction. Echocardiography is the primary modality for diagnosing cardiac tamponade. However, the increasing complexity of invasive cardiac procedures and their potential association with tamponade necessitates familiarity with the identification and treatment of tamponade in the cardiac catheterization laboratory.

### Pathophysiology

The pericardium consists of an external layer of fibrous connective tissue (ie, fibrous pericardium) and an internal double-layered sac (ie, serous pericardium) that typically contains 15 to 50 mL of fluid. The intrapericardial pressure normally approximates the intrapleural pressure ($-5$ to $+5$ cm $H_2O$) and is lower than the

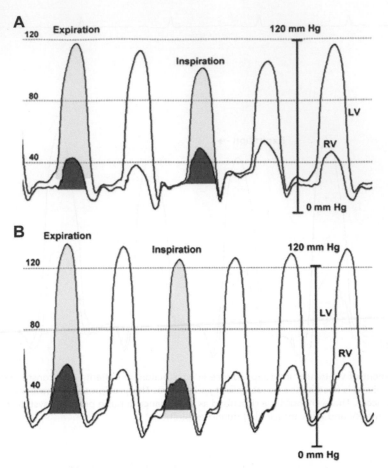

**Fig. 4.** The systolic area index for differentiating constrictive pericarditis from restrictive cardiomyopathy. (*A*) In a patient with constrictive pericarditis, there is an increase in the area of the RV pressure curve (*orange-shaded area*) during inspiration compared with expiration. The area of the left ventricular (LV) pressure curve (*yellow-shaded area*) decreases during inspiration as compared with expiration. (*B*) Conversely, in a patient with restrictive cardiomyopathy, there is a decrease in the area of the RV pressure curve (*orange-shaded area*) as compared with expiration. The area of the LV pressure curve (*yellow-shaded area*) is unchanged during inspiration as compared with expiration. (*Reprinted from* Talreja DR, Nishimura RA, Oh JK, et al. Constrictive pericarditis in the modern era: novel criteria for diagnosis in the cardiac catheterization laboratory. J Am Coll Cardiol 2008;51:317; with permission.)

diastolic filling pressure of the cardiac chambers. Fluid accumulation in the pericardial space in tamponade raises the intrapericardial pressure in an exponential pattern that follows a J-shaped pressure volume curve.[9] Initially, fluid accumulation occurs at the expense of the pericardial reserve volume, with minimal increase in intrapericardial pressure (flat segment of the J-shaped pericardial pressure volume curve). Further accumulation of pericardial fluid produces a sharp increase in intrapericardial pressure (ascending limb of the *J*). The elbow of the *J* represents the beginning of pericardial restraint to cardiac filling. Rapidly accumulating effusions reach the point of pericardial restraint

at smaller volumes.[10,11] This evolving sequence of the hemodynamic effects of cardiac tamponade has been described as 3 phases.[12] In phase I, intrapericardial pressure increases but does not equilibrate with ventricular pressure. Phase II occurs when the intrapericardial pressure equilibrates with the RV filling diastolic pressure. Further accumulation of pericardial fluid leads to phase III, in which the intrapericardial pressure equilibrates with the left ventricular filling pressure. Impairment of ventricular filling by the elevated intrapericardial pressure precipitates a reduction in cardiac stroke volume and output, leading to arterial hypotension. On echocardiography, diastolic collapse

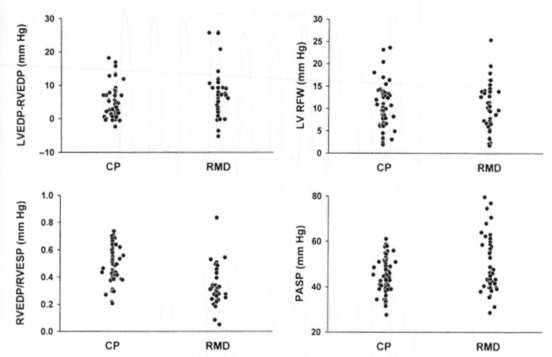

Fig. 5. Utility of the systolic area index for differentiating constrictive pericarditis from restrictive cardiomyopathy. A scatter plot of the ratio of RV to left ventricular (LV) area during expiration versus inspiration. CP, constrictive pericarditis; RMD, restrictive cardiomyopathy. LVEDP, left ventricular end-diastolic pressure; PASP, pulmonary artery systolic pressure; RFW, rapid filling wave; RVEDP, right ventricular end-diastolic pressure; RVESP, right ventricular end-systolic pressure. (*Reprinted from* Talreja DR, Nishimura RA, Oh JK, et al. Constrictive pericarditis in the modern era: novel criteria for diagnosis in the cardiac catheterization laboratory. J Am Coll Cardiol 2008;51:318; with permission.)

of the free wall of the cardiac chambers is visible once the intrapericardial pressure exceeds the intracardiac pressure, with collapse of the free walls of the right atrium preceding that of the RV.

Pulsus paradoxus is a hallmark of cardiac tamponade that is due to exaggerated ventricular interdependence. The pericardial fluid reduces the pericardial space for cardiac chamber expansion (ie, mechanical compartmentalization). Expansion of the RV chamber during inspiration and RV volume loading, therefore, occurs at the expense of the left ventricle. The manifestation of pulsus paradoxus is an inspiratory decline in left ventricular stroke volume and consequently a decrease in the aortic pulse pressure (>10 mm Hg).[13]

## INVASIVE HEMODYNAMICS

Cardiac catheterization is usually not needed to make the diagnosis of cardiac tamponade. In these patients, the atrial pressure tracing is typically elevated with prominent x descents and blunted or absent y descents (Fig. 8). Preservation of the x descent occurs because systolic ejection leads to a decrease in intracardiac

volume and a temporary reduction in intrapericardial pressures. During the remainder of the cardiac cycle, elevated intrapericardial pressure impairs ventricular filling leading to blunting or obliteration of the y descent. Corresponding changes are also seen in ventricular pressure tracings with elevated diastolic pressures and loss or blunting of early diastolic pressure (or ventricular minimum pressure). Other hemodynamic findings include equalization of end-diastolic pressures, reduced cardiac output, and alterations in the systolic ejection period or pulse pressure that result from decreased stroke volume, analogous to the bedside finding of pulsus paradoxus. In order to maintain the cardiac output, compensatory tachycardia occurs. During pericardiocentesis, intrapericardial pressure may be sampled and found to be elevated and equal to the ventricular end-diastolic pressure.

There are uncommon clinical presentations of cardiac tamponade. Localized cardiac tamponade occurs when a loculated pericardial effusion is tactically located to impair ventricular filling. This manifestation may occur after cardiac surgery or other postoperative settings. The loculated effusion may be present

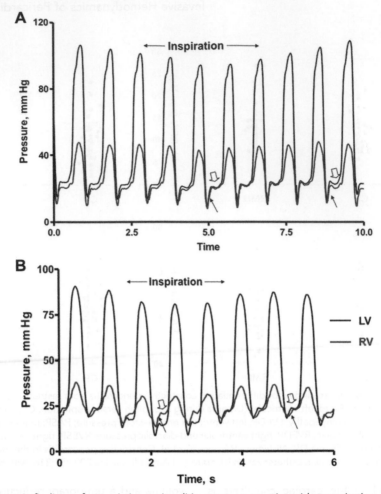

Fig. 6. Hemodynamic findings of constrictive pericarditis versus severe tricuspid regurgitation. Enhanced ventricular interdependence may be present in both disorders. (A) In a patient with severe tricuspid regurgitation, deep inspiration leads to separation of the diastolic pressures with a higher RV diastolic pressure (*arrowhead*), and the rapid filling wave in the RV (*arrows*) becomes deeper and steeper. (B) In a patient with constrictive pericarditis, there is elevation and equalization of diastolic pressures. However, the RV rapid filling wave (*arrowheads*) is not accentuated on inspiration. Black arrows indicate the portion of hemodynamic recording that corresponds to the inspiratory phase of respiration. (*Reprinted from* Jaber WA, Sorajja P, Borlaug BA, et al. Differentiation of tricuspid regurgitation from constrictive pericarditis: novel criteria for diagnosis in the cardiac catheterization laboratory. Heart 2009;95:1451; with permission.)

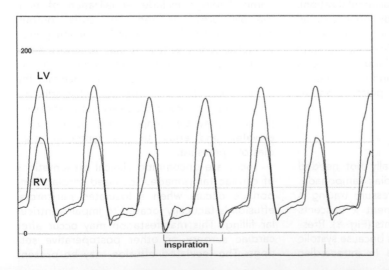

Fig. 7. Pressure recordings from a patient with restrictive cardiomyopathy. The left ventricular (LV) and RV pressures move concordantly with respiration.

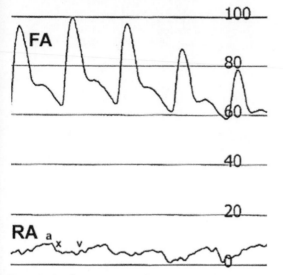

**Fig. 8.** Cardiac tamponade. Hypotension in the femoral artery (FA) pressure with loss of the y descent in the RA pressure tracing is evident. With inspiration, there is a decrease in the aortic pulse pressure.

in the posterior pericardial space adjacent to the atria, which poses challenges for detection by echocardiography. Posterior loculated effusion should be suspected in postoperative patients with hemodynamic instability. Low-pressure tamponade occurs without elevated jugular venous pressure because the intracardiac filling pressures are low.[14] Examples of this manifestation are patients with tuberculosis or malignancy complicated by severe dehydration.

## REFERENCES

1. McCaughan BC, Schaff HV, Piehler JM, et al. Early and late results of pericardiectomy for constrictive pericarditis. J Thorac Cardiovasc Surg 1985;89(3): 340–50.

2. Ammash NM, Seward JB, Bailey KR, et al. Clinical profile and outcome of idiopathic restrictive cardiomyopathy. Circulation 2000;101(21):2490–6.

3. Gentry J, Klein AL, Jellis CL. Transient constrictive pericarditis: current diagnostic and therapeutic strategies. Curr Cardiol Rep 2016;18(5):41.

4. Vaitkus PT, Kussmaul WG. Constrictive pericarditis versus restrictive cardiomyopathy: a reappraisal and update of diagnostic criteria. Am Heart J 1991;122(5):1431–41.

5. Talreja DR, Nishimura RA, Oh JK, et al. Constrictive pericarditis in the modern era: novel criteria for diagnosis in the cardiac catheterization laboratory. J Am Coll Cardiol 2008;51(3):315–9.

6. Hurrell DG, Nishimura RA, Higano ST, et al. Value of dynamic respiratory changes in left and right ventricular pressures for the diagnosis of constrictive pericarditis. Circulation 1996;93(11):2007–13.

7. Bush CA, Stang JM, Wooley CF, et al. Occult constrictive pericardial disease. Diagnosis by rapid volume expansion and correction by pericardiectomy. Circulation 1977;56(6):924–30.

8. Jaber WA, Sorajja P, Borlaug BA, et al. Differentiation of tricuspid regurgitation from constrictive pericarditis: novel criteria for diagnosis in the cardiac catheterisation laboratory. Heart 2009;95(17): 1449–54.

9. Janicki JS, Weber KT. The pericardium and ventricular interaction, distensibility, and function. Am J Physiol 1980;238(4):H494–503.

10. Spodick DH. Acute cardiac tamponade. N Engl J Med 2003;349(7):684–90.

11. Shabetai R. The pathophysiology of cardiac tamponade. Cardiovasc Clin 1976;7(3):67–89.

12. Reddy PS, Curtiss EI. Cardiac tamponade. Cardiol Clin 1990;8(4):627–37.

13. Takata M, Harasawa Y, Beloucif S, et al. Coupled vs. uncoupled pericardial constraint: effects on cardiac chamber interactions. J Appl Physiol (1985) 1997; 83(6):1799–813.

14. Antman EM, Cargill V, Grossman W. Low-pressure cardiac tamponade. Ann Intern Med 1979;91(3):403–6.

# Invasive Hemodynamics of Valvular Heart Disease

Michele Pighi, MD, Anita W. Asgar, MD, MSc*

---

**KEYWORDS**

• Valvular heart disease • Hemodynamics • Stenosis • Regurgitation

**KEY POINTS**

- Invasive hemodynamics assessment is an important diagnostic tool in the management of patients with valvular heart disease.
- Proper tools, technique, and understanding pitfalls are important.
- Appropriate diagnosis and treatment are necessary for optimal patient outcomes.

---

## INTRODUCTION

The evaluation of valvular heart disease has made a dramatic shift in the past several decades with the evolution of 2-dimensional echocardiography and Doppler echocardiography. These noninvasive techniques have become the mainstay of the evaluation and follow-up of valvular heart disease. The 2014 American Heart Association/American College of Cardiology Valvular Heart Disease Guidelines recommend transthoracic echocardiography as a class I indication for the diagnosis, to determine prognosis and for the timing of intervention in valvular heart disease.[1] Despite this recommendation, invasive hemodynamic assessment remains an essential tool in equivocal cases. The interventional cardiologist remains the expert in hemodynamic evaluation and a thorough understanding of the tools, interpretation of data and pitfalls is fundamental. This article reviews the indications, technique, and interpretation of hemodynamic assessments in valvular heart disease.

### General Principles of Invasive Hemodynamic Assessment of Valvular Heart Disease

A thorough, systematic approach to the hemodynamic assessment of valvular heart disease should begin with a review of the noninvasive imaging to understand the question being asked and the diagnostic dilemma requiring clarification. Once this has been identified, a plan of the necessary measurements and assessments should be made and vascular access and tools required determined. In general, high quality pressure measurements often require either 6-Fr or 7-Fr vascular access and rebalancing and zeroing of the baseline should be done to ensure accurate values. Ideally, all catheters should undergo periodic flushing with heparinized saline during the procedure to prevent the formation of microthrombi. In some cases, operators use doses of systemic unfractionated heparin for longer procedures or complex anatomies.

### Valvular stenosis

The evaluation of valve stenosis requires the measurement of the valve gradient and calculation of valve area.[2] In the cardiac catheterization laboratory, valve areas are calculated using the transvalvular pressure gradient and cardiac output by way of the Gorlin or Hakki equation (Table 1).

Valve gradients are best measured with catheters positioned on both sides of the valve being evaluated and simultaneous pressure measurement. Peak valve gradients have traditionally been measured in the catheterization laboratory; however, these "artificial" gradients are now recognized to be nonphysiologic and have

---

Department of Medicine, Montreal Heart Institute, Universite de Montreal, 5000 Rue Bélanger, Montreal, Quebec H1T 1C8, Canada
* Corresponding author.
E-mail address: anita.asgar@gmail.com

Intervent Cardiol Clin 6 (2017) 319–327
http://dx.doi.org/10.1016/j.iccl.2017.03.003
2211-7458/17/© 2017 Elsevier Inc. All rights reserved.

**Table 1**
**Equations used to calculate valve area in the catheterization laboratory**

| | Formula |
|---|---|
| Gorlin | $AVA = (CO/HR \times SEP)/44.5 \times \sqrt{\Delta P}$ |
| | $AVA$ = aortic valve area (cm$^2$); |
| | $CO$ = cardiac output (L/min); |
| | $HR$ = heart rate (beats/min); |
| | $SEP$ = systolic ejection period (s); |
| | 44.5 = constant; $\Delta P$ = mean systolic pressure gradient |
| Hakki | $AVA = CO/\sqrt{\Delta P}$ |
| | $AVA$ = aortic valve area (cm$^2$); |
| | $CO$ = cardiac output (L/min); |
| | $\Delta P$ = peak systolic pressure gradient |

been largely replaced by the measurement of mean gradients over the systolic ejection period, which is felt to be a better indicator of valve stenosis severity.[3]

The cardiac output is ideally measured for each patient. The gold standard for estimating cardiac output is the Fick principle, in which cardiac output is $O_2$ consumption divided by the difference between arterial and venous $O_2$, although many sites rely on the thermodilution method. Care must be taken when using thermodilution because it may be less accurate in the setting of intracardiac shunts, low cardiac output states, significant tricuspid regurgitation, or arrhythmia.

The Gorlin equation incorporates cardiac output, heart rate, systolic ejection period (or diastolic filing period), an empirical constant, acceleration of gravity factor, and the pressure difference across the stenotic valve to calculate valve area. The simplified Hakki equation uses the cardiac output and pressure gradient to arrive at a valve area with similar accuracy to that of the Gorlin equation.[4]

## AORTIC STENOSIS
### Indication
Invasive hemodynamic assessment of aortic stenosis is recommended when the results of noninvasive tests are equivocal or when the patient's symptoms are out of proportion to gradients and valve area measured noninvasively. In fact, underestimation of valve gradients may occur by echocardiography if the Doppler beam is not aligned parallel to the aortic jet; the Doppler velocity and, therefore, the true transvalvular gradient may be underestimated. In addition, calculation of the aortic valve area by echo uses the continuity equation, which may be subject to inaccuracies related to the assumption of a circular left ventricular (LV) outflow tract and the measurement of the LV outflow tract diameter.

### Technique
A simultaneous assessment of LV and ascending aortic pressures[5] is required for the evaluation of aortic stenosis to measure the mean aortic transvalvular gradient. This is ideally performed using a catheter with side holes such as a pigtail catheter and can be performed using either a retrograde or an anterograde (transseptal) technique.

The retrograde technique requires the use of a dual lumen pigtail catheter measuring pressure above and below the aortic valve, in the ascending aorta and left ventricle, respectively. This technique does require retrograde crossing of the aortic valve to position a catheter in the LV, which may be best accomplished by the use of an Amplatz or Judkins Right catheter and straight-tip wire as shown in Table 2. Once in position in the left ventricle, the catheter should be changed using an exchange wire for a dual lumen pigtail catheter. In the absence of a dual lumen catheter, measurement may be performed using a pigtail in the left ventricle and pressure from the femoral artery, or via a second arterial access point with a second pigtail in the ascending aorta. A realignment of the pressure tracing will be necessary when using the femoral artery owing to delays in arterial wave transmission to the extremities.

**Table 2**
**Evaluation of aortic stenosis**

| Approach | Vascular Access | Equipment |
|---|---|---|
| Retrograde | Arterial 6 Fr | Amplatz AL1 Judkins Right (JR4) Straight-tip wire 150 cm Exchange wire (J-tip) 260 cm Pigtail catheter 6 Fr (dual or single lumen) |
| Anterograde | Venous 7 Fr | Mullins sheath and dilator 0.032 inch J-tip wire Brockenborough needle (BRK or BRK1) Pigtail 7 Fr |
| | Arterial 6 Fr | Pigtail 6 Fr |

The anterograde approach consists of simultaneous evaluation of LV and aortic pressures with 2 catheters: one is positioned in the ascending aorta just above the aortic valve and the other in the left ventricle via a transseptal puncture. The transseptal puncture is performed in the usual fashion and the needle and dilator are removed as the Mullins catheter is advanced into the left atrium. A pigtail catheter is then advanced via the Mullins into the left ventricle. This technique may be more difficult in the case of mitral stenosis (MS); however, it would permit evaluation of both mitral and aortic stenosis in those patients with combined valve disease.

### Hemodynamic findings and interpretation

Evaluation of hemodynamic data begins with a qualitative assessment of the pressure tracings obtained in both the aorta and LV. In the case of fixed valvular obstruction seen in aortic stenosis, there is a delay and reduction in the upstroke of the central aortic pressure that begins at aortic valve opening and correlates with the well-known physical findings of parvus and tardus (Fig. 1A).

This may also be reflected as a slow ventricular upstroke on the LV pressure tracing. Quantitative evaluation of the hemodynamic data may reveal a normal or increased LV "a" wave, and commonly an elevated LV end-diastolic pressure owing to reduced compliance of the hypertrophied LV. Simultaneous pressure measurement in aortic stenosis reveals a pressure gradient as shown in Fig. 1B, and valve area is calculated, as previously described.

### Challenges in hemodynamic assessment

**Carabello sign.** During the pullback technique, the transvalvular gradient may be slightly increased by the presence of a catheter across the stenotic aortic valve, thereby reducing the effective orifice area. In this context, it is possible to observe the so-called Carabello sign,[6] an increase in arterial blood pressure during left heart catheter pullback in patients with severe

**A**

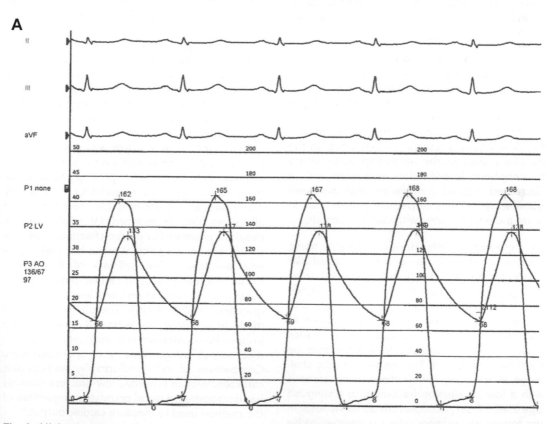

**Fig. 1.** (A) Aortic pressure tracings in an 82-year-old patient with severe aortic stenosis. (a) Aortic pressure tracing demonstrating delayed upstroke in the setting of severe obstruction. (b) Aortic pressure tracing immediately after transcatheter aortic valve replacement demonstrating improvement following relief of the obstruction. (B) Simultaneous LV and aortic pressure measurements in aortic stenosis. A slight delay can be seen in the upstroke of both the aortic and left ventricular pressure tracing with the presence of mean transvalvular gradient of 32 mm Hg for a calculated valve area of 0.86 cm² in the setting of a cardiac output of 4.0 L/min.

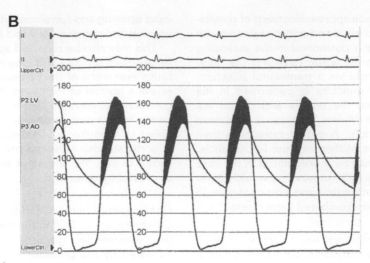

**Fig. 1.** (*continued*)

aortic stenosis (in particular in valve areas of 0.7 cm² or smaller, when 7-Fr or 8-Fr catheters are used to cross the valve). This effect is proportional to the severity of the underlying aortic stenosis and is only observed with very severe stenosis.

**Aortic pressure.** When evaluating aortic stenosis, the location for aortic pressure measurement is important, because there are differences between a true central aortic pressure and a peripheral artery pressure, which shows a delay in aortic pressure upstroke of 80 to 120 ms and a higher peak systolic aortic pressure. Moreover, the peak arterial pressure is often higher in the periphery than in the ascending aorta owing to peripheral amplification associated with a decreased arterial compliance and increased pulse wave velocity (especially problematic in older patients or those with calcified vessels).

**Low gradient aortic stenosis.** Severe aortic stenosis is defined as a mean transvalvular gradient of 40 mm Hg or greater[1]; however, small changes in transvalvular flow can result in significant reductions in the valve gradient and lead to the recognition of the clinical entity described as low-flow, low-gradient aortic stenosis. In such cases, the ventricular systolic function may be decreased or normal. The main diagnostic challenge in low-flow, low-gradient aortic stenosis with a low LV ejection fraction is to distinguish true severe from pseudosevere aortic stenosis. In the former, the primary culprit is deemed to be the valve disease, and the LV dysfunction is a secondary or concomitant phenomenon. Conversely, the predominant factor in pseudosevere aortic stenosis is deemed to be myocardial disease, and aortic stenosis severity is overestimated owing

to incomplete opening of the valve in relation to the low-flow state.[7]

The Gorlin equation is flow dependent and may underestimate the valve area when the cardiac output is reduced (ie, <3 L/min). For those patients with reduced cardiac output or severe LV dysfunction, recalculation of the aortic valve area after a pharmacologic stimulation of cardiac output, using dobutamine, may be performed. An increase in the transvalvular gradient with subsequent decrease in the calculated aortic valve area confirms the diagnosis of severe aortic stenosis.

In the setting of low-flow, low-gradient aortic stenosis with a normal ejection fraction, there is a low-flow state as a result of pronounced or exaggerated concentric LV remodeling, reduced LV cavity size and decreased LV compliance and filling resulting in reduced LV stroke volume despite a preserved LV ejection fraction. These patients have severe aortic stenosis but their gradients are lower. The hallmark of this clinical presentation is a reduced cardiac output (stroke volume index <35 mL/m² and low transvalvular gradients [<40 mm Hg]). The diagnosis can be made noninvasively by echocardiography or by invasive hemodynamics with measurement of cardiac output using oximetry or thermodilution. Comparison of echocardiography and cardiac catheterization in low-flow, low-gradient stenosis has demonstrated good correlation regardless of the method used to measure cardiac output.[8]

## MITRAL STENOSIS
### Indication
The widespread availability of echocardiography has led to a limited role for cardiac catheterization

in the diagnosis of MS. Nevertheless, invasive pressure measurements have a role when noninvasive tests are not conclusive; there is a discrepancy between noninvasive tests and clinical findings or symptoms, or in the setting of pulmonary arterial hypertension that is out of proportion to the severity of MS as determined by echocardiography. In such cases, cardiac catheterization is important to further characterize the pulmonary hypertension by determining whether it is secondary to MS, LV diastolic or systolic dysfunction, or intrinsic pulmonary disease.

Invasive catheterization is also of importance in monitoring hemodynamic status during a transcatheter balloon mitral valvuloplasty.

## Technique
In the cardiac catheterization laboratory, the severity of MS is reflected by the mean mitral valve gradient measured during diastole by the simultaneous comparison of the LV pressure (obtained with a LV catheter positioned retrogradely from the aorta), and the left atrial (LA) pressure (measured directly and more precisely using a transseptal catheter or indirectly with a pulmonary artery catheter in the wedged position). The equipment required is outlined in **Table 3**.

## Hemodynamic Findings and Interpretation
In pure MS, qualitative evaluation of the left ventricle is normal unless there is coexisting coronary artery disease or LV dysfunction from other causes. Quantitative assessment of LA or wedge pressure tracings demonstrates an increased LA pressure with a prominent "a" wave in patients in sinus rhythm and a decreased "y" descent, which is proportional to the severity of MS (**Fig. 2**). There may be a coexisting increase in the v wave in the case of coexistent mitral regurgitation (MR) or significant elevation of filling pressures. Pulmonary hypertension is also frequently present in those patients with significant MS.

The mitral valve gradient is calculated as the difference between the mean LA pressure (measured either directly or indirectly), and the mean LV pressure during diastole. This diastolic gradient is affected by the length of diastole, decreasing at low heart rates and increasing at higher rates. During atrial systole, the gradient increases and is markedly higher than the LV end-diastolic pressure. The mean pulmonary artery wedge pressure usually reflects the mean LA pressure; however, the pulmonary artery wedge pressure/LV pressure gradient frequently overestimates the true severity of MS owing to a phase shift in the pulmonary artery wedge pressure and a delay in transmission of the change in pressure contour through the pulmonary circulation.

## Pitfalls
### Atrial fibrillation
In patients with atrial fibrillation, the severity of MS as assessed via the pulmonary capillary wedge pressure may differ from that obtained with the direct measurement of the LA pressure. Patients who are in atrial fibrillation require planimetry and the average of valve gradients over at least 10 cardiac cycles.

### Wedge pressure versus left atrial pressure measurement
Accurate wedge tracings may be difficult to obtain in patients with MS because of pulmonary hypertension or dilated right heart chambers. The pulmonary capillary wedge pressure tracing must also be realigned with the LV tracing to account for the time delay. Although it is generally accepted that the pulmonary capillary wedge pressure provides a satisfactory estimate of LA pressure, some studies show that PCW pressure may overestimate the LA pressure by 2 to 3 mm Hg, thereby increasing the measured mitral valve gradient.

### Limitations of the Gorlin formula
The mitral valve area is derived using the Gorlin formula. Because the square root of the mean gradient is used, the calculated valve area is more strongly influenced by the cardiac output

| Table 3 Evaluation of mitral stenosis and mitral regurgitation | | |
|---|---|---|
| **Approach** | **Vascular Access** | **Equipment** |
| Indirect (pulmonary capillary wedge pressure) | Venous 6 Fr | Multipurpose or pulmonary artery balloon-tip pressure catheter |
| | Arterial 6 Fr | Pigtail catheter 6 Fr |
| Direct (left atrial pressure) | Venous 7 Fr | Mullins sheath and dilator 0.032 inch J-tip wire |
| | Arterial 6 Fr | Brockenborough needle (BRK or BRK1) Pigtail 6 Fr |

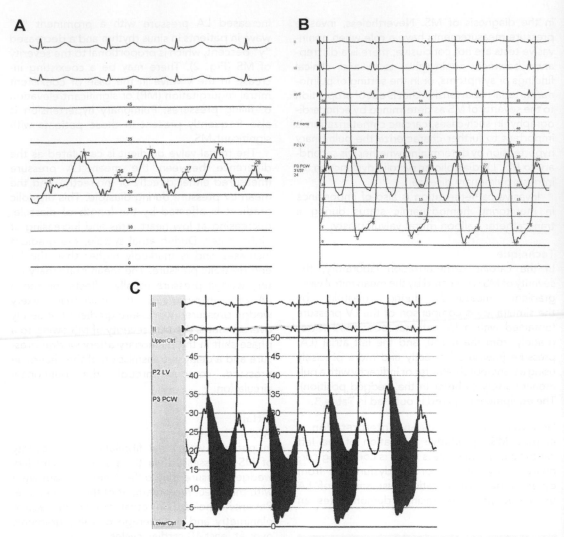

Fig. 2. Simultaneous left ventricular and pulmonary capillary wedge pressure tracings in mitral stenosis. (A) The "a" wave is prominent and measures approximately 28 to 30 mm Hg with an increased "v" wave as well. (B, C) The mean mitral valve gradient is 17 mm Hg for a calculated valve area of 0.92 cm² in the setting of a cardiac output of 4.0 L/min.

than the pressure gradient. Accordingly, errors in measuring cardiac output may have profound effects on the calculated valve area, particularly in patients with low cardiac outputs. In patients with stenosis and regurgitation of the same valve, the net forward flow, as determined by the Fick or thermodilution method, overestimates the severity of the valvular stenosis because the Gorlin formula is based on total forward flow across the stenotic valve, not net forward flow. Therefore, if valvular regurgitation is present, an angiographic cardiac output is the appropriate value to use as the cardiac output. In low-output states, calculation using the Gorlin equation may result in smaller valve areas.

## Valvular Regurgitation

In the majority of cases, patients with valvular regurgitation can be fully evaluated noninvasively only requiring coronary angiography before intervention. In some cases, however, as in the case of valve stenosis, the clinical presentation may not be congruent with the echocardiographic findings. In particular, patients with MR may be difficult to evaluate if the jet is eccentric and seems out of proportion with the severity of pulmonary hypertension. For regurgitant lesions, a semiquantitative assessment using angiography is used traditionally to grade severity of regurgitation (Table 4). Additional important information includes the assessment of pulmonary hypertension for mitral valve

**Table 4**
Sellers angiographic criteria for severity of aortic and mitral regurgitation

| Grade | Aortic Regurgitation | Mitral Regurgitation |
|-------|---------------------|---------------------|
| 1+ | Contrast refluxes from the aortic root into the left ventricle but clears on each beat | Contrast refluxes into the left atrium but clears on each beat |
| 2+ | Contrast refluxes into the left ventricle with a gradually increasing density of contrast in the left ventricle that never equals contrast intensity in the aortic root | Left atrial contrast density gradually increases but never equals left ventricle density |
| 3+ | Contrast refluxes into the left ventricle with a gradually increasing density such that left ventricle and aortic root density are equal after several beats | The density of contrast in the atrium and ventricle equalize after several beats |
| 4+ | Contrast fills the left ventricle resulting in an equivalent radiographic density in the left ventricle and aortic root on the first beat | The left atrium becomes as dense as the left ventricle on the first beat and contrast is seen refluxing into the pulmonary veins |

disease and evaluation of LV end-diastolic pressures in aortic regurgitation.

## MITRAL REGURGITATION

MR is a common valvular disorder that can arise from abnormalities of any part of the mitral valve apparatus. MR may be owing to a primary abnormality (often referred to as organic MR) of 1 or more components of the valve apparatus (leaflets, chordae tendineae, papillary muscles, and/or annulus) or may be secondary (previously referred to as functional MR) to another cardiac disease (such as coronary heart disease or a cardiomyopathy).

### Indication
The widespread availability of echocardiography has led to a limited role for cardiac catheterization in the diagnosis of MR. Nevertheless, invasive pressure measurements have a role when noninvasive tests are not conclusive; there is a discrepancy between noninvasive tests and clinical findings or between clinical symptoms and hemodynamics at rest, or severe pulmonary arterial hypertension is out of proportion to the severity of MR as determined by noninvasive tests. Invasive catheterization remains important in monitoring hemodynamics during percutaneous procedures for the reduction of the MR (ie, edge-to-edge mitral repair).

### Technique
Quantitative analysis of valve regurgitation can be performed in the catheterization laboratory by subtracting forward flow (cardiac output) from the total LV output (angiographic volumes), although this method is laborious and rarely used. Most commonly, the severity of MR is assessed in the catheterization laboratory by angiographically evaluating the degree of MR[9] (see Table 4) as well as assessing the LA v wave and degree of pulmonary hypertension. The equipment required is identical to that used for the evaluation of MS (see Table 3).

In addition to the evaluation of MR severity by angiography, assessment of pulmonary hypertension is paramount. In cases of discrepancy between the severity of MR and magnitude of pulmonary hypertension, care must be taken to measure the pulmonary pressures, and transpulmonary gradient. In the setting of precapillary pulmonary hypertension, reversibility should be evaluated to assess for further treatment decisions.

### Hemodynamic Findings and Interpretation
Qualitative assessment of the LA or wedge pressure tracing in significant MR demonstrates increased mean pressures with a prominent "v" wave (Fig. 3). The height of the 'v' wave is a sensitive but not a specific marker for MR (eg, possible association with ventricular septal defect and disorders associated with altered compliance and pressure–volume relationships) and does not necessarily reflect disease severity. It is reflective of LA compliance hence the "v" wave may not be elevated even with severe MR in a compliant left atrium. The LV pressure waveforms in systole and diastole are often normal, but may be associated with an increase in filling pressure owing to volume overload (although the LV stroke volume is increased, the forward stroke volume is normal because a part of the stroke volume regurgitates back into the left atrium).

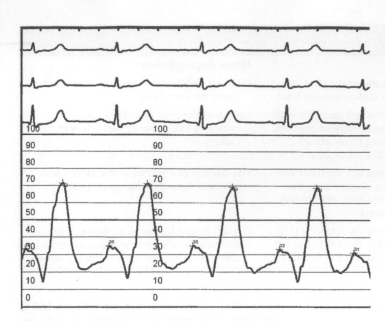

Fig. 3. Left atrial pressure tracing in a patient with severe mitral regurgitation referred for a MitraClip procedure. The patient is in sinus rhythm, there is an elevation of the mean left atrial pressure with a prominent "v" wave measuring 70 mm Hg.

## Pitfalls

The height of the "v" wave is not a specific and sensitive marker for MR, in particular, when severe (ie, 3 or 4+)[10] (Table 5). The amplitude of the "v" wave does not reflect precisely the degree of severity of the MR because its morphology depends on the pressure–volume relationship. Indeed, the pressure–volume curve produces different "v" waves depending on volume and LA compliance. With a left atrium of low compliance, such as in acute severe MR, increasing pressure is obtained with increasing flow or volume in the left atrium; in this setting, a large "v" wave can be associated with a small increase in pressure. By comparison, a higher compliance of the left atrium, such as in chronic MR, would yield a much smaller "v" wave.

## AORTIC REGURGITATION

### Indication

The 2014 American Heart Association/American College of Cardiology guidelines[1] recommend cardiac catheterization if noninvasive data are nondiagnostic or if there is a discrepancy between clinical and echocardiographic evaluation.

### Technique

The assessment of the aortic regurgitation in the catheterization laboratory is performed using angiography (see Table 4). This should be performed using a side hole catheter such as a pigtail placed above the valve so as not to interfere with normal valve function. It is important to inject a sufficient amount of contrast (45–50 mL) to opacify the cardiac chambers. After angiography, the valve is crossed retrogradely to evaluate the LV pressures.

### Hemodynamic Findings and Interpretation

The aortic pressure tracing in aortic regurgitation reveals a rapid upstroke (owing to augmented LV contractility) and an increased systolic pressure (owing to increased stroke volume), associated with a rapid decrease in the

| Table 5 | | | |
|---|---|---|---|
| Use of the pulmonary arterial wedge V wave to identify 3 or 4 + angiographic mitral regurgitation | | | |
| | V-Wave Peak Pressure (≥40 mm Hg) | V-Wave Mean PCWP Difference (≥10 mm Hg) | V-Mean PCWP (≥2.0) |
| Sensitivity | 0.44 | 0.66 | 0.10 |
| Specificity | 0.94 | 0.87 | 0.97 |

Abbreviation: PCWP, pulmonary capillary wedge pressure.
Modified from Snyder RW, Glamann DB, Lange RA, et al. Predictive value of prominent pulmonary arterial wedge V waves in assessing the presence and severity of mitral regurgitation. Am J Cardiol 1994;73(8):568–70.

aortic pressure (owing to the regurgitation). At the end of diastole, there is near equalization of the aortic and LV pressures owing to the valvular incompetence. The pulse pressure, which is defined as the systolic minus the diastolic pressure, is increased, because the systolic and diastolic pressures are increased and decreased, respectively. Additional findings may include an elevated LV end-diastolic pressure if the regurgitation is acute or more normalized pressure if the disease is chronic and compensated.

## SUMMARY

Cardiac catheterization remains an invaluable tool for the assessment and management of complex cases of valvular heart disease in which noninvasive testing is inconclusive. In this setting, the ability of the interventional cardiologist to perform an appropriate evaluation that addresses the clinical questions and provides the required answers is paramount. This somewhat "lost" art, in the era of a dependence on echocardiography, must be maintained and practiced to ensure the optimal treatment of patients.

## REFERENCES

1. Nishimura RA, Otto CM, Bonow RO, et al. 2014 AHA/ACC guideline for the management of patients with valvular heart disease: a report of the American College of Cardiology/American Heart Association Task Force on Practice Guidelines. J Am Coll Cardiol 2014;63(22):e57–185.

2. Carabello BA, Usher BW, Hendrix GH, et al. Predictors of outcome for aortic valve replacement in patients with aortic regurgitation and left ventricular dysfunction: a change in the measuring stick. J Am Coll Cardiol 1987;10(5):991–7.

3. Carabello BA. What is new in the 2006 ACC/AHA guidelines on valvular heart disease? Curr Cardiol Rep 2008;10(2):85–90.

4. Hakki AH, Iskandrian AS, Bemis CE, et al. A simplified valve formula for the calculation of stenotic cardiac valve areas. Circulation 1981;63(5): 1050–5.

5. Assey ME, Zile MR, Usher BW, et al. Effect of catheter positioning on the variability of measured gradient in aortic stenosis. Cathet Cardiovasc Diagn 1993;30(4):287–92.

6. Carabello BA, Barry WH, Grossman W. Changes in arterial pressure during left heart pullback in patients with aortic stenosis: a sign of severe aortic stenosis. Am J Cardiol 1979;44(3):424–7.

7. Pibarot P, Dumesnil JG. Low-flow, low-gradient aortic stenosis with normal and depressed left ventricular ejection fraction. J Am Coll Cardiol 2012; 60(19):1845–53.

8. Lauten J, Rost C, Breithardt OA, et al. Invasive hemodynamic characteristics of low gradient severe aortic stenosis despite preserved ejection fraction. J Am Coll Cardiol 2013;61(17):1799–808.

9. Sellers RD, Levy MJ, Amplatz K, et al. Left retrograde cardioangiography in acquired cardiac disease: technic, indications and interpretations in 700 cases. Am J Cardiol 1964;14(4):437–47.

10. Snyder RW, Glamann DB, Lange RA, et al. Predictive value of prominent pulmonary arterial wedge V waves in assessing the presence and severity of mitral regurgitation. Am J Cardiol 1994;73(8):568–70.

# Invasive Hemodynamics of Pulmonary Disease and the Right Ventricle

David Silber, DO*, Justine Lachmann, MD

---

## KEYWORDS

- Pulmonary arterial hypertension • Pulmonary hypertension • Right heart failure
- Pulmonary vascular resistance • Pressure-volume loop • Conductance catheter

---

## KEY POINTS

- The hemodynamic definitions of pulmonary hypertension (PH) at rest and with vasodilatory challenge provide an ability to categorize the etiology of PH and guide treatment.
- A conductance catheter can provide additional information on the ability of the right ventricle (RV) to increase stroke volume in acutely and chronically increased pulmonary vascular resistance.
- Understanding of the RV maladaptations to increased pulmonary vascular resistance facilitates understanding of the chronicity of the RV response to increase PH and/or increase pulmonary vascular resistance.

---

## INTRODUCTION

Pulmonary arterial hypertension (PAH) is a progressive disease characterized by an increase in the pulmonary artery pressure (PAP) and pulmonary vascular resistance, leading ultimately to right ventricular (RV) failure and death.[1] PH is defined as a mean PAP of greater than 25 mm Hg, or a peak pressure of greater than 35 mm Hg.[2] PH and its associated right heart failure exhibits particular hemodynamic values seen during a right heart catheterization (RHC). However, the values typically obtained do not describe the hemodynamic perturbations that the RV experiences with chronic PH. The relation of the pressure and volume in the RV can provide the conceptual framework needed to understand the reason why a failing RV can be a deadly consequence of chronic PH with or without a chronically elevated pulmonary vascular resistance. This article reviews the concepts of PH as they relate to the construction and understanding of pressure–volume loops in healthy and diseased RVs.

## HISTORY OF PULMONARY HYPERTENSION AND THE RIGHT VENTRICLE

The elusive definition and name of PH has had several different iterations over the past century. PAH was first described during the late 1800s by a German physician Ernst Von Rombery calling it primary vascular sclerosis. It was not until 1951 that David Dresdale called it primary PH, accompanied by actual hemodynamic detail.[3–5] This was an important discovery because it helped to contribute a key concept of the role of vasoconstriction in the pathophysiology of PH.

With the basic hemodynamic map set forth by Dresdale, advances in the field of invasive hemodynamics emerged rapidly.[6] Paul Wood's work with valvular heart disease, congenital heart disease, and PH helped to establish the first important physiologic concepts, including that of pulmonary vascular resistance. In 1966, he developed the hemodynamic parameter to diagnose PH, which was a pulmonary blood pressure of greater than 30/15 mm Hg. Other key contributors to PH can be seen in **Table 1**.

---

Winthrop Cardiology Associates, PC, NYU-Winthrop Hospital, 212 Jericho Turnpike, Mineola, NY 11501, USA
* Corresponding author.
E-mail addresses: dsilber@winthrop.org; drdavidsilber@gmail.com

Intervent Cardiol Clin 6 (2017) 329–343
http://dx.doi.org/10.1016/j.iccl.2017.03.004
2211-7458/17/© 2017 Elsevier Inc. All rights reserved.

**Table 1**
**Early contributors of pulmonary hypertension**

| | |
|---|---|
| William Harvey, 1628 | Publication of his book *Exercitatio Anotomica de Motu Cordis et sanguinis in Animabilus* |
| Ernst von Romberg, 1891 | Description of abnormal findings in autopsy as pulmonary vascular sclerosis, first name given for pulmonary hypertension |
| Abel Ayerza, 1913 | Key lecture integrating cyanosis and right heart failure, names the condition as "cardiac negro" |
| Werner Forssman, 1929 | Demonstrated that it was possible to perform a right-sided catheterization in humans by performing catheterization on himself |
| David Dresdale, 1951 | Coined the term primary pulmonary hypertension |
| Forssman, Cournand, Richards, 1956 | Awarded Nobel Prize for their contribution to the discovery of circulatory and cardiopulmonary systems |
| Paul Wood, 1958 | Published pulmonary hypertension with special references to vasoconstrictive factor |

The RV has also been the stepchild of the ever more popular left ventricle (LV) with regard to research and knowledge. In antiquity, Galen described the RV as the primary ventricle to eject the already oxygenated blood that came from the liver to the vital organs of the body.[7] This notion was not challenged until the early 16th century by Michael Servetus of Spain, in which he stipulated that blood was actually continuously produced rather than consumed and then recirculated.[7] He was later killed for his heretical notion, but it was a notion that helped William Harvey to set up his first experiments on pulmonary circulation nearly 50 years later. This established the framework for the current understanding of RV and pulmonary circulation.[8] Nearly 500 years later, we now understand that the RV is not merely a capacitor for pulmonary circulation, but a highly efficient pump, similar to the LV.

## ANATOMY OF THE RIGHT VENTRICLE AND PULMONARY CIRCULATION

Believed to be the less muscular ventricle needing only to supply blood to 1 organ, much has been learned about the RV and its intricate relationship to the pulmonary circulation and, thus, the entire heart's cardiac output (CO). With the advances in mechanical circulatory support and heart transplantation, it is now known that one of the largest barriers to functional hemodynamics is impairment of the RV.[9] Understanding and predicting how the RV will perform when a LV assist device is inserted helps to guide physicians on whether or not LV assist device or even transplantation is possible for their patient.[10]

The RV and its outflow tract develop from the anterior heart field, whereas the LV derives from the primary heart field.[11] The sinus part of the RV comes from the primitive ventricle portion, and the infundibulum derives its tissue from the conus cordis.[12–14]

There are many anatomic differences between the LV and RV. The RV is the most anterior portion of the heart, lying under the sternum. It can be divided into 3 parts: (1) the inlet, which consists of the tricuspid valve, chordae tendineae, and papillary muscles, (2) the trabeculated apical myocardium, and (3) the infundibulum or conus, which consists of the smooth outflow tract region. There are often overlooked muscular components consisting of the parietal, septomarginal, and moderator bands, which will eventually attach to the anterior papillary muscle.

Anatomic differences between the LV and RV are not trivial when comparing the overall shape of the RV to the LV. The LV is an elliptical muscular pump whereas the RV is a triangular, thin-walled pump.[12–15] The muscle mass of the RV is 1/6th of the LV. With both COs remaining the same, the difference between RV and LV is their respective stroke work index, which is about 25% of the LV owing to the lower pulmonary vascular resistance and increased RV compliance.[9,16]

RV stroke work index = (PAm − CVP) × SVI

where PAm is the pulmonary artery mean pressure (mm Hg), CVP is the central venous pressure (mm Hg), and SVI is the stroke volume index (stroke volume/cardiac index; $mL/m^2$).

The LV and RV are connected by an interventricular septum which accounts for about one-third of RV CO, but also by epicardial fibers that are aligned longitudinally on the RV and circumferentially on the LV.[16] These 2 can become pathologic when PH develops. The last two-thirds of the RV CO is contributed by its longitudinal shortening versus the elliptical squeezing of the LV.[17]

RV anatomy sets up the hemodynamics seen on RHC, which is a low pulmonary vascular resistance.[16] In utero, pulmonary vascular resistance is much higher compared with the systemic vascular resistance (SVR) and their equations can be seen in Table 2.[18] The increased pulmonary vascular resistance is owing to the alveoli being filled with fluid. The high pulmonary vascular resistance then allows oxygenated blood from the mother to be shunted to the systemic circulation via the ductus arteriosus and foramen ovale.[19] The decrease in pulmonary vascular resistance after birth with the closure of the patent ductus arteriosus and increased SVR establishes the normal hemodynamic parameters needed in adult life (Fig. 1).

The thin-walled and crescent-shaped RV wraps around the more muscle-bound LV. The thin wall generates less ventricular pressure as compared with the LV owing to Laplace's Law (tension $\propto$ pressure $\times$ radius). Even with this difference in anatomy, the CO of the RV and LV must equal each other for each cardiac cycle.

## PULMONARY HYPERTENSION

PH today, as defined by the 4th World Symposium on Pulmonary Hypertension held in 2008 again is a mean PAP of greater than 25 mm Hg, or a peak pressure of greater than 35 mm Hg.[1,2] As seen in Box 1,[2] the newest classification with groups

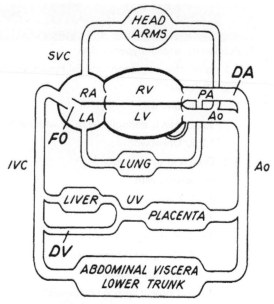

Fig. 1. In the fetal circulation the ductus venosus (DV) serves as a bypass for umbilical venous blood to enter the inferior vena cava directly. The foramen ovale (FO) carries well-oxygenated blood from the inferior vena cava into the left atrium and left ventricle. The ductus arteriosus (DA) carries the major portion of blood ejected from the right ventricle to the descending aorta and mainly to the placenta. Ao, aorta; IVC, inferior vena cava; LA, left atrium; LV, left ventricle; PA, pulmonary artery; RA, right atrium; RV, right ventricle; SVC, superior vena cava; UV, umbilical vein.

| Table 2 Pulmonary vascular resistance relationship to the transpulmonary gradient across the pulmonary vascular bed to the cardiac output generated by the right ventricle | |
|---|---|
| **Hemodynamic Parameters** | **Normal Value** |
| Mean arterial pressure(MAP)$=\frac{SBP+(DBP\times2)}{3}$ | 70–100 mm Hg |
| Heart rate (HR) | 60–100 bpm |
| Right atrial pressure (RA) | $\leq$6 mm Hg |
| Right ventricular (RV) | Systolic 15–30 mm Hg Diastolic 1–8 mm Hg |
| Pulmonary artery (PA) | Systolic 15–30 mm Hg Mean 9–18 mm Hg Diastolic 6–12 mm Hg |
| Pulmonary capillary wedge pressure (PCWP) | $\leq$12 mm Hg |
| Cardiac output (CO) | 4–8 L/min |
| Cardiac index(CI)$=\frac{CO}{BSA}$ | 2.6–4.2 L/min/m$^2$ |
| Stroke volume(SV)$=\frac{CO}{HR}$ | 60–120 mL/contraction |
| Stroke volume index(SVI)$=\frac{CI}{HR}$ | 40–50 mL/contraction/m$^2$ |
| Systemic vascular resistance(SVR)$=\frac{MAP-mean\ RA}{CO}\times80$ | 800–1200 dyn $\times$ s/cm$^5$ |
| Pulmonary vascular resistance(PVR)$=\frac{mean\ PA-mean\ PCWP}{CO}\times80$ | 120–250 dyn $\times$ s/cm$^5$ |

---

**Box 1**
**Updated clinical classification of pulmonary hypertension**

1. Pulmonary arterial hypertension
   1.1. Idiopathic pulmonary arterial hypertension
   1.2. Heritable[a]
       1.2.1. BMPR2[a]
       1.2.2. ALK1, endoglin (with or without hereditary hemorrhagic telangiectasia)[a]
       1.2.3. Unknown[a]
   1.3. Drug and toxin induced
   1.4. Associated with
       1.4.1. Connective tissue diseases
       1.4.2. HIV infection
       1.4.3. Portal hypertension
       1.4.4. Congenital heart diseases
       1.4.5. Schistosomiasis[a]
       1.4.6. Chronic hemolytic anemia[a]
   1.5. Persistent pulmonary hypertension of the newborn
1'. Pulmonary venoocclusive disease and/or pulmonary capillary hemangiomatosis[a]
2. Pulmonary hypertension owing to left heart disease
   2.1. Systolic dysfunction[a]
   2.2. Diastolic dysfunction[a]
   2.3. Valvular disease
3. Pulmonary hypertension owing to lung diseases and/or hypoxia
   3.1. Chronic obstructive pulmonary disease
   3.2. Interstitial lung disease
   3.3. Other pulmonary diseases with mixed restrictive and obstructive pattern[a]
   3.4. Sleep-disordered breathing
   3.5. Alveolar hypoventilation disorders
   3.6. Chronic exposure to high altitude
   3.7. Developmental abnormalities
4. Chronic thromboembolic pulmonary hypertension[a]
5. Pulmonary hypertension with unclear multifactorial mechanisms[a]
   5.1. Hematologic disorders: myeloproliferative disorders, splenectomy[a]
   5.2. Systemic disorders: sarcoidosis, pulmonary Langerhans cell histiocytosis, lymphangioleiomyomatosis, neurofibromatosis, vasculitis[a]
   5.3. Metabolic disorders: glycogen storage disease, Gaucher disease, thyroid disorders[a]
   5.4. Others: tumoral obstruction, fibrosing mediastinitis, chronic renal failure on dialysis[a]

[a] Main modifications to the previous Venice classification.
*Abbreviations:* ALK1, activin receptor-like kinase type 1; BMPR2, bone morphogenetic protein receptor type 2; HIV, human immunodeficiency virus.
*Data from* Dana Point, 2008.

---

1 through 5 is represented with their respective subgroups. Patients afflicted with PH have common symptoms of dyspnea on exertion, chest pain, peripheral edema, and syncope.

PAH is what is seen in group 1. The key feature to this group is an elevation in PAP with normal pulmonary capillary wedge pressure.[2] Group 1 includes genetic or heritable causes, such as idiopathic PAH, and can correspond with either sporadic disease or a nondefined risk factor. Genetic causes stemming from the bone morphogenic protein receptor type 2 gene (BMPR2) is present in close to 70% of such patients.[20] Other diseases such as connective tissue disorders, human immunodeficiency virus, congenital shunts, human immunodeficiency virus infection, and portal hypertension are included in this group.

Group 2 PH consists of an elevation in the PAP and in the pulmonary capillary wedge pressure. This group is the most common etiology PH and is owing to left heart disease.[21] This includes left-sided atrial/ventricular heart disease, left-sided valvular disease, pulmonary venous obstruction, and pulmonary venoocclusive disease.[2] Mitral stenosis was once the prevalent cause of pulmonary venous congestion in this subgroup of PH; however, LV dysfunction predominates in present-day medicine.[22]

The next most common, group 3, consists of patients with chronic hypoxia with increased PAP. This is seen in diseases of the lung parenchyma, or at elevated altitudes, with resultant impaired gas exchange. Airway obstruction, severe hypoxemia, hypercapnia, and low diffusion capacity for carbon monoxide are observed. The chronic hypoxia has been known to be a potent vasoconstrictor of the pulmonary arterial bed, increasing the PAP in response.[23]

Venous thromboembolic disease is a frequent and deadly cardiovascular disease that has an estimated incidence of 100 to 200 per 100,000 people.[24] If patients survive the initial thromboembolic event, they can develop group 4 PH as chronic thromboembolic PH. The formal diagnosis is an elevated PAP with a previous history of pulmonary embolism more than 3 months earlier.[25] This insult leads to elevated PAP by further progressive vascular remodeling. Although thrombus is considered the more common cause of this, other occlusive disorders that are nonthrombotic include tumor or foreign body.[26]

Last, group 5 PH is derived from conditions with uncertain mechanisms. The key feature here is an increase in the PAP associated with a systemic disease in which a causal relationship has not been established.[27] Least is known about this group, which includes sarcoidosis, chronic anemia, histiocytosis X, schistosomiasis, and lymphangiomatosis.[28]

## RIGHT HEART CATHETERIZATION

RHC allows us to measure and analyze the pressures of the right atrium (RA), RV, and pulmonary

artery. The Swan-Ganz catheter also allows for inference of the left atrium pressures by examination of the pulmonary capillary wedge pressure reading. From these locations and pressures, the CO, cardiac index, SVR, pulmonary vascular resistance, and stroke work index can be calculated. All of these measurements are paramount in the diagnosis and management of pulmonary diseases and RV diseases.[29]

The initial development of RHC began in 1844, when Claude Bernard performed the first successful animal cardiac catheterization. In 1929, Werner Forssmann performed his own self-RHC while accessing his RA and standing for some time in front of an x-ray machine for confirmation of catheter placement.[30] Forssmann, along with Andre Frederic Cournand and Dickinson Woodson Richards, would later receive the Nobel Prize in Medicine and Physiology in 1956 for their advancement and achievements in the field of the RHC.[31,32]

Initial access to the right heart can either be from the inferior or superior vena cava. An inferior vena cava approach tends to be the more common approach when the patient is in the catheterization laboratory, whereas the superior vena cava via the internal jugular vein is the more common approach at the bedside. Both are nonexclusive to each location, with the latter being done with ultrasound guidance.[33] Using the Seldinger technique from 1921, the desired vessel or cavity is punctured with a sharp hollow needle called a trocar and ultrasound guidance can be used. A round-tipped guidewire is then advanced through the lumen of the trocar, and the trocar is withdrawn. A sheath can now be passed over the guidewire into the cavity or vessel with the guidewire then removed after placement.[34–36]

After access, the most common catheter used today is the Swan-Ganz Catheter (Fig. 2). The

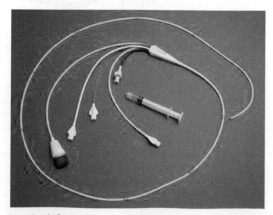

Fig. 2. A Swan-Ganz catheter.

balloon tip catheter helps to navigate the many turns it must encounter when entering the right heart. Fig. 3 shows the Swan-Ganz Catheter traversing the caval system into the right heart. When coming from the inferior vena cava

approach, twisting and torquing the catheter can be used for the balloon to traverse the RA, tricuspid valve, RV, and then through the pulmonic valve. Less manipulation is required typically with the superior vena caval

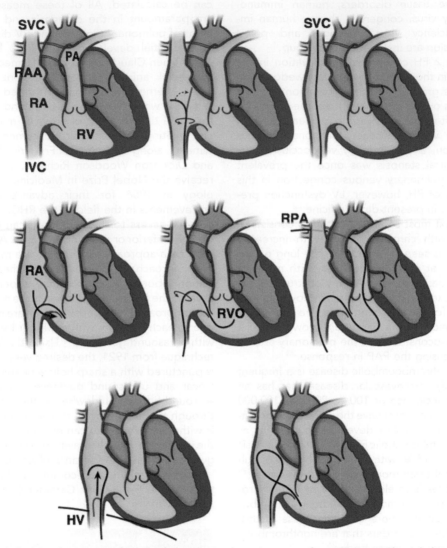

Fig. 3. Right heart catheterization from the femoral vein, shown in cartoon form. (*Top row*) The right heart catheter is initially placed in the right atrium (RA) aimed at the lateral atrial wall. Counterclockwise rotation aims the catheter posteriorly and allows advancement into the superior vena cava (SVC). Although it is not evident in the figure, clockwise catheter rotation into an anterior orientation would lead to advancement into the right atrial appendage (RAA) and thereby preclude SVC catheterization. (*Center row*) The catheter is then withdrawn back into the right atrium and aimed laterally. Clockwise rotation causes the tip of the catheter to sweep anteromedially and cross the tricuspid valve. With the catheter tip in a horizontal orientation just beyond the spine, it is positioned below the right ventricular (RV) outflow (RVO) tract. Additional clockwise rotation causes the catheter to point straight up and allows advancement into the main pulmonary artery and from there into the right pulmonary artery (RPA). (*Bottom row*) Two maneuvers useful in catheterization of a dilated right heart. A larger loop with a downward-directed tip may be required to reach the tricuspid valve and can be formed by catching the tip of the catheter in the hepatic vein (HV) and advancing the catheter quickly into the right atrium. The reverse loop technique (*bottom right*) gives the tip of the catheter an upward direction, aimed toward the outflow tract. PA, pulmonary artery. (*From* Baim DS, Grossman W. Percutaneous approach, including transseptal and apical puncture. In: Baim DS, Grossman W, editors. Cardiac catheterization, angiography, and intervention. 7th edition. Philadelphia: Lea & Febiger; 2006. p. 86.)

approach.[37–39] Other catheters, such as a more stiff multipurpose Goodale-Lubin or Cournand catheters, can also be used in difficult cases.

Pressure tracings and normal values obtained from RHC can be seen in Table 2. The RA pressure is characterized by a and v waves with 2 descents called x and y. The a wave corresponds with the pressure increase within the RA during atrial contraction and can be seen following the P wave on electrocardiograph. The x descent represents the pressure decay after the a wave, which is analogous to atrial relaxation after it produces the atrial kick. Sometimes, a c wave can be seen just after the a wave. This is owing to the movement of the tricuspid annulus returning toward the RA just at the beginning of RV contraction. Following the closure of the tricuspid valve, the v wave represents the pressure increase in the atria during atrial diastole and its peak pressure corresponds to the T wave on the electrocardiograph. Finally, the y descent represents the rapid decrease in pressure seen in the atrium when the tricuspid valve opens, emptying its contents passively into the RV.[37,39,40]

The RV waveform is more robust in size while having both a systolic and diastolic pressure. It has a distinctive ventricular waveform of rapid pressure increase during contraction and pressure decay as ventricular relaxation occurs. In most conditions, the RV end-diastolic pressure should be close to the RA pressure in normal loading and compliance conditions. Seeing a wave on an RV tracing can be indicative of a poorly compliant condition, which can be seen in PH.[37,39,40]

Like most arterial waveforms, the pulmonary artery tracing will have a rapid increase in pressure with a systolic peak, a pressure decay, and a defined dicrotic notch. The peak systolic pressure should correlate with the T wave on an electrocardiograph. When comparing the systolic pressure of the RV with the pulmonary artery, there should not be a gradient seen unless there is pulmonary valve stenosis present. Variations in PAP can be seen whether looking during inspiration (decreasing intrathroacic pressure) or expiration (increasing intrathroacic pressure). This is most important when checking pressures on mechanically ventilated patients because end-expiratory pressure is the correct point in time to measure the PAP (where the intrathoracic pressure is believed to be closest to zero).[37,39,40]

Last, the left atrial pressure can be estimated by using the pulmonary capillary wedge pressure. With the balloon of the catheter inflated in the lung zone 3, it is believed that there is no antegrade flow for its ports to measure. The only pressure that is being measure is the retrograde pressure from the left atrium. The pulmonary capillary wedge pressure acts as a surrogate of LA pressure. As with RA pressure tracings, a and v waves are also present, along with their x and y descents. The a wave is normally smaller when compared with the v wave and is more delayed when lining it up with an electrocardiograph, because the pressure is a transmitted pressure and not a direct pressure that is seen when the catheter tip is in the RA. Typically, the a wave is after the QRS, whereas the v wave is seen after the T wave.

Obtaining a proper pulmonary capillary wedge pressure can be challenging. When transducing the LA pressure to the tip of the Swan-Ganz catheter, it must be placed in the correct lung zone. The lung can be divided into 3 zones: zone 1 at the apex of the lung, zone 2 at the central portion of the lung, and zone 3 at the base of the lung. These zones are for the upright patient, and while supine, the zones will correlate more typically from anterior to posterior locations of the thorax owing to the change in blood distribution while supine. Zone 3 is the preferred area to obtain an accurate pulmonary capillary wedge pressure. This is owing to zones 1 and 2 exhibiting physiologic capillary collapse and a true column of pressure coming from the left atrium may not be obtained in these zones. In zone 3, however, the alveolar pressure is lower than the pulmonary venous pressure and, therefore, will not interrupt the pressure gradient that can be obtained from the left atrium. Tracings that help to confirm a high-quality pulmonary capillary wedge pressure are well-defined a and v waves and a pulmonary capillary wedge pressure saturation of greater than 90%. Additionally, the pulmonary capillary wedge pressure should be slightly lower than the pulmonary artery diastolic pressure, unless, as is seen in PH, they have an increased pulmonary vascular resistance.[37,39,40]

## EXPECTED RIGHT HEART CATHETERIZATION FINDINGS BASED ON PULMONARY HYPERTENSION GROUP

The pulmonary vascular resistance relates the transpulmonary gradient across the pulmonary vascular bed to the CO generated by the RV. This relationship is written in Table 2 and is illustrated with the following equation:

$$PVR = \frac{PAm - PCWPm}{CO} = \frac{TPG}{CO}$$

where PAm is the pulmonary artery mean pressure, PCWPm is the mean pulmonary capillary wedge pressure and TPG is the transpulmonary gradient.

Patients with PH are expected to have an increased pulmonary artery mean pressure in all groups of PH. As listed in Table 4, the mean pulmonary capillary wedge pressure is typically normal, which defines precapillary PH. This increases the transpulmonary pressure gradient across the pulmonary vascular bed, and proportionally increases the pulmonary vascular resistance if the RV CO remains unchanged. Postcapillary PH is defined as group 2 PH, in which the mean pulmonary capillary wedge pressure is increased owing to increased left-heart filling pressures. Although the pulmonary artery mean pressure and mean pulmonary capillary wedge pressure are increased, the resultant transpulmonary pressure gradient seems to be normal. Thus, for any given RV CO, the resultant pulmonary vascular resistance will be smaller in a patient with postcapillary/group 2 PH compared with a precapillary/nongroup 2 PH patient.

## PRESSURE–VOLUME LOOPS AND HEMODYNAMICS SEEN IN PULMONARY HYPERTENSION ON THE RIGHT VENTRICLE

Most of our current literature in cardiac physiology concentrates on the LV. With many of our advanced therapies geared toward left-sided mechanical assist devices for severe LV dysfunction, more has been learned about the other and equally important RV.[9] Without the RV, which is designed to accommodate an entire systemic venous return, there would be difficulty in having an adequate LV CO. Systemic organs need oxygen for the plethora of metabolic activities that are needed to remain in a homeostatic balance. With the RV's ability to accommodate a large volume of blood to be passed to the lungs for oxygenation, it requires a lower pulmonary vascular resistance for this thin-walled structure to pump forward.[41] When the pulmonary vascular resistance increases in PH, altered RV mechanics and CO can have deleterious effects on the body. Animal models and complex congenital heart defects demonstrate normal and abnormal RV hemodynamics. Similar to LV pressure–volume loops, RV pressure–volume loops are helpful in describing the normal and abnormal hemodynamic states of the RV.[42]

A ventricular pressure–volume loop displays instantaneous relationship of the intraventricular pressure and the volume throughout one cardiac cycle. Common terminology and their definitions can be seen in Table 3.[43] Classic LVpressure–volume loops can be seen in Fig. 4.[44]

The end-diastolic pressure–volume relationship (EDPVR) helps to form the boundary on which the pressure–volume loop falls at the end of a cardiac cycle. Its nonlinear slope shows the relations of pressure and volume and also diastolic, lusitropic compliance of the ventricle. The end-systolic pressure–volume relationship (ESPVR) is when the myocytes are at their maximal contraction. Its slope is linear, unlike the EDPVR, and the slope end-systolic elastance ($E_{es}$) defines the LV's elastance, which is change in pressure divided by change in volume ($\Delta P/\Delta V$). Elastance is inversely proportional to compliance, such that the stiffer the ventricular wall (owing to ischemia, LV hypertrophy, and/or infiltrative disease), the greater the ventricle's elastance. Shifts in the ESPVR and EDPVR will occur with changes in ventricular contractility and diastolic lusitropy, respectively. Increased contractility shifts the ESPVR upward; decreased contractility shifts the line down. Increased lusitropy decreases the EDPVR and lower lusitropy increases the EDPVR.

The peripheral or SVR determines the LV end-systolic pressure for a given contractile state. The SVR is described as the afterload on the LV and is represented by the aortic elastance, which is LV end-systolic pressure divided by LV stroke volume. The elastance line starts at the EDV and intersects at the ESPVR. Thus, the SVR is depicted as the slope of the elastance line on an LV pressure–volume loop. The intersection of the elastance and $E_{es}$ help estimate the LV's stroke volume for a given contractile state and a particular cardiac cycle.[43–45]

The thin-walled, high-capacity RV is represented as a PV loop that is different in shape (Fig. 5).[46] The pressure–volume loop of the RV looks more trapezoidal or triangular in shape versus the more sharply defined rectangular shape of the LV pressure–volume loop.[46–49]

This may be owing to the physical difference in their anatomy. Whereas the LV must serve the systemic circulation, the RV serves the pulmonary circulation. Pulmonary circulation has much shorter arteries and veins that are also larger and more compliant, as compared with the systemic circulation.[50] This produces a lower pulmonary vascular resistance and RV afterload with a higher compliance compared with the systemic circulation. Compared with the LV pressure–volume loop, which is enclosed by both the ESPVR and EDPVR, the RV pressure–volume loop exhibits a less visible and much lower RV end-systolic pressure, as well as less-defined isovolumic relaxation and contraction periods.[51]

| Table 3 Common terminology and their definitions | |
|---|---|
| **Term** | **Definition** |
| Afterload | The mechanical load on the ventricle during ejection period. This is determined by the arterial system variables, such as aortic pressure, ejection wall stress, total peripheral (or systemic) resistance, and arterial impedance. |
| Compliance | Describes the diastolic property of stiffness seen in the ventricle. Mathematically it is the reciprocal of the EDPVR $(dP/dV)^{-1}$. |
| Contractility | Strength of the ventricle; determined by afterload and preload conditions. |
| Ea | Effective arterial elastance, the slope of the line extending from the EDV to the ESV. Its slope is defined as the total peripheral resistance (TPR or systemic vascular resistance). |
| EDPVR | End-diastolic pressure–volume relationship. The relationship between pressure and volume in the ventricle at the instant point of time of complete relaxation (end-diastole) |
| $E_{es}$ | End-systolic elastance: the slope of the ESPVR (mm Hg/mL); an index of contractility. |
| $E_{max}$ (elastance) | The maximum value of the ratio of ventricular pressure to volume during the cardiac cycle, surrogate for ventricular contractility in pressure–volume loops. |
| EF | Ejection fraction: ratio between the stroke volume (SV = EDV − ESV) and EDV. Most common metric of ventricular contractility. Limited by preload and afterload. |
| Elastance | The changes in pressure for a given change in volume within a chamber and is an indication of the stiffness of the chamber (mm Hg/mL). Higher the elastance, the stiffer the ventricle. |
| ESPVR | End-systolic pressure–volume relationship. Relationship between the ventricular pressure and volume at the instant moment in time of maximal activation (end-systole) during one cardiac cycle. A linear relationship, independent of loading conditions. |
| Preload | The load the ventricle is given at the end of diastole |

Ventricles regulate their contraction in response to different afterload and preload conditions. When a muscle fiber is stretched during diastole for a given preload, the contracting fiber develops a tension that depends on that initial stretch on that muscle fiber. As stated in the Frank-Starling principle, when a fiber is stretched farther, the fiber will contract faster and stronger than a muscle fiber that is stretched less.[43] Myocardial fibers contractile responses can also change independent of their initial fiber length.

For any given preload, greater tension on the myocardium will increase the inotropic response of that muscle fiber.[43] Inotropic state of the LV and RV are depicted by the ventricle's $E_{es}$.

The RV uses these 2 principles when it encounters unique afterloads and preloads per cardiac cycle by 2 additional autoregulation principles, heterometric and homeometric autoregulation. Heterometric autoregulation is based on changes in preload, that is, an increase in RV end-diastolic volume produces an increase in

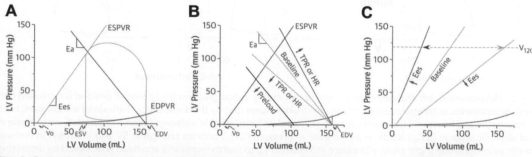

**Fig. 4.** Pressure volume loop. Ea, aortic elastance; EDV, end-diastolic volume; $E_{es}$, maximum elastance; EDPVR, end-diastolic pressure–volume relationship; ESV, end-systolic volume; ESPVR, end-systolic pressure–volume relationship; HR, heart rate; LV, left ventricular; TPR, total peripheral resistance.

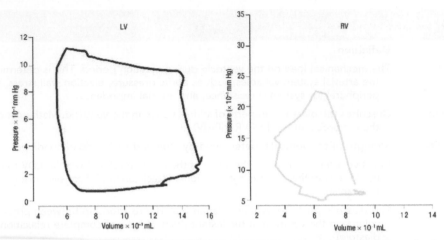

Fig. 5. The thin-walled, high-capacity right ventricle is represented as a pressure–volume loop that is different in shape.

RV stroke volume to achieve a normal RV end-systolic volume; this response is length dependent, as described.[41,51] Homeometric autoregulation is the inotropic mechanism (contractile) reaction to increased afterload, without a concomitant change in preload. This is also known as the Anrep effect, in which the ventricle responds to an increased afterload with an increase in myocardial inotropy.[43,51–53] When the afterload is increased in the setting of increased preload, heterometric autoregulation yields an increase in RV end-systolic pressure without a change in RV

stroke volume or RV inotropy, whereas a pure afterload increase on the RV causes the homeometric autoregulation to yield an increase in RV $E_{es}$, without a change in RV stroke volume or RV preload. These principles are depicted in Fig. 6.[51]

The RV produces less pressure as compared with the LV to achieve the same stroke volume. The RV stroke work is comparatively less compared with that of the LV. Stroke work is the stroke volume produced by the ventricle multiplied by the mean arterial pressure resulting from this stroke volume (stroke volume × mean

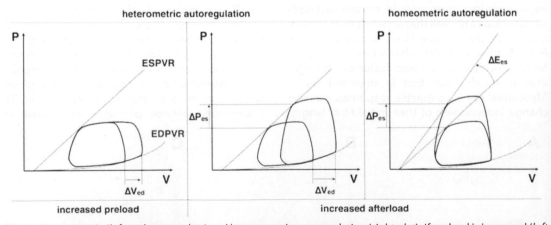

Fig. 6. Heterometric (left and center plots) and homeometric autoregulation (right plot). If preload is increased (left plot), heterometric autoregulation increases the stroke volume (SV) by the same $\Delta V_{ed}$. If afterload is increased, both heterometric and homeometric responses are activated. In heterometric autoregulation (center plot), an increase in end-diastolic volume ($\Delta V_{ed}$) leads to an increase in pressure ($\Delta P_{es}$) with no change in SV and inotropy. In homeometric autoregulation (right plot), a pressure increase ($\Delta P_{es}$) to match increased afterload is achieved by increasing right ventricular (RV) contractility ($\Delta E_{es}$) with no change in SV and preload. The baseline loop is sketched in red. The end-systolic pressure–volume relationship (ESPVR) line and the end-diastolic pressure–volume relationship (EDPVR) line define the limits of RV working conditions.

arterial pressure). This can be calculated by measuring the area under the pressure–volume loop curve. The RV depends on the LV fiber anatomic orientation to generate a bellowslike contraction; this is known as ventricular coupling. With each simultaneous contraction of the LV, the anchoring effect of the LV contracting myocardial fibers allow the intracameral RV pressure to increase by 20% to 40%, thereby augmenting the RV stroke volume.[9,16,46,49,51] The combination of a low pulmonary vascular resistance and longitudinal contractile effort by the RV myocardial fibers allow the RV to generate a stroke volume that parallels the stroke volume of the LV.

The RV is less able to adapt to greater changes in pulmonary vascular resistance. In the acute setting, a pulmonary embolism can greatly increase the pulmonary vascular resistance and precipitate acute RV failure owing to the RV's dependence on a low pulmonary vascular resistance for adequate RV stroke volume (Fig. 7).[25] When PH is present and the mean PAP exceeds 25 mm Hg at rest, the pulmonary vascular resistance is increased. The RV autoregulatory mechanisms are activated, so that adequate stroke volume is preserved and delivered to the LV. With chronic PH, the RV remodels and hypertrophies, thereby mimicking the LV contractile behavior.[53,54] The RV loses the bellowslike action typically seen in RV's exposed to low pulmonary vascular resistance and dilates significantly to shift the interventricular septum and compress the LV. This causes the LV to lose its ellipsoid shape, and remove the anchoring effect the RV needs to contract in a longitudinal direction. This nonphysiologic RV is not well-tolerated, owing to the resultant poor LV stroke volume

and CO.[19,49] Overall, the RV architecture maladapts with a prolonged increase in the pulmonary vascular resistance, leading to RV failure.[55,56]

## TOOLS USED TO ASSESS RIGHT VENTRICULAR AND LEFT VENTRICULAR PRESSURE–VOLUME LOOPS

Our ability to assess the RV with invasive hemodynamics can be done by 2 different methods—a conductance catheter or a conventional right heart Swan-Ganz catheter. Conductance catheters are not commonly used on human subjects in vivo, although they can produce pressure–volume loops for each ventricle in patients with PH and/or RV failure. The use of a Millar catheter (https://millar.com/products/research/pressure) is an example of a commercially available conductance catheter.

The catheter plots in vivo recordings beat by beat to create a patient-specific RV pressure–volume loop. Multiple RV pressure–volume loops over various loading conditions need to be performed to construct the ESPVR and resultant RV elastance and RV $E_{es}$ values. This is achieved with derivation of the pressure–volume loops before, during, and after simultaneous occlusion of the inferior vena cava during RHC.

The catheter tip with its end holes at the apex can be placed in an RV for data recording. The pressure–volume loop is constructed by the catheter by measuring voltage differences in conductance at different locations in the RV.[47,48,57] Because blood has a known conductance, an algorithm has been devised to calculate the volume this catheter has encountered with its known pressure. The single-beat recording method is a

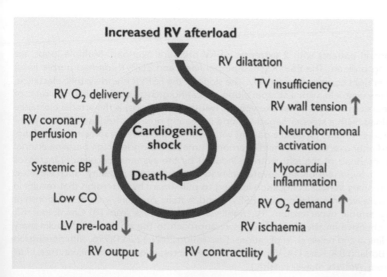

Fig. 7. In the acute setting, a pulmonary embolism can greatly increase the pulmonary vascular resistance (PVR) and precipitate acute RV failure owing to the RV's dependence on a low PVR for adequate RV stroke volume. BP, blood pressure; CO, cardiac output; LV, left ventricular; RV, right ventricular; TV, tricuspid valve.

known technique that is preferred for acquisition of the pressure–volume loop datasets.[47,48,58,59] Fig. 8 shows an example of these in vivo recordings in a normal RV with different loading conditions when the inferior vena cava is occluded and a pressure–volume loop in a patient with PAH.

In PAH, the higher the afterload encountered by the RV (increased pulmonary vascular resistance), the less triangular and/or ellipsoid the RV pressure–volume loop becomes, and the more the pressure–volume loop mimics the rectangular shape of an LV pressure–volume loop.

RV failure in the context of the PH disease spectrum can then be defined as the right heart's inability to maintain forward systolic flow for a particular metabolic demand without heterometric dimension adaptation (ie, the RV is unable to increase its RV end-diastolic volume further to maintain an adequate RV stroke volume).[55] Using conductance catheters may not be feasible; therefore, traditional RHCs with a Swan-Ganz catheter can be used. Table 4 displays the hemodynamic parameters that define the group of PH.[60]

## REVERSIBILITY STUDY IN PULMONARY HYPERTENSION

Demonstration of pulmonary vasoreactivity during a RHC can identify patients who may benefit from calcium channel blocker use, particularly those with idiopathic or drug-induced PH (ie, group 1 PH).[61] Group1 PH patients typically exhibit pulmonary vasoconstriction that may respond to oral vasodilators, particularly calcium channel blockers. Inhaled nitric oxide or intravenous epoprostenol can be used to induce pulmonary vasodilation. A significant response is a reduction of the mean PAP by 10 mm Hg or greater, while maintaining a mean PAP of 40 mm Hg or less and a simultaneously unchanged or increased CO.

Acute vasoreactivity testing is not recommended in nongroup 1 PH patients owing to the nonvasoreactive mechanisms that cause the PH in these patients. Therefore, the vasoreactivity testing with inhaled nitric oxide or intravenous epoprostenol is not expected to produce a significant change in the patient's pulmonary vascular resistance. Nitric oxide is dissolved in

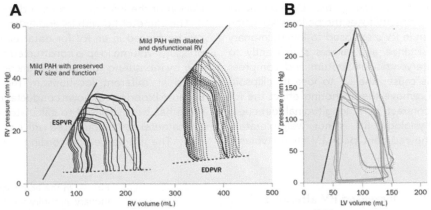

Fig. 8. (A) RV pressure–volume loops in patients with 2 extremes of RV pressure overload. Multiple loops are generated for each patient by altering preload. The ESPVR (*solid purple lines*) and EDPVR (*dashed purple lines*) are defined by the upper left and lower right corners, respectively. The slope of the ESPVR is end-systolic elastance, which represents the contractility of the ventricle, with a steeper slope indicating greater contractility. The ratio of end-systolic pressure (upper left corners of the loops) to stroke volume (width of the loops) is the arterial elastance (*blue lines*) and is a measure of afterload, with a steeper negative slope indicating greater afterload (greater pressure per volume ejected). (B) LV pressure–volume loops in a patient with heart failure with preserved systolic function (diastolic dysfunction) before and after exertion. With mild exertion (isometric handgrip), high baseline arterial elastance (in this case representing afterload of the left ventricle induced by the systemic circulation) increases markedly (*arrow*), with notable systemic hypertension and severely elevated end-diastolic pressure. Such elevated LV end-diastolic pressure causes pulmonary venous congestion leading to pulmonary hypertension that results in dyspnea. EDPVR, end-diastolic pressure–volume relationship; ESPVR, end-systolic pressure–volume relationship; LV, left ventricular; PAH, pulmonary arterial hypertension; RV, right ventricular. (*Data from* [A] Champion HC, Michelakis ED, Hassoun PM. Comprehensive invasive and noninvasive approach to the right ventricle-pulmonary circulation unit: state of the art and clinical and research implications. Circulation 2009;120(11):996, with permission from Wolters Kluwer Health; and [B] Borlaug BA, Kass DA. Ventricular-vascular interaction in heart failure. Heart Fail Clin 2008;4(1):28, with permission from Wolters Kluwer Health.)

**Table 4**
**Hemodynamic definitions of PH as assessed by right heart catheterization**

| Definition | Characteristics | Clinical Group(s)[a] |
|---|---|---|
| PH | mPAP ≥25 mm Hg | All |
| Precapillary PH | mPAP ≥25 mm Hg<br>PAOP ≤15 mm Hg<br>CO N or reduced[b] | 1 Pulmonary arterial hypertension<br>3 PH owing to lung diseases<br>4 Chronic thromboembolic PH<br>5 PH with unclear and/or<br>   multifactorial mechanisms |
| Postcapillary PH | mPAP ≥25 mm Hg<br>PAOP >15 mm Hg<br>CO N or reduced[b] | 2 PH owing to left heart disease |
| Passive | TPG ≤12 mm Hg | |
| Reactive ("out of proportion") | TPG >12 mm Hg | |

*Abbreviations:* CO, cardiac output; mPAP, mean pulmonary artery pressure; PAP, pulmonary arterial pressure; PAOP, pulmonary artery occlusion pressure; PH, pulmonary hypertension; TPG, transpulmonary pressure gradient (mPAP – PAOP).
[a] DanaPoint classification.
[b] High cardiac output can be present in cases of hyperkinetic conditions such as systemic-to-pulmonary shunts (only in the pulmonary circulation), anemia, hyperthyroidism, and so on.

$N_2$ gas, and upon exposure to $O_2$ gas, nitrogen dioxide is formed. Nitrogen dioxide can induce oxidative injury to lung epithelial linings. The nitrogen dioxide gas can be codelivered with inhaled nitrous oxide to patients during vasodilator testing and can place patients with postcapillary PH at greater risk for alveolar edema.[62]

## SUMMARY

PH falls into 5 groups, as defined by the World Health Organization. The hemodynamic definitions of PH at rest and with vasodilatory challenge provide an ability to categorize the etiology of PH and to guide treatment. Use of a conductance catheter can help to provide additional information on the ability of the RV to increase the stroke volume in the setting of acutely and chronically elevated pulmonary vascular resistance. Understanding of the RV maladaptations to increased pulmonary vascular resistance facilitates understanding of the chronicity of the RV response to increased PH and/or pulmonary vascular resistance. Use of the conductance catheters may guide the clinician to inform and treat the patient who may be at high risk for death from pulmonary illnesses. Swan-Ganz catheters can help to determine precapillary versus postcapillary PH and help to determine the usefulness of vasodilator studies.

## REFERENCES

1. Barst RJ. Pulmonary hypertension: past, present and future. Ann Thorac Med 2008;3(1):1–4.
2. Simonneau G, Robbins IM, Beghetti M, et al. Updated clinical classification of pulmonary hypertension. J Am Coll Cardiol 2009;54(1 Suppl):S43–54.
3. Romberg E. Ueber Sklerose der Lungenarterie: Aus der medicinischen Klinik zu Leipzig. Dtsch Arch Klin Med 1891;48:197–206 [in German].
4. Monckeberg JG. Ueber die genuine Arteriosklerose der Lungenarterie. Dtsch Med Wochenschr 1907;33(31):1243–6.
5. Winters WL, Joseph RR, Learner N. "Primary" pulmonary hypertension and Raynaud's phenomenon: case report and review of the literature. Arch Intern Med 1964;114(6):821–30.
6. Park MH. Historical perspective on the classification of pulmonary hypertension. In: Maron BA, Zamanian RT, Waxman AB, editors. Pulmonary hypertension: basic science to clinical medicine. New York: Springer International Publishing; 2016.
7. Schultz SG. William Harvey and the circulation of the blood: the birth of a scientific revolution of modern physiology. News Physiol Sci 2002;17:175–80.
8. Cattermole GN. Michael Servetus: physician, Socinian and victim. J R Soc Med 1997;90:640–4.
9. Slaughter MS, Pagani FD, Rogers JG, et al. Clinical management of continuous-flow left ventricular assist devise in advanced heart failure. J Heart Lung Transplant 2010;29(4 Suppl):S1–39.
10. Kormos RL, Teuteberg JJ, Pagani FD, et al. Right ventricular failure in patients with the HeartMate II continuous-flow left ventricular assist device: incidence, risk factors, and effect on outcomes. J Thorac Cardiovasc Surg 2010;139(5):1316–24.
11. Zaffran S, Kelly RG, Meilhac SM, et al. Right ventricular myocardium derives from the anterior heart field. Circ Res 2004;95(3):261–8.
12. Jiang L. Right ventricle. In: Weyman AE, editor. Principle and practice of echocardiography. Baltimore (MD): Lippincott Williams & Wilkins; 1994. p. 901–21.
13. Haddad F, Hunt SA, Rosenthal DN, et al. Right ventricular function in cardiovascular disease,

part I: anatomy, physiology, aging, and functional assessment of the right ventricle. Circulation 2008; 117:1436–48.

14. Goor DA, Lillehei CW. Congenital malformations of the heart. Congenital malformations of the heart: embryology, anatomy, and operative considerations. New York: Grune & Stratton; 1975.

15. Li JK. Comparative cardiac mechanics: Laplace's law. J Theor Biol 1986;118(3):339–43.

16. Sadeghpour A, Alizadehasl A. The right ventricle: a comprehensive review from anatomy, physiology, and mechanics to hemodynamic, functional, and imaging evaluation. Arch Cardiovasc Imaging 2015;3(4):e35717.

17. Lang RM, Badano LP, Mor-Avi V, et al. Recommendations for cardiac chamber quantification by echocardiography in adults: an update from the American Society of Echocardiography and the European Association of Cardiovascular Imaging. J Am Soc Echocardiogr 2015;28(1): 1–39.

18. Sabatine SA, editor. Pocket medicine: the Massachusetts General Hospital handbook of internal medicine. 6th edition. Philadelphia: Wolters Kluwer; 2017.

19. Rudolf AM. The fetal circulation after birth: their importance in congenital heart disease. Circulation 1970;41:343–59.

20. Sztrymf B, Coulet F, Girerd B, et al. Clinical outcomes of pulmonary arterial hypertension in carriers of BMPR2 mutation. Am J Respir Crit Care Med 2008;177(12):1377–83.

21. Oudiz RJ. Pulmonary hypertension associated with left-sided heart disease. Clin Chest Med 2007;28: 233–41.

22. Moraes DL, Colucci WS, Givertz MM. Secondary pulmonary hypertension in chronic heart failure: the role of endothelium in pathophysiology and management. Circulation 2000;102:1718–23.

23. Behr J, Ryu JH. Pulmonary hypertension in interstitial lung disease. Eur Respir J 2008;31(6):1357–67.

24. Heit JA. The epidemiology of venous thromboembolism in the community. Arterioscler Thromb Vasc Biol 2008;28(3):370–2.

25. Konstantinides SV. 2014 ESC guidelines on the diagnosis and management of acute pulmonary embolism. Eur Heart J 2014;35(45):3145–6.

26. Auger WR, Fedullo PF. Chronic thromboembolic pulmonary hypertension. In: Klinger JR, Frantz RP, editors. Diagnosis and management of pulmonary hypertension. New York: Humana Press; 2015. p. 115–42.

27. Kalantari S, Gomberg-Maitland M. Group 5 pulmonary hypertension: the orphan's orphan disease. Cardiol Clin 2016;34(3):443–9.

28. Dingli D, Utz JP, Krowka MJ, et al. Unexplained pulmonary hypertension in chronic myeloproliferative disorders. Chest 2001;120:801–8.

29. Ragosta M. Introduction to hemodynamic assessment in the cardiac catheterization laboratory. In: Ragosta M, editor. Textbook of clinical hemodynamics. Philadelphia: Saunders; 2008. p. 01–15.

30. Mueller RL, Sanborn TA. The history of interventional cardiology: cardiac catheterization, angioplasty, and related interventions. Am Heart J 1995;129(1):146–72.

31. Cournand A, Ranges HA. Catheterization of the right auricle in man. Exp Biol Med (Maywood) 1941;46(3):462–6.

32. Kern MJ, Sorajja P, Lim MJ, editors. Cardiac catheterization handbook. 6th edition. Philadelphia: Elsevier, Inc; 2016.

33. Binanay C, Califf R, Hasselblad V, et al. Evaluation study of congestive heart failure and pulmonary artery catheterization effectiveness: the ESCAPE trial. JAMA 2005;294(13):1625–33.

34. Higgs ZC, Macafee DA, Braithwaite BD, et al. The Seldinger technique: 50 years on. Lancet 2005; 366(9494):1407–9.

35. Swan HJ, Ganz W, Forrester J, et al. Catheterization of the heart in man with use of a flow-directed balloon-tipped catheter. N Engl J Med 1970; 283(9):447–51.

36. Sharkey SW. A guide to interpretation of hemodynamic data in the coronary care unit. Philadelphia: Lippincott-Raven Publishers; 1997. p. 22.

37. Grossman W. Pressure measurement. In: Baim DS, editor. Grossman's cardiac catheterization, angiography, and intervention. Philadelphia: Lippincott Williams & Wilkins; 2006. p. 137–44.

38. Harvey S, Harrison DA, Singer M, et al. Assessment of the clinical effectiveness of pulmonary artery catheters in management of patients in intensive care (PAC-Man): a randomised controlled trial. Lancet 2005;366(9484):472–7.

39. Cotter G, Cotter OM, Kaluski E. Hemodynamic monitoring in acute heart failure. Crit Care Med 2008;36(1 Suppl):S40–3.

40. Spiller P, Webb-Peploe MM. Blood flow. Eur Heart J 1985;6(Suppl C):11–8.

41. Kovacs G, Berghold A, Scheidl S, et al. Pulmonary arterial pressure during rest and exercise in health subjects: a systemic review. Eur Respir J 2009; 34(4):888–94.

42. Gewillig M. The Fontan circulation. Heart 2005; 91(6):839–46.

43. Burkhoff D. Mechanical Properties of the Heart and its Interaction with the Vascular System. New York: Columbia Graduate School of Arts and Sciences. Columbia.edu [Internet]; 2003. Available at: http://www.columbia.edu/itc/gsas/g6001/BasicLV-Mechanics.pdf. Accessed April 20, 2017.

44. Burkhoff D, Sayer G, Doshi D, et al. Hemodynamics of mechanical circulatory support. J Am Coll Cardiol 2015;66(23):2663–74.

45. Maurer MS, Kronzon I, Burkhoff D. Ventricular pump function in heart failure with normal ejection fraction: insights from pressure-volume measurements. Prog Cardiovasc Dis 2006;49(3):182–95.

46. Redington AN, Gray HH, Hodson ME, et al. Characterisation of the normal right ventricular pressure-volume relation by biplane angiography and simultaneous micromanometer pressure measurements. Br Heart J 1988;59(1):23–30.

47. Naeije R, Brimioulle S, Dewachter L. Biomechanics of the right ventricle in health and disease (2013 Grover Conference series). Pulm Circ 2014;4(3):395–406.

48. Maughan WL, Shoukas AA, Sagawa K, et al. Instantaneous pressure-volume relationship of the canine right ventricle. Circ Res 1979;44(3):309–15.

49. Greyson CR. The right ventricle and pulmonary circulation: basic concepts. Rev Esp Cardiol 2010;63(1):81–95.

50. Saouti N, Westerhof N, Postmus PE, et al. The arterial load in pulmonary hypertension. Eur Respir Rev 2010;19(117):197–203.

51. Bellofiore A, Chesler N. Methods for measuring right ventricular function and hemodynamic coupling with the pulmonary vasculature. Ann Biomed Eng 2013;41(7):1384–98.

52. Monroe RG, Gamble WJ, LaFarge CG, et al. The Anrep effect reconsidered. J Clin Invest 1972;51(10):2573–83.

53. Santamore WP, Dell'Italia LJ. Ventricular interdependence: significant left ventricular contributions to right ventricular systolic function. Prog Cardiovasc Dis 1998;40(4):289–308.

54. Sagawa K, Maughan L, Suga H, et al. Cardiac contraction and the pressure-volume relationship. New York: Oxford University Press; 1998.

55. Naeije R, Manes A. The right ventricle in pulmonary arterial hypertension. Eur Respir Rev 2014;23(134):476–87.

56. Wauthy P, Naeije R, Brimioulle S. Left and right ventriculo-arterial coupling in a patient with congenitally corrected transposition. Cardiol Young 2005;15(06):647–9.

57. Porterfield JE, Kottam AT, Raghavan K, et al. Dynamic correction for parallel conductance, GP, and gain factor, alpha, in invasive murine left ventricular volume measurements. J Appl Physiol (1985) 2009;107(6):1693–703.

58. Champion HC, Michelakis ED, Hassoun PM. Comprehensive invasive and noninvasive approach to the right ventricle–pulmonary circulation unit: state of the art and clinical and research implications. Circulation 2009;120(11):992–1007.

59. Borlaug BA, Kass DA. Invasive hemodynamic assessment in heart failure. Heart Fail Clin 2009;5(2):217–28.

60. Grignola JC. Hemodynamic assessment of pulmonary hypertension. World J Cardiol 2011;3(1):10–7.

61. Galiè N, Humbert M, Vachiery JL, et al. 2015 ESC/ERS Guidelines for the Diagnosis and Treatment of Pulmonary Hypertension: the Joint Task Force for the Diagnosis and Treatment of Pulmonary Hypertension of the European Society of Cardiology (ESC) and the European Respiratory Society (ERS): endorsed by: Association for European Paediatric and Congenital Cardiology (AEPC), International Society for Heart and Lung Transplantation (ISHLT). Eur Heart J 2016;37(1):67–119.

62. Petit PC, Fine DH, Vásquez GB, et al. The pathophysiology of nitrogen dioxide during inhaled nitric oxide therapy. ASAIO J 2017;63:7–13.

# Invasive Hemodynamics of Adult Congenital Heart Disease: From Shunts to Coarctation

Surendranath R. Veeram Reddy, MD,
Alan W. Nugent, MBBS, Thomas M. Zellers, MD,
V. Vivian Dimas, MD*

---

## KEYWORDS

- Adults with congenital heart disease • Shunting lesions • Repaired congenital heart disease
- Cardiac catheterization • Fontan procedure • Cyanosis

---

## KEY POINTS

- Adults living with congenital heart disease (ACHD) now exceed the pediatric (CHD) population.
- Calculation of resistance and flows is required before occlusion/closure of shunting lesions to assess suitability for closure.
- Obstructions in series (right and left sided) commonly occur in these ACHD patients and should be carefully evaluated because significant distal obstructions can be underestimated.
- Cyanotic, single-ventricle CHD represents the most complex and heterogeneous subset of ACHD patients. Complete understanding of anatomy and goals of catheterization are necessary to perform a complete assessment and determine candidacy for intervention.
- Minor hemodynamic aberrancies are often significant and underestimated in single-ventricle patients.

---

## INTRODUCTION

The population of adults with congenital heart disease (ACHD) continues to grow, with this population now exceeding the living population of children with congenital heart disease (CHD).[1,2] Improvements in diagnosis, medical care, surgery, and transcatheter technologies have resulted in longer life expectancy for children with CHD. As the population ages, increasing numbers of ACHD patients are in need of adult specialists for ongoing care. Based on this need, the American Board of Internal Medicine created a sub-board and training track for physicians who desire to take care of these patients.[2] Unfortunately, the demand for practitioners who are able to care for these complex patients far exceeds the physician pool, and undoubtedly most physicians will encounter adults with CHD both repaired and unrepaired during their practice.[1] Interventional Cardiologists are likely to be asked to assist in evaluating this complex patient group; therefore, understanding intracardiac hemodynamics is critical for a complete assessment of these patients. Although not exhaustive, this article serves to provide a basic understanding of the hemodynamic nuances and aberrancies encountered for some of the more common lesions likely to be encountered. The 2008 American Heart Association and 2010 European Society of Cardiology guidelines articles delineate the indications for cardiac catheterization in ACHD.[3,4]

---

Disclosures: None of the authors have disclosures, financial or otherwise, to report relevant to this article.
Division of Cardiology, Department of Pediatrics, University of Texas Southwestern Medical Center, Children's Health System of Texas, 1935 Medical District Drive, Dallas, TX 75235, USA
* Corresponding author.
E-mail address: Vivian.Dimas@childrens.com

Intervent Cardiol Clin 6 (2017) 345–358
http://dx.doi.org/10.1016/j.iccl.2017.03.005
2211-7458/17/© 2017 Elsevier Inc. All rights reserved.

## BIVENTRICULAR CONGENITAL HEART DISEASE

### Shunting Lesions

All patients with hemodynamically significant shunting lesions should undergo a complete hemodynamic assessment before any intervention to assess the clinical significance of the shunt and rule out comorbid conditions such as pulmonary hypertension, coronary artery disease (in older patients), or ventricular dysfunction in attempts to determine candidacy for closure (transcatheter or surgical).[3,5] Understanding the concepts of how pulmonary and systemic blood flow affect calculations of resistance allows one to understand that absolute numbers alone do not necessarily apply, that is, mean pulmonary artery pressure (PAp) or transpulmonary gradient alone. In adult patients with shunt lesions where there is echocardiographic documentation of pulmonary hypertension (PAp >50% systemic), catheterization is essential for decision making.[4] Correct assessment of pulmonary vascular resistance (PVR) requires an accurate assessment of flows.

Cardiac output calculations are based on indicator dilution techniques, with the most common indicator being oxygen. The Fick calculation uses the difference in oxygen content (a product of oxygen carried on the hemoglobin plus dissolved blood oxygen if applicable) across a vascular bed. Specifically, the Fick principle states that "a substance will diffuse through an area at a rate that is dependent upon the difference in concentration of the substance at two given points."[3,6] To calculate the $O_2$ content, one must remember that 1 g of hemoglobin (Hb) carries 1.36 mL of $O_2$ and that the coefficient of solubility for $O_2$ in the blood is 0.003. Thus:

Oxygen content ($CaO_2$) = $SaO_2$ × Hb × 1.36 × 10 + 0.003($PaO_2$)

If oxygen is being used as the indicator, the operator must know the oxygen consumption ($VO_2$) (the amount of oxygen extracted from the air per unit time) and the quantity (saturation) of oxygen in the upstream (mixed venous) and downstream (mixed arterial) blood. The difference between these values represents the arteriovenous difference (A − $VO_2$ difference). This principle can be applied to the pulmonary or systemic circulation in the absence of intracardiac shunting. The $VO_2$ represents the difference in concentration of oxygen in room air and the concentration of oxygen in the expired air multiplied by the volume of gas flow in milliliter per minute, which is then indexed to body surface area (BSA)

to obtain the absolute $VO_2$ (mL/min/m²). It can be measured but is typically assumed, as it is particularly cumbersome to measure in the nonintubated patient. Unfortunately, assuming $VO_2$ can introduce up to 40% error in output calculations,[7–9] newer devices now allow $VO_2$ to be measured in the intubated patient with reliable accuracy.[6,10] Oxygen consumption cannot be accurately measured if supplemental oxygen is being used. Once determination of the above factors is made, then cardiac output (CO) can be calculated via the Fick equation below:

CO = $VO_2$ (mL/min)/(SA % sat − MV % sat) × Hb × 1.36 × 10

By indexing the $VO_2$ to BSA, cardiac index (CI) can be obtained using the same calculation:

CI = $VO_2$ (mL/min/m²)/(SA % sat − MV % sat) × Hb × 1.36 × 10

Because of errors associated with the assumption of $VO_2$, many catheterization laboratories use thermodilution with cold saline as the indicator. This method has proven unreliable in patients with significant tricuspid insufficiency, low cardiac output, arrhythmias, or the presence of intracardiac shunts.[11,12]

In the presence of intracardiac shunting, calculation of flow in each of the separate circuits is required. Calculation of pulmonary blood flow (Qp) requires determination of oxygen content in pulmonary venous and pulmonary arterial blood. Calculation of systemic blood flow (Qs) requires determination of oxygen content in the systemic arterial and mixed venous blood. The shunt is the difference in total flow between the 2 circuits.

Qp = $VO_2$ (mL/min/m²)/(PV % Sat − PA % Sat) × 1.36 × Hb × 10

Qs = $VO_2$ (mL/min/m²)/(SA % Sat − MV % Sat) × 1.36 × Hb × 10

If $VO_2$ is assumed, estimates of absolute flows are calculated.

Shunt calculations become more difficult to assess if multiple levels of shunting exist. A basic premise is that the best assessment of a shunt's contribution is noted in the most distal chamber possible rather than the receiving chamber. To calculate a shunt, saturations must be measured in the chamber before the shunt and the most distal chamber to shunt to allow for adequate mixing. In situations where there is essentially only left-to-right flow, then a standard Qp-to-Qs ratio may be calculated. In the presence of bidirectional shunting, one may choose to calculate the effective Qp or Qs depending on the clinical scenario. Significant right-to-left shunting is often presumed absent with systemic arterial saturations greater than 96%.

Historically, in the pediatric literature, patients with a calculated PVR greater than 6 Wood units on 100% oxygen defined a patient as an unsuitable candidate for closure and those with PVR greater than 8 Wood units were deemed inoperable. There are emerging data in older patients with high PVR undergoing successful transcatheter closure.[13,14] If during baseline hemodynamics the calculated PVR on room air exceeds 5 to 6 Wood units, pulmonary vasodilator testing to assess reactivity of the vascular bed is recommended. If pulmonary vasodilator testing is performed, it is critical to obtain blood gas measurements in all required locations to accurately assess dissolved oxygen to avoid underestimation of the resistance. In addition, a complete repeat hemodynamic catheterization should be performed to assess for changes in pressures related to vasodilator administration.

### Atrial septal defects

In the presence of ventricular dysfunction, shunts may be overestimated or underestimated; however, it should be noted that even small (<1.5 Qp:Qs) shunts may be more hemodynamically significant in the presence of ventricular dysfunction. This finding can be seen commonly in older patients with atrial septal defects (ASDs) where shunting can be decreased in the presence of right ventricular dysfunction and/or increased right atrial pressure or increased in the presence of left ventricular dysfunction and/or elevated left atrial pressure. Hemodynamic and anatomic assessment should be performed in all patients in whom closure is anticipated. Diastolic dysfunction can have significant implications on therapy before and immediately after closure. The impact of the acute removal of the atrial level shunt or "pop off" resulting in changes to ventricular preload in the setting of ventricular dysfunction has been described and can be anticipated if full hemodynamic assessment is completed before closure.[5,15]

### Ventricular septal defects

With advancing age, even small ventricular septal defects (VSDs) may become problematic. Increased left-to-right shunting can occur due to an increase in left ventricular systolic and/or diastolic pressure; aortic insufficiency may occur related to VSD location to the aortic valve, and development of double-chambered right ventricle (RV) may occur. Finally, the development of

Eisenmenger syndrome with associated cyanosis may occur.[3,4] As with all shunting lesions, accurate assessment of flows and resistances is used to guide management. Right ventricular hypertension itself does not always confer the diagnosis of pulmonary hypertension. Causes of RV hypertension can include the presence of unrecognized or underestimated right ventricular outflow tract (RVOT) obstruction as well as contamination of the pressure waveform related to the VSD flow. Once elevated PVR is confirmed, pulmonary vasodilator testing should be performed as discussed previously to assess suitability for closure.

### Patent ductus arteriosus

The presentation of patent ductus arteriosus (PDA) in the adult population can vary from an asymptomatic heart murmur to Eisenmenger syndrome. Catheterization is not necessary for diagnostic purposes unless closure is being considered.[3,4] As with VSDs (high-pressure shunting lesions), careful assessment of flows and PVR is critical to decision making. Generally, it is reasonable to perform closure of a PDA in patients with elevated PVR with a net left-to-right shunt. As noted previously, a calculated PVR greater than 8 had historically been deemed inoperable; however, this concept may be evolving as there are emerging data that PDAs can be successfully closed in patients with significantly elevated PVR. These patients remain exceedingly high risk, and long-term follow-up data do not yet exist; therefore, one should exercise caution in this population.[13] Test occlusion in these patients in addition to pulmonary vasodilator testing can be considered to attempt to assess hemodynamic response to closure.[14]

### Repaired Congenital Heart Disease

Three cyanotic heart defects, d-transposition of the great arteries (d-TGA), tetralogy of Fallot (TOF), and truncus arteriosus (TA), account for most infants born with cyanosis who will undergo a 2-ventricle repair. Most of these patients survive their infant surgery and live well into adulthood, but many will develop hemodynamic sequelae as they age (Table 1).

### D-transposition of the great arteries

There are several anatomic associations with d-TGA, including VSD, a spectrum of pulmonary valve and subvalvar stenosis, coarctation of the aorta, and PDA. The following surgical repairs can be encountered. The Senning and Mustard operations are "atrial switch operations," rerouting blood from the inferior vena cava (IVC) and

**Table 1**
Commonly encountered hemodynamic sequelae in repaired CHD

| Defects | Sequelae | Hemodynamics/ Pressure Measurements | Angiography |
|---|---|---|---|
| d-TGA s/p Mustard/Senning | SVC or IVC obstruction, pulmonary venous baffle obstruction, residual VSD, pulmonary stenosis | SVC, systemic venous atrium, LV, PA, and PA wedge, RVEDp Shunt calculations | SVC or IVC: stenosis/ decompression LV: sub-PS and PS PA: PV baffle obstruction |
| d-TGA s/p Rastelli/Nikaidoh | Residual VSD, LVOT baffle obstruction, conduit obstruction, conduit regurgitation, branch PA stenosis | SVC, right atrium (RA), RV, MPA, branch PA, LV, and aorta Shunt calculations | LV: residual VSD and LVOTO RV or MPA: residual PS, PI, or branch PS |
| d-TGA s/p Arterial Switch | Coronary artery stenosis, MPA or branch PA stenosis, aortic dilation | SVC, RA, RV, MPA, branch PA, LV, and aorta Shunt calculations | Aorta: aortic dilation and coronaries MPA: MPA and branch pulmonary stenosis |
| TOF repair | Residual VSD, residual pulmonary valve or conduit stenosis or regurgitation, branch PA stenosis/hypoplasia, aortic dilation, coronary abnormalities | SVC, RA, RV, conduit, MPA, branch PA, LV, and aorta Shunt calculations | LV: residual VSD RV: conduit or subvalvar PS MPA: conduit or MPA regurgitation and branch PA stenosis Aorta: coronaries |
| TA repair | Residual VSD, residual pulmonary valve or conduit stenosis or regurgitation, branch PA stenosis/hypoplasia, aortic dilation, coronary abnormalities | SVC, RA, RV, conduit, MPA, branch PA, LV, and aorta Shunt calculations | LV: residual VSD RV: conduit or subvalvar PS MPA: conduit or MPA regurgitation and branch PA stenosis Aorta: coronaries |

superior vena cava (SVC) to the mitral valve, left ventricle (LV), and PAs. In turn, the pulmonary venous blood is redirected across the baffle to the tricuspid valve, systemic RV, and aorta. Some patients have a VSD and/or some degree of pulmonary stenosis (PS). If the PS is mild, the Mustard or Senning operation may be accompanied by a simple VSD closure.

Cardiac catheterization must determine anatomically if SVC or IVC baffle obstruction is present; the SVC limb is the most common site, but it may be accompanied by azygous vein decompression to the IVC. Thus, a pressure gradient across this limb of the baffle may not be significant or present. Angiography in the SVC is the key to this diagnosis.[16] Pulmonary venous obstruction can occur less frequently, most often presenting as a pathway obstruction, not as an individual pulmonary vein narrowing. Wedge to right ventricular end diastolic pressure (RVEDp) differences combined with pulmonary angiography with recirculation or angiography in the

pulmonary venous baffle (via transseptal approach) is needed. Residual VSDs can occur and are usually diagnosed by echocardiography, but shunt calculations determine significance. Pulmonary valve and subvalve stenosis must be evaluated in those patients born with this association; LV and main pulmonary artery (MPA) pressure measurements and LV angiography determine the extent of the stenosis. Finally, RVEDp measurements are necessary to document because RV dysfunction, both systolic and diastolic, is common with increasing age.

The Rastelli or Nikaidoh procedures are offered to patients with d-TGA, VSD, and pulmonary stenosis/atresia. In the Rastelli operation, the VSD is baffled from the LV to the aorta, and a valved conduit is placed between the RV and the PA; no atrial baffle is needed in this scenario. The Nikaidoh procedure involves moving the aortic root (including coronary transfer) from the RV to the LV and closing the VSD to the aorta and again creating an RV to PA pathway, classically with a nonvalved conduit. The sequelae seen with these procedures are similar, including residual VSDs, LVOT pathway obstruction, conduit obstruction, and regurgitation with subsequent RV dilation. Proximal PA narrowing or stenosis may also be found, adding an additional level of obstruction to the RVOT.[17] Hemodynamic measurements across these pathways, shunt calculations to determine significance of residual VSD, and angiography in the RV and LV, at a minimum, are needed for assessment.

The arterial switch operation is currently the operation of choice for uncomplicated d-TGA. In this procedure, the great arteries are transected and "switched"; the aorta is sewn to the native pulmonary trunk, and the PA is sewn to the native aortic trunk. The coronary arteries are removed using a "button" technique and sewn to the neoaortic (former pulmonary) sinuses of Valsalva, allowing oxygenated aortic blood to enter the coronaries. If a VSD is present, the VSD is closed in the normal fashion. The sequelae associated with the arterial switch include main and proximal branch PA anastomotic stenoses, supravalvar AS, stenosis related to coronary button harvest, and stretching of the pulmonary arteries across the aortic root (LeCompte maneuver).[18] Pressure measurements in the RV, MPA, and branch pulmonary arteries and angiography in the MPA should be performed. Coronary abnormalities after reimplantation are expected in some patients.[19]

### Tetralogy of Fallot and truncus arteriosus

TOF and TA repairs both involve VSD repair and creation of, or augmentation of, the RVOT, including transannular patch, pulmonary valve dilation, or RV-to-PA conduit placement (in all cases of TA and TOF with pulmonary atresia/hypoplasia). The most common sequelae in patients status post repair of TOF and TA include RVOT obstruction and/or regurgitation. This may be at the subvalvar, valvar, or supravalvar location.[20] Conduit calcification with stenosis can add an additional level of complexity to the RVOT obstruction. Hemodynamic measurement in the RV, conduit (if present), MPA, and branch pulmonary arteries determines the severity of RVOT and branch PA obstruction. Angiography in the RV can delineate position and extent of obstruction, but angiography in the MPA or distal conduit delineates the degree of pulmonary regurgitation, supravalvar, and branch PA stenosis/hypoplasia. Angiography in the LV can locate residual VSDs, but left-to-right shunt calculations determine the

significance of the residual VSD. Aortic angiography delineates congenital coronary abnormalities (usually the left coronary from the right coronary in TOF) and aortic root size (although MRI and computed tomography are accurate and noninvasive).

Rarely, one might encounter a patient with residual surgical shunts, such as a Blalock Taussig (BT; subclavian to pulmonary artery), Waterston (ascending aorta to right pulmonary artery [RPA]), or Potts (descending aorta to left pulmonary artery [LPA]) shunt, all of which may be associated with PA stenosis or hypoplasia. Shunt calculations, hemodynamic assessment, and angiography are essential to evaluate the PA pressures, shunt flow, and patency, as well as PA distortion.

### Left-Sided Obstructive Lesions
### Mitral stenosis

Whether congenital or secondary to a prosthetic mitral valve, mitral stenosis (MS) creates a diastolic gradient between the left atrium (LA) and LV. In the setting of a normal mitral valve, the LA and LV tracing in diastole override one another, and the end-diastolic pressure of the LV is best and most consistently recorded at the point where the tracings cross. In the setting of MS, the LA is generally noncompliant, thus creating a large "a" wave. Measuring the mitral valve gradient is best achieved with a simultaneous LA and LV pressure recording. The PA wedge pressure can be used in place of the LA tracing, but the timing of the wedge pressure is slightly delayed, thus decreasing the accuracy of the gradient measurement. There will be a separation between the 2 curves in diastole with a peak gradient measured at the site of maximum distance (usually at the timing of the "a" wave) and a mean gradient that is the area between the 2 curves.[21]

### Valvar aortic stenosis

Aortic stenosis (AS) is most commonly at the level of the valve. If the obstruction is at the level of the valve, a sudden decrease in systolic pressure will occur at the same time as a sudden increase in diastolic pressure to indicate the catheter is no longer in the ventricle. The peak-to-peak gradient is a simple subtraction from the LV systolic pressure to the ascending aorta systolic pressure. However, if the pressures are recorded simultaneously, the peak pressure in the aorta is slightly delayed compared with the LV, and thus the measured peak-to-peak gradient never actually occurs in real time. This is one of the reasons for the differing measurement of the gradient with catheterization and echocardiography (which measures in real time).

### Valve area

In both mitral and valvar AS in pediatrics, the cardiac output is assumed to be maintained. Thus, in valvar AS, a peak-to-peak gradient on pullback is the standard measurement for management decisions. The reason for this assumption is that in pediatrics the LV function is in fact almost always maintained. The main exception is critical valvar AS in a newborn with ductal-dependent systemic circulation and poor LV function. However, in the ACHD population, or in the elderly with valvar AS, maintenance of cardiac output cannot be assumed and in fact is commonly reduced. This leads to the need to correct the gradient for the cardiac output and heart rate and the concept of valve area.

Measurement of valve area requires the measurement of cardiac output (using either the Fick method or thermodilution). There are sources of error in cardiac output measurement, and thus, the most accurate valve area calculations require attention to detail in cardiac output measurement and simultaneous pressure recordings.

### Left ventricular outflow tract obstruction

Because of either a congenital subaortic membrane or a hypertrophic cardiomyopathy, there is a space underneath the aortic valve that has a ventricular waveform that is lower than rest of the ventricle. The size of the subaortic ventricular region may be too small for a pigtail with multiple side holes and an end-hole catheter may be needed. If there is instability of the catheter, and inability to record the outflow tract pressure, an over-the-wire pullback can be performed. This is achieved by placing a small-diameter wire in the apex of the LV and advancing a catheter with a much larger lumen over the wire. Connecting the catheter to a Tuohy device enables a controlled pullback from LV to LV outflow tract to aorta over the stabilizing wire, even enabling angiography if needed to verify the location of the obstruction.

If a ventricular ectopic beat occurs, the pause causes an increase in LV pressure from longer filling time and from increased contraction. Therefore, the next ventricular systole after the delay has an increase in stroke volume. In congenital subaortic membrane, this causes an increase in LV pressure and an increase in aortic pressure (with an overall increase in the gradient). In hypertrophic cardiomyopathy, with dynamic obstruction, there is an increase in LV pressure, but because of an increase in dynamic subaortic obstruction, the aortic pressure decreases. This phenomenon has previously been described as the Brockenbrough-Braunwald-Morrow sign.[22]

### Supravalvar aortic stenosis

During a pullback, there will be the same systolic pressure in the aorta as in the LV, with the only change being the diastolic pressure. With further withdrawal of the catheter, a systolic gradient will be recorded as the catheter exits the aortic root, passes the sinotubular junction, and enters the ascending aorta. This is sometimes difficult to record as the aortic valve can open to the sinotubular junction, removing space between aortic root and ascending aorta. In this case, the catheter needs to be placed in the aortic root (take care when placing a catheter into a coronary cusp of supravalvar AS because this may compromise coronary artery perfusion) for pressure measurement.

### Coarctation of the aorta

Obstruction to the aorta can be discrete with a sudden change in systolic and diastolic pressure on pullback, but there can also be obstruction at multiple levels. Typically, discrete obstruction is at the level of the aortic isthmus, after the takeoff of the left subclavian artery. The next most common site is the distal transverse arch, which is between the takeoff of the left common carotid artery and left subclavian artery. Clearly identifying the location of the gradient is extremely important before proceeding with an intervention. In longstanding aortic obstruction, collateral circulation can develop, "decompressing" the obstruction. This decompression can result in a decreased pressure gradient across the stenosis. In these circumstances, absolute gradients may not be a reliable indicator of the degree of obstruction. In the presence of obstructions in series, the operator must do their best to evaluate the contribution of each obstruction with the understanding that the distal obstructions will be underestimated.

## UNIVENTRICULAR CONGENITAL HEART DISEASE

All complex CHDs not amenable for complete biventricular repair are grouped under "univentricular" or "single-ventricle" physiology and include hypoplastic right and left heart syndromes, tricuspid atresia, mitral atresia, double inlet LV, and so forth. Invasive hemodynamic assessment of symptomatic adults with single-ventricular physiology is a critical step in overall treatment strategy.

Adults with single ventricle physiology can be broadly classified into 2 categories:

### Partial/Shunt Palliated

Patients who continue to be "shunt dependent" for pulmonary blood flow fall into this category. There are 3 different types of shunt-dependent patients.

*Palliative pulmonary artery banding surgery*
Certain univentricular hearts (eg, tricuspid atresia with large VSD, unbalanced atrioventricular septal defect, and so forth) are palliated with a PA band in infancy to prevent pulmonary overcirculation and achieve a "balanced circulation." As children with initial PA banding procedure grow into adulthood, they may present with cyanosis (band too tight or PA distortions) or symptoms of pulmonary vascular disease (from an inadequate banding leading to pulmonary hypertension).

*Systemic artery to pulmonary artery shunts*
These types of shunts are also known as aorto-pulmonary shunts and are primarily performed to provide pulmonary blood flow.

i. *Classic Blalock-Taussig Shunt* (**Fig. 1**): End-to-side subclavian artery to ipsilateral PA anastomosis.

ii. *Modified Blalock-Taussig Shunt* (see **Fig. 1**): Side-to-side small Gore-Tex tube connection between innominate/subclavian artery to ipsilateral PA.

iii. *Pott Shunt* (see **Fig. 1**): Side-to-side descending aorta to LPA anastomosis.

iv. *Waterston Shunt* (see **Fig. 1**): Side-to-side ascending aorta to RPA anastomosis.

v. *Central Shunt* (**Fig. 2**): Side-to-side small Gore-Tex tube connection between ascending aorta and PA.

vi. *Melbourne Shunt* (**Fig. 3**): End-to-side central MPA to aorta connection.

It is standard practice to avoid traversing the central and BT shunts during catheterization to avoid triggering coagulation cascade and thrombus formation. The PA pressures can be measured indirectly by advancing the diagnostic catheter across the ASD to the pulmonary vein wedge position for pulmonary vein wedge pressures. If the BT shunt has to be traversed to obtain hemodynamics and/or perform angiography/interventions, extreme care should be taken to maintain patency of the BT/central shunt to prevent

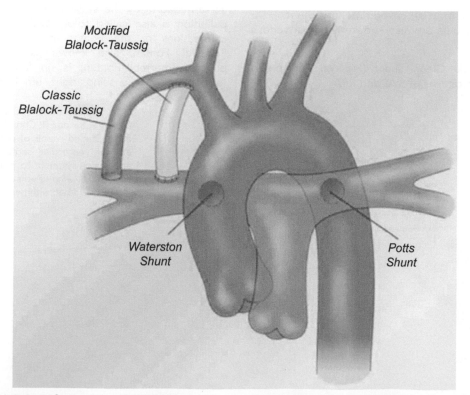

**Fig. 1.** Variations of systemic to pulmonary shunts. (*From* Romfh A, Pluchinotta FR, Porayette P, et al. Congenital heart defects in adults: a field guide for cardiologists. J Clin Exp Cardiolog 2012;S8:1–24; with permission.)

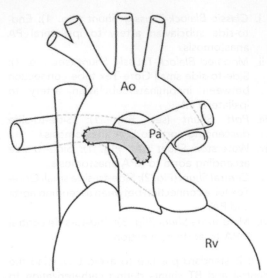

Fig. 2. Central shunt. (*From* Biglino G, Giardini A, Hsia TY, et al; MOCHA Collaborative Group. Modeling single ventricle physiology: review of engineering tools to study first stage palliation of hypoplastic left heart syndrome. Front Pediatr 2013:30;1:31; with permission.)

clotting. It is standard practice to intensify anticoagulation therapy or start the patient on heparin drip for the first 1 to 2 days after catheterization.

### Superior (partial) cavopulmonary shunt

These shunts are also known as partial venous shunts.

i. Classic Glenn Shunt (**Fig. 4**): End-to-end anastomosis of SVC and RPA.

ii. Bidirectional Glenn Shunt (**Fig. 5**): End-to-side anastomosis of SVC and RPA. After SVC disconnection, the right atrial end is sewn off.

iii. Hemi-Fontan (**Fig. 6**): Side-to-side anastomosis of SVC and RPA, and the superior cavoatrial junction is closed with a dam of homograft tissue.

Diagnostic cardiac catheterization of a Glenn pathway patient is typically performed with 2 venous accesses (femoral vein and internal jugular vein) and one arterial access primarily for monitoring blood pressures during the procedure and to intervene on the aorta/collaterals. Pressures and saturations should be obtained in the Glenn circuit as well as in the pulmonary veins, atria and systemic ventricle, and great arteries to assess Qp:Qs and hemodynamically significant stenosis throughout the venous and systemic pathways.

### Fully Palliated (Fontan)

Patients who undergo complete separation of the pulmonary and systemic circulation have passive flow of deoxygenated blood from the SVC and IVC (including hepatic venous blood) to the lungs, with return of oxygenated blood to the pulmonary venous atrium and out the aorta/neoaorta by the systemic ventricle. Such palliation is also called total caval pulmonary connections or the Fontan procedure. The "classic" Fontan, also known as an atrial-pulmonary artery Fontan, is no longer performed due to ensuing right atrial dilation

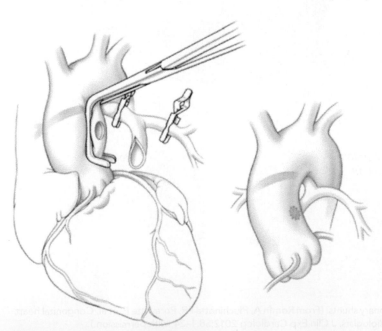

Fig. 3. Melbourne shunt. (*From* Talwar S, Saxena R, Choudhary SK, et al. Staged repair of pulmonary atresia, ventricular septal defect and major systemic to pulmonary collaterals. Ann Pediatr Cardiol 2010;3(2):136–9; with permission.)

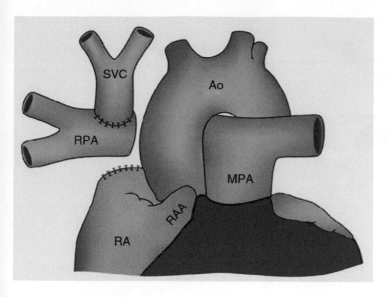

Fig. 4. Glenn shunt. (*From* Siegel MJ, Miszalski-Jamka T, Pelberg R. Systemic Vein to Pulmonary Artery Shunts: Glenn, Fontan and Kawashima Procedures. In: Siegel MJ, Miszalski-Jamka T, Pelberg R, editors. CT Atlas of Adult Congenital Heart Disease. New York: Springer; 2013. p. 289–98; with permission.)

resulting in arrhythmias and reduced pulmonary blood flow due to kinetic energy loss in the compliant circuit (failed Fontan pathway). In the current era, 2 types of Fontan palliation are performed with or without fenestration based on anatomy and surgeon preference: (1) intracardiac lateral tunnel Fontan (a tunnel created within the right atrium connecting the IVC to the RPA/central PAs) and (2) extracardiac Fontan (Gore-Tex conduit connecting the IVC to the RPA/central PAs).

The following represents the most common indications for referral for catheterization of single-ventricle patients:

1. Cyanosis, new or worsening
2. Exercise deterioration or worsening fatigue at rest

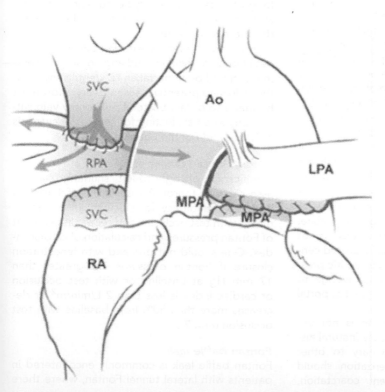

Fig. 5. Bidirectional Glenn shunt. (*From* Neema PK, Sethuraman M, Krishnamanohar SR, et al. Superior vena cava syndrome after pulsatile bidirectional Glenn shunt procedure: perioperative implications. Ann Card Anaesth 2008;12(1): 53–6; with permission.)

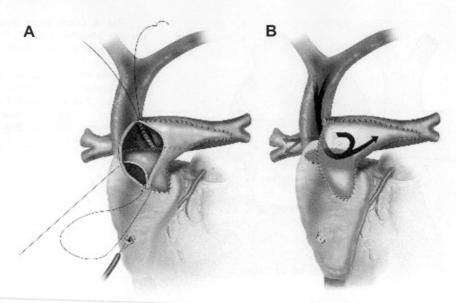

Fig. 6. Hemi-Fontan procedure. (*From* Spray TL. Hemi-Fontan procedure. Oper Tech Thorac Cardiovasc Surg 2013;18(2):124–37; with permission.)

3. Unexplained ascites, edema
4. Oxygen unresponsive hypoxemia
5. New onset or recurrent arrhythmias
6. Hemoptysis
7. Transplant evaluation, for "failing" univentricular hearts

Understanding the postoperative anatomy is critical to performing a thorough catheterization. To complete a full hemodynamic assessment, saturations should be obtained in the following locations to accurately calculate Qp and Qs: SVC, bilateral pulmonary arteries, bilateral pulmonary veins (when accessible), and femoral artery/aorta. Pressures should be measured throughout the Fontan circuit. Because of the nonpulsatile nature of the Glenn and Fontan pathways, even significant obstructions will only generate gradients of 1 to 4 mm Hg. If decompressing collaterals are present, a further reduction in gradient can occur. Thus, clinical symptoms and angiographic findings are important in determining indications for intervention, rather than pressure gradient alone. In adult Fontan patients, hepatic disease is not uncommon because of chronically elevated central venous pressures; thus, a transhepatic pressure gradient from hepatic venous wedge to hepatic vein is useful for the assessment of portal vein hypertension.

Systemic ventricular dysfunction is not uncommon and may occur intrinsically (natural history of systemic RV) or secondary to other complicating features. Catheterization should include evaluation for recurrent coarctation,

anastomotic narrowing of the reconstructed aortic arch, volume overload secondary to aortopulmonary collaterals from brachiocephalic branches, or trachea-bronchial tree; in patients 40 years or older, coronary artery disease should be excluded. When evaluating arch obstruction in single-ventricle patients, typical standards for gradients do not apply because hemodynamically significant obstructions can be present despite a low gradient.

In cyanotic patients with Fontan physiology, detailed hemodynamic and angiographic assessment should be undertaken to identify and treat the following potential causes. Every effort must be made to obtain bilateral pulmonary vein saturations when evaluating for sources of cyanosis in Glenn and Fontan patients.

### Patent Fontan fenestration
Significance of right-to-left shunting can be assessed with thorough assessment of flows (Qp and Qs). Candidacy for closure can be determined with test occlusion and repeat assessment of Fontan pressures and calculation of cardiac index. One should not proceed with fenestration closure if Fontan pressures are greater than 17 mm Hg at baseline or with test occlusion or cardiac index is less than 2 L/min/m$^2$ or decreases more than 50% from baseline with test occlusion (Fig. 7).[23]

### Fontan baffle leak
Fontan baffle leak is commonly encountered in patients with lateral tunnel Fontan, where there

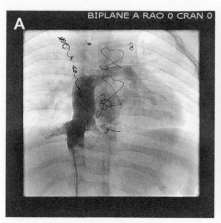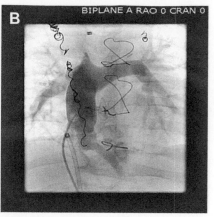

Fig. 7. (A) Angiographic appearance of a small patent Fontan fenestration in an extracardiac fenestrated Fontan patient. (B) Angiogram post–device closure of fenestration with resolution of right to left shunt.

is a leak at the suture lines with the atrial muscle resulting in right-to-left shunting and cyanosis. Calculation of Qp/Qs is performed to assess significance. Unless there is a very small leak, it is typically hard to perform test occlusion to assess candidacy of closure and/or close with standard closure devices. Covered stents are typically used to close the large lateral tunnel baffle leaks (Fig. 8).

### Venovenous collaterals
Venovenous collaterals originate from small primordial connections between the systemic veins and the pulmonary veins and develop secondary to venous hypertension and become engorged in patients with elevated Fontan pressures. These tortuous channels act as right-to-left shunts and often arise from 3 to 4 distinct locations in the Fontan pathway: left internal jugular vein and innominate vein junction, anterolateral surface of the SVC, caudal Fontan anastomosis with the hepatic veins, right innominate veins, and subclavian veins. Once identified, these collaterals should be selectively imaged to delineate the entire course of the vessel to determine candidacy for occlusion (Fig. 9).

### Pulmonary arteriovenous malformations
Lack of hepatic intrinsic factor has been associated with the development of microscopic/macroscopic pulmonary arteriovenous malformations (AVMs) in patients with classic Glenn, in older patients with long-standing bidirectional Glenn pathway, and in the few heterotaxy syndrome patients who survive to adulthood. When one encounters pulmonary vein desaturation during the hemodynamic part of the study,

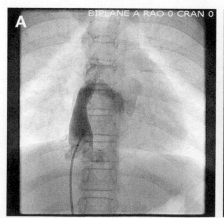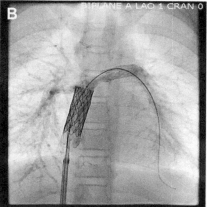

Fig. 8. (A) Angiogram demonstrating large baffle leak in a patient with a lateral tunnel Fontan. (B) Angiogram following covered stent exclusion of the baffle leak.

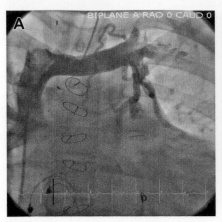
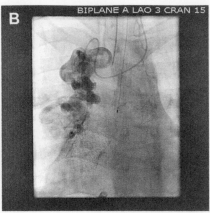

Fig. 9. Angiograms demonstrating venovenous collaterals from left innominate vein (A) and right SVC (B), which drain caudally to the pulmonary veins, resulting in cyanosis.

care must be taken to perform PA angiograms with or without the use of echocardiographic bubble study to assess for PAVMs. Patients with heterotaxy, long-standing Glenn palliation, classic Fontan, and lateral tunnel or extracardiac Fontan patients with IVC flow selectively flowing to one lung distribution are at high risk of developing significant PAVMs. This will lead to impaired gas exchange with resultant pulmonary venous desaturations in the affected lung (Fig. 10).

### Aortopulmonary collaterals

Competitive collateral blood supply to the lungs from branches of the ipsilateral brachiocephalic arteries (most commonly from the internal mammary arteries) acts as a source of left-to-right shunting, eventually causing elevated single-ventricle pathway pressures and volume overload of the single ventricle. A detailed evaluation for identification and occlusion of aortopulmonary collaterals should be undertaken in single-ventricle patients with evidence of volume

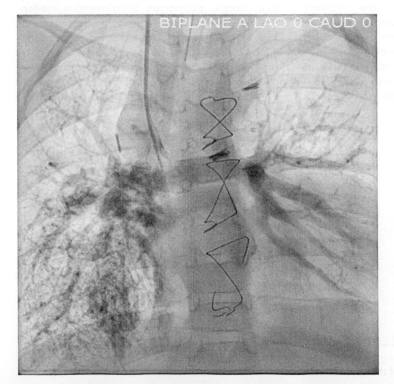

Fig. 10. Angiographic appearance of PAVMs in the right lower lobe with rapid pulmonary venous return.

overload and elevated ventricular filling pressures and/or systemic venous pathway pressures.

## SUMMARY

Adults with CHD are increasing in number. There is a growing need for physicians to help manage this complex group of patients. This is ideally performed in centers where expertise in the management of ACHD patients exists. Careful preprocedure planning with clear goals will help the interventional cardiologist provide the most complete catheterization. The role of a thorough hemodynamic assessment cannot be emphasized enough in the evaluation of patients with CHD. There is significant heterogeneity across defects and palliations; thus, careful attention to detail is required to assure complete data are obtained without omission of critical information needed for decision making. A complete understanding of intracardiac hemodynamics, including pressure relationships, flow calculations, and pitfalls associated with each component, allows the interventionalist to minimize error by limiting assumptions and gathering clear and interpretable data.

## REFERENCES

1. Gilboa SM, Devine OJ, Kucik JE, et al. Congenital heart defects in the United States: estimating the magnitude of the affected population in 2010. Circulation 2016;134:101–9.
2. Madan P, Kim YY. Training in adult congenital heart disease. J Am Coll Cardiol 2015;65(20):2254–6.
3. Warnes CA, Wiliams RG, Bashore TM, et al. ACC/AHA 2008 guidelines for the management of adults with congenital heart disease. Executive summary. A report of the American College of Cardiology/American Heart Association task force on practice guidelines (writing committee to develop guidelines for the management of adults with congenital heart disease). Circulation 2008; 118:2395–451.
4. Baumgartner H, Bonhoeffer P, De Groot NM, et al. ESC Guidelines for the management of grown-up congenital heart disease (new version 2010). The Task Force on the Management of Grown-up Congenital Heart Disease of the European Society of Cardiology (ESC). Eur Heart J 2010;31(23):2915–57.
5. Webb G, Gatzoulis MA. Atrial septal defects in the adult. Recent progress and overview. Circulation 2006;114:1645–53.
6. Shaddy RE, Webb G. Applying heart failure guidelines to adult congenital heart disease patients. Expert Rev Cardiovasc Ther 2008;6(2):165–74.
7. Feltes TF, Bacha E, Beekman RH III, et al. Indications for cardiac catheterization and intervention in pediatric cardiac disease. A scientific statement from the American Heart Association. Circulation 2011;123:2607–52.
8. Myers PO, Tissot C, Beghetti M. Assessment of operability of patients with pulmonary arterial hypertension associated with congenital heart disease. Circ J 2014;78(1):4–11.
9. Giglia TM, Humpl T. Preoperative pulmonary hemodynamics and assessment of operability: is there a pulmonary vascular resistance that precludes cardiac operation? Pediatr Crit Care Med 2010;11(2 Suppl):S57–69.
10. Masutani S, Senzaki H. Left ventricular function in adult patients with atrial septal defect: implication for development of heart failure after transcatheter closure. J Card Fail 2011;17(11):957–63.
11. Webb G, Gatzoulis MA. Congenital heart disease for the adult cardiologist. Circulation 2006;114: 1645–53.
12. Nishimura RA, Carabello BA. Hemodynamics in the cardiac catheterization laboratory of the 21st century. Circulation 2012;125:2138–50.
13. Rigby ML. Closure of a large patent ductus arteriosus in adults: first do no harm. Heart 2007;93(4): 417–8.
14. Zhang D, Zhu X, Lv B, et al. Trial occlusion to assess the risk of persistent pulmonary arterial hypertension after closure of a large patent ductus arteriosus in adolescents and adults with elevated pulmonary artery pressure. Circ Cardiovasc Interv 2014;7:473–81.
15. Ermis P, Franklin W, Venkatachalam M, et al. Left ventricular hemodynamic changes and clinical outcomes after transcatheter atrial septal defect closure in adults. Congenit Heart Dis 2014;10: E48–53.
16. Poterucha JT, Taggart NW, Johnson JN, et al. Intravascular and hybrid intraoperative stent placement for baffle obstruction in transposition of the great arteries after atrial switch. Catheter Cardiovasc Interv 2016;89(2):306–14.
17. Lee HP, Bang JH, Baek JS, et al. Aortic root translocation with artery switch for transposition of the great arteries or double outlet right ventricle with ventricular septal defect and pulmonary stenosis. Korean J Thorac Cardiovasc Surg 2016;49(3):190–4.
18. Morgan CT, Mertens L, Grotenhuis H, et al. Understanding the mechanism for branch pulmonary artery stenosis after the arterial switch operation for transposition of the great arteries. Eur Heart J Cardiovasc Imaging 2016;18(2):180–5.
19. Quarrie R, Kopf GS, Hashim S. Left main coronary artery occlusion in an asymptomatic patient: late complication after arterial switch operation. J Card Surg 2016;31(9):599–600.

20. Cheung MM, Konstantinov IE, Redington AN. Late complication of repair of tetralogy of Fallot and indications for pulmonary valve replacement. Semin Thorac Cardiovasc Surg 2005; 17(2):155–9.

21. Keane JF, Lock JE. Hemodynamic evaluation of congenital heart disease. In: Lock JE, Keane JF, Perry SB, editors. Diagnostic and interventional catheterization in congenital heart disease. 2nd edition. Norwell (MA): Kluwer Academic Publishers Group; 2000. p. 50.

22. Pollock SG. Pressure tracings in obstructive cardiomyopathy. N Engl J Med 1994;331:238.

23. Bridges ND, Mayer JE, Lock JE, et al. Effect of baffle fenestration on outcome of the modified Fontan operation. Circulation 1992;86:1762–9.

# Hemodynamics of Cardiogenic Shock

Ariel Furer, MD[a],*, Jeffrey Wessler, MD[b], Daniel Burkhoff, MD, PhD[b,c]

| KEYWORDS |
|---|
| • Cardiogenic shock • Hypoperfusion • Hemodynamic • Pressure-volume loops • Right heart catheterization |

| KEY POINTS |
|---|
| • Treatment of cardiogenic shock remains a clinical challenge. |
| • Greater understanding of the pathophysiology of cardiogenic shock from different causes and of the available treatment strategies is leading to new treatment concepts. |
| • If the left ventricular dysfunction is based on ischemia or infarction, changes in myocardial perfusion occurring at different stages of the process can play pivotal roles. |
| • It is important that clinicians appreciate and understand the physiologic meaning of these measurements and take them into account when treating patients with cardiogenic shock. |

## INTRODUCTION

Cardiogenic shock (CS) represents an advanced state of morbidity along the pathophysiologic pathway of end-organ hypoperfusion caused by reduced cardiac output (CO) and blood pressure (Table 1). Acute coronary syndromes (ACSs) remain the most common cause of CS, with an estimated 100 to 120,000 patients in the United States and Europe subsequently having CS after ACS each year.[1] The spectrum of hypoperfusion states caused by low CO ranges from pre-CS to refractory CS and can be characterized by an array of hemodynamic parameters. This review provides the foundation for a hemodynamic understanding of CS including the use of hemodynamic monitoring for diagnosis and treatment, the cardiac and vascular determinants of CS, and a hemodynamic approach to risk stratification and management of CS.

## DEFINITIONS

The spectrum of CS can be divided into pre-CS, CS, and refractory CS—whereby each state is characterized by increasing levels of tissue hypoperfusion and poorer response to treatment but have in common an underlying reduction in CO. Although several different parameters have been used to define CS, the most widely used definitions focus on hemodynamic parameters based on blood pressure and cardiac index (CI).[2] Abnormalities of central venous pressure, pulmonary capillary wedge pressure (PCWP), and systemic vascular resistance (SVR) are typically involved but not always included in CS definitions owing to variability in measurement, and serum lactate is often included to provide objective evidence of end-organ hypoperfusion. For each of these parameters, it is well recognized that there is a continuum ranging from the completely normal condition to a state of refractory CS. Current management strategies rely on this continuum, in particular by drawing attention to patients who are on the verge of significant end-organ dysfunction development in whom early intervention can be particularly effective.

In this regard, the state of pre-CS, also referred to as *nonhypotensive cardiogenic shock*, has been

Disclosures: D. Burkhoff is a consultant to Medtronic, Corvia Medical. Cardiovascular Research Foundation is recipient of an unrestricted educational grant from Abiomed.

[a] Internal Medicine T, Tel-Aviv Sourasky Medical Center, 6 Wiezmann street, Tel Aviv 64239, Israel; [b] Division of Cardiology, Columbia University, 161 Fort Washington Avenue, New York, NY 10032-3784, USA; [c] Cardiovascular Research Foundation, 1700 Broadway, New York, NY 10019, USA
* Corresponding author.
E-mail address: furera@gmail.com

**Table 1**
Definitions of pre–cardiogenic shock, cardiogenic shock, and refractory cardiogenic shock according to clinical and hemodynamic criteria and response to therapy

|  | Pre-CS (Nonhypotensive) | CS | Refractory CS |
|---|---|---|---|
| Clinical criteria | Signs of peripheral hypoperfusion: Oliguria (urine output <30 mL/h) Cold extremities Altered mental status Increased serum lactate | Signs of peripheral hypoperfusion | Signs of peripheral hypoperfusion |
| Hemodynamic criteria | SBP ≥90 mm Hg without circulatory support[3] | SBP <90 for >30 min or the need for pharmacologic or intra-aortic balloon pump support to maintain a systolic blood pressure >90 mm Hg or mean arterial pressure 30 mm Hg lower than baseline. Cardiac index <2.2 L/min/m². Elevated filling pressures of the left, right, or both ventricles | Same as CS |
| Response to treatment |  |  | Ongoing evidence of tissue hypoperfusion despite administration of adequate doses of 2 vasoactive medications and treatment of the underlying etiology.[9] |

discussed and defined as clinical evidence of peripheral hypoperfusion with systolic blood pressure (SBP) more than 90 mm Hg without vasopressor circulatory support. Compared with patients with CS, patients with pre-CS had similar CI, left ventricular ejection fraction (LVEF), and PCWP but higher SVR (1753 ± 675 vs 1389 ± 689 dyn/cm/sec$^{-5}$, $P$ = .07).[3] Notably, patients with pre-CS are often difficult to identify because of subtle signs of hypoperfusion; however, proper diagnosis can be important because of high rates of in-hospital mortality (as high as 43%).[3]

CS has been defined clinically as (1) SBP less than 90 mm Hg for greater than 30 minutes or use of vasopressors to achieve those levels; (2) evidence of pulmonary edema or elevated left ventricle (LV) filling pressures (LV end diastolic pressure or PCWP); (3) evidence of organ hypoperfusion including at least one of the following: (a) change in mental status; (b) cold, clammy skin; (c) oliguria; (d) increased serum lactate.[4,5] Finally, refractory-CS can be defined as CS unresponsive to medical or mechanical support.

The use of invasive hemodynamic measurements is important for definitive diagnosis and for characterizing the extent and site of the cardiac pathologic condition through the measurement of right-sided filling pressures, pulmonary pressures, wedge pressures, and CO.

## ETIOLOGY

A multitude of processes can lead to CS. CS can occur acutely in a patient without prior cardiac history or progressively in a patient with long-standing chronic heart failure. The most prevalent etiology of CS remains ACS (including ST-segment elevation myocardial infarction [MI] and non–ST-segment elevation acute coronary system), which accounts for nearly 80% of cases. Despite advances in treatment and revascularization, CS remains the most lethal complication of MI, with mortality rates ranging from 38% to 65% in different cohorts.[6–8] CS in ACS results most commonly from myocardial dysfunction caused by ischemia or infarct but can also be caused by mechanical complications including acute mitral regurgitation from papillary muscle rupture, ventricular septal rupture, and free wall rupture. Non-ACS causes of CS, although less frequent, can result from abnormalities or as a consequence of a primary cardiac, valvular, electrical, or pericardial abnormality[4,9] including decompensated valvular disease, acute myocarditis, left ventricular outflow obstruction in hypertrophic obstructive cardiomyopathy, cardiomyopathy, pericardial tamponade, arrhythmias, mechanical (traumatic) injury to the heart, postcardiotomy syndrome, uncontrolled arrhythmia, and progression of congenital lesions. The prevalence of these various non-ACS causes of CS has been estimated as follows: progression of chronic heart failure (11%), valvular and other mechanical causes (6%), stress-induced/Takotsubo cardiomyopathy (2%), and myocarditis (2%).[10] Among heart failure patients, CS was the presenting clinical feature of 7.7% of patients with either new-onset heart failure or decompensated chronic heart failure patients.[11]

## DIAGNOSIS AND EVALUATION OF CARDIOGENIC SHOCK PATIENTS

Although physical examination and laboratory, electrocardiographic, and echocardiographic testing remain the mainstay in the initial evaluation of a patient suspected of having CS, increasing emphasis on hemodynamic evaluation has the potential for earlier recognition and more appropriate management of CS with subsequent improvement on outcomes. The initial clinical evaluation in CS is difficult in unstable patients owing to rapidly changing hemodynamics and the frequent contribution of multiple comorbid processes.[12] Traditional signs of heart failure, including pulmonary congestion and jugular venous distention, may be misleading in a patient with right ventricular (RV) failure, pulmonary embolism, chronically compensated heart failure, arrhythmias, and mechanical complications—thus reducing the specificity of these signs to diagnose CS. Invasive hemodynamic assessment using pulmonary artery catheterization (PAC) provides an important adjunct in the diagnosis and continuous evaluation of a patient with CS. This technique allows bedside direct and indirect measurement of major determinants of cardiac performance (such as preload, afterload, and CO) supplying additional data to support clinical decision making.[13] Right heart catheterization additionally offers information regarding fluid status and right heart filling pressures, adequacy of oxygen delivery, and the

degree of pulmonary vascular resistance. These hemodynamic data in turn can guide the therapeutic choices through volume optimization, vasodilators, vasopressors, and inotropes as appropriate and the critical decision regarding whether to provide mechanical circulatory support (MCS). In fact, invasive hemodynamic measurements are often necessary for the proper selection, timing, and settings of medical and mechanical support. Finally, hemodynamic changes throughout treatment course and follow-up have shown prognostic importance.[14,15]

The use of invasive hemodynamic assessment is in decline,[16] primarily because of data from studies such as the ESCAPE trial,[17] in which an overall neutral impact of PAC-guided therapy was seen in heart failure patients compared with therapy guided by clinical evaluation alone. However, this study was limited by several potential confounders, including the possibility that the neutral results actually reflected a negation of the benefit of aggressive reduction in filling pressures by the harmful effects of therapies such as inotropes that were used based on the hemodynamic profile extracted from the use of PAC. In fact, high-volume centers in the ESCAPE trial along with patients in CS may have shown outcome benefit with PAC compared with non-PAC use. Other studies have examined the use of PAC in the treatment of ACS patients, finding associations with PAC use and increased 30-day mortality, although CS patients have shown a notable exception whereby the harmful effect of PAC was diminished.[18–20] In the retrospective SUPPORT study,[20] although higher mortality rates were observed in intensive care unit patients and related to PAC, it is difficult to determine whether these effects were not simply caused by PAC use in sicker patients compared with non-PAC use. A second study by Murdoch and colleagues[21] confirms this suspicion, as PAC insertion was not predictive of death (odds ratio, 1.08; 95% confidence interval, 0.87–1.33) after correcting for treatment bias, suggesting that higher mortality in PAC-guided patients may be owing to worse baseline condition rather than the effect of hemodynamic measurement or the invasive nature of the procedure.

The debate about the necessity of PAC use is further fueled by findings from studies examining physician ability to predict hemodynamic findings without the use of PAC compared with invasive measures that showed only half of the estimations were correct.[22] Additionally, in a reported series of patients treated for circulatory shock, 63% of cases underwent a change in treatment plan after insertion of PAC.[23] No study yet has used PAC-derived variables to drive treatment protocols to determine whether invasive hemodynamic-guided data result in better outcomes than do data derived from noninvasive methods such as echocardiography.[24] Although noninvasive measurements are commonly used to gain proxy information regarding hemodynamic changes in critically ill patients, in the setting of CS, these measures are hampered by lack of accuracy and may not identify dynamic changes that can only be assessed invasively.[25]

Filling pressures are a necessary but often overlooked component of PAC measurements. In a recent analysis of the ESCAPE trial of patients treated for acute decompensated heart failure, last recorded CI was not associated with clinical outcomes, whereas PCWP was associated with long-term morbidity and mortality. These findings argue further that treatment goals should focus not only on improving cardiac function but also hemodynamic assessment and reduction of filling pressures, which can only reliably be achieved through invasive measurement.[26] This finding has been substantiated by recent literature from patients with mechanical circulatory support (MCS) arguing that direct hemodynamic evaluation of patients with left ventricular assist devices is required for optimization and determination of ventricular-vascular device interactions.[27]

Invasive hemodynamic measurement is not without risk—including complications, inaccuracies, and interpretation ambiguity. Complications include insertion site hematoma, arterial puncture, arrhythmias, infections, pulmonary infarction, pulmonary hemorrhage, and pulmonary artery puncture.[24] Inaccuracies in measurement include temporal, positional, and volumetric variation, and interpretation can be different according to patient characteristics and overall clinical contextualization as well as conflicting measurements.[28] Each of these limitations is heavily influenced by the experience level of the operating physician. With PAC insertion done by junior physicians along with the decline in overall volume of PAC procedures, it is expected that higher rates of complications and misinterpretation may occur.[29]

## PATHOPHYSIOLOGY AND HEMODYNAMICS

CS shock stemming from myocardial ischemia and infarction provides a useful model to illustrate the pathophysiologic and hemodynamic effects of CS. Beginning with an incident MI of sufficient size to significantly reduce ventricular chamber contractility, the cascade of events that culminates in CS starts with initial decline of CO and subsequent increase of left and RV diastolic pressures that eventually leads to further decline of coronary perfusion and a resulting cycle of myocardial impairment. End-organ damage develops with pulmonary congestion, tissue hypoxia, and further myocardial ischemia.

Several compensatory mechanisms are activated in response to these hemodynamic changes, including increased sympathetic tone (yielding both positive inotropic and chronotropic effects), activation of the renin angiotensin aldosterone system (yielding increases in preload as a result of fluid retention and afterload as a result of vasoconstriction), and subsequent activation by the natriuretic peptide system that responds to myocardial stretch and attempts to counteract the renin angiotensin aldosterone system through natriuresis, diuresis, and vasodilation.

It can be difficult to clearly ascertain whether certain changes are beneficial or detrimental. One such example is afterload reduction with decreased arterial blood pressure, whereby the unloading of the ventricle has a protective effect while coronary perfusion declines even further, worsening myocardial ischemia and necrosis.[5] Similarly, the increased sympathetic tone and the release of catecholamines is essential to maintain adequate CO by increasing contractility, but at the same time this increases myocardial oxygen consumption and puts the patient at higher risk of arrhythmias and additional myocardial necrosis.

The following provides a useful model for a hemodynamic understanding of CS by examining the cardiac and vascular determinants of CS.

### Decreased Contractility

Although impaired contractility is a primary driver of CS owing to ischemia, impaired contractility does not necessarily mean the patient will have CS after an acute ischemic event. Rather, it is the degree of cardiovascular adaptability both before the event and immediately afterward that will determine the hemodynamic outcome and whether the patient will subsequently have CS. Moreover, LVEF is probably not sensitive enough to express the degree of cardiac impairment observed in CS. This finding shown in the SHOCK trial whereby LVEF of CS patients was approximately 30%, and nearly one-quarter of patients had LVEF greater than 40%, a proportion similar to that reported in other MI trials that included reduced LVEF patients without evidence of CS.[30] Additionally, patients who recovered and had improvement in their functional status showed no change in their LVEF compared with values recorded during the acute phase of CS.[5] Several groups have reported that nearly half of CS nonsurvivors died with a normal CI[31]; despite this, among CS patients, LVEF was found to be a reliable predictor of mortality.[30] Lastly, because CS is a proinflammatory state that has important effects on preload and afterload, the correlation between contractility and CO may be particularly variable in the CS population.[32]

For purposes of illustrating and understanding the pathophysiology of CS, pressure-volume (PV) analysis can be particularly helpful. Fig. 1A depicts the PV loop of a normal person;

the loop is contained within the boundaries of the end-systolic and end-diastolic pressure volume relationships (ESPVR and EDPVR, respectively). With the incident MI, the ESPVR shifts downward and rightward, signifying the abrupt reduction of ventricular contractility (**Fig. 1**B). This reduction is accompanied by immediate and profound reductions in blood pressure (indexed by the height of the PV loop), stroke volume (SV, indexed by the width of the PV loop) and cardiac output (the product of SV and heart rate). Mild elevations of LV end-diastolic pressure and PCWP may also be seen.

## Autonomic Response to Decreased Contractility

Decreases in blood pressure are sensed by the baroreceptors, which activate efferent autonomic nerve fiber firing to heart and vascular structures and activate adrenal release of epinephrine. These factors act to increase

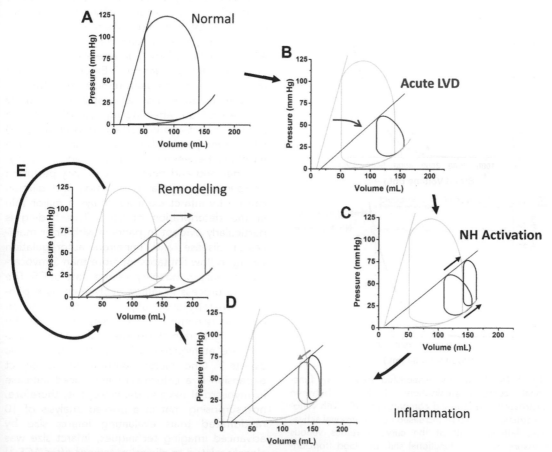

**Fig. 1.** The pathophysiology of CS illustrated by use of PV loops. (A) Normal state. (B) PV loop shows changes after acute MI (*red*); (C) PV loop shows changes caused by autonomic response to decreased contractility (*blue*); (D) PV loop shows changes caused by release of inflammatory mediators (*green*); (E) PV loop shows manifestation of cardiac remodeling (*pink*) with changes in both ESPVR and EDPVR relationship. See text for further details. LVD, left ventricular dysfunction; NH, neurohormonal.

heart rate (CO), attempt to increase cardiac contractility, and cause systemic vasoconstriction, which increases SVR and induces venoconstriction. Venoconstriction plays a critical role in the pathophysiology of CS[33] and results in a leftward shift of the venous pressure-volume curve, which functionally shifts blood from an unstressed to a stressed compartment (Fig. 2), thus increasing functional circulating blood volume and causing elevations of central venous and pulmonary venous pressures. In aggregate, these effects cause further rightward shifts of the PV loop, increases in blood pressure, and inconsequential effects on cardiac output (increased heart rate tending to increase CO and increased SVR tending to decrease CO) as illustrated in Fig. 1C.

## Inflammatory Response

An essential consequence of CS, with or without primary myocardial injury is the accompanying

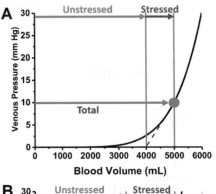

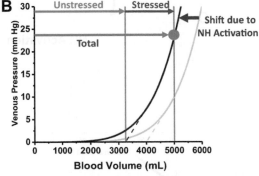

Fig. 2. (A) Venous PV relationship (blue) shows functional compartmentalization of blood between unstressed and stressed compartment. (B) With venoconstriction caused by increased neurohormonal activation, leftward shift of the curve increases venous pressure owing to functional shift of blood from unstressed to stressed blood volume despite constant total blood volume. Because of the steepness of the curve, relatively small shifts can cause large increases of venous pressure. Further discussion in Burkhoff and Tyberg.[33] NH, neurohormonal.

inflammatory process, which manifests in release of several inflammatory mediators. From a hemodynamic standpoint this inflammation causes pronounced nitric oxide mediated vasodilation. This has been seen in CS patients initially considered due to impaired myocardial function that have prominent declines in SVR.[1,9] Among the explanations for this observation are (1) the pronounced cytokine-mediated response seen in CS after acute MI,[34,35] (2) sepsis or bacteremia (eg, gut bacterial transmigration),[36] and (3) oxygen free radicals buildup and amplified nitric oxide synthesis as part of ischemia-reperfusion syndrome.[35,37] Regardless of the mechanism, these inflammatory mediators counteract certain aspects of the neurohormones, resulting in reduction in SVR and the potential for venodilation, both of which can decrease blood pressure (Fig. 1D).

## Remodeling

Persistent neurohormonal activation and elevated filling pressures drive the process of remodeling,[38] characterized by progressive increases in LV size and reductions in function. Furthermore, in the setting of infarction, remodeling is mediated by 2 interrelated processes: extension and expansion.[35] Extension involves areas of the myocardium remote from the primary infarct zone and was explained previously by the CS state affecting myocardial perfusion by (1) infarct-related artery re-occlusion, (2) intracoronary thrombus propagation, or (3) a mismatch between the elevated myocardial oxygen demand and decline in coronary perfusion pressures. Ventricular dysfunction and dilation caused by infarct extension plays a major role in the deterioration of CS.[39] This finding is particularly evident in patients with prior multivessel disease and impaired autoregulation owing to flow limitation in more than 1 myocardial territory in the low pressure state of CS. The second process in infarct evolvement is expansion, whereby areas adjacent to the infarction become ischemic. This process occurs as the cells neighboring the border zone of an infarction are at higher risk for additional ischemic events.[40] One factor contributing to infarct expansion is a catecholamine-induced increase in myocardial oxygen demand. It is, therefore, not surprising that in a pooled analysis of 10 randomized trials evaluating infarct size by advanced imaging techniques, infarct size was closely related to clinical outcomes after ACS.[41]

Infarct extension, expansion, and, more generally, remodeling, manifest on the pressure-volume diagram as rightward shifts of both the ESPVR and the EDPVR and reflect in the global changes in LV size, structure, and function characteristic of chronic heart failure (Fig. 1E).

## Right Ventricular Failure Involvement in Cardiogenic Shock

The RV has several unique characteristics compared with the LV that are important in understanding the pathway by which RV failure can cause CS on its own or contribute to CS during primary LV dysfunction. First, compared with the LV, the RV differs substantially in terms of size, structure, metabolism, and afterload. Second, the RV has remarkable recovery abilities after RV infarct. Involvement of the RV in CS is less common compared with LV involvement (~5% vs ~95%, respectively, in the SHOCK trial),[42] yet patients with CS caused by RV failure have mortality rates similar to those in patients with CS caused by LV failure. Furthermore, patients with CS caused by involvement of both LV and RV have worse outcomes than patients with LV involvement alone.

Most patients with isolated RV failure have suffered inferior or posterior MI and present with CS earlier (>3 hours earlier) compared with LV-failure patients.[42] This finding emphasizes the fact that the RV is prone to rapid decline in function because of its formation and thin walls, and indeed a short time span is needed for transition from stable conditions to development of right heart failure.[43,44] Elevated right atrial pressures with similar LV filling pressures, CO and CI, are found in patients with RV CS. Finally, because the septal wall is responsible for an important part of the contractile force generated by the RV,[45] septal ischemia involvement of LV infarction can have a marked impact on RV function because of RV-LV interactions.[46]

Fortunately, several studies found an impressive recovery of RV function in survivors of CS caused mainly by RV dysfunction.[47,48] This observation underscores the importance of early recognition of RV failure as a cause of CS and the need for treatment aimed at prompt relief of RV ischemia. Notably, there are some early promising results seen with the use of temporary mechanical unloading with percutaneous RV assist devices[47] allowing patients to bridge through the period of RV failure.

## MECHANICAL COMPLICATIONS OF ACUTE MYOCARDIAL INFARCT PRESENTING AS CARDIOGENIC SHOCK

In patients with CS after acute MI (AMI; especially first or nonanterior MI) a high index of suspicion should be kept for mechanical complications as the source of CS rather than LV dysfunction.[9] Mechanical complications include ventricular septal rupture, contained free wall rupture, and papillary muscle rupture. In most of such cases, rapid echocardiographic evaluation will reveal the mechanism of CS, and because prognosis is dismal in mechanical CS, urgent intervention (usually surgical) should be delivered promptly.[49]

## RISK STRATIFICATION AND PROGNOSIS

The prognosis of CS remains poor despite advances in treatment options and improved understanding of the pathophysiologic mechanisms. Risk stratification models in CS, in principle, allow for early identification and direction of aggressive treatment of those at highest risk. Age, SBP, heart rate, and presenting Killip class were found to be predictive of adverse outcomes in the GUSTO I and III trials.[50,51] In the PURSUIT cohort, presenting ST depressions, height, and rales on physical examination showed additional prognostic value; however, positive predictive values remained less than 50%.[51] In the TRIUMPH study, which included vasopressor-dependent CS patients after revascularization, only SBP and creatinine clearance were found to be predictive of mortality (variables that have since been validated in the SHOCK-II trial[52]).

A severity score system derived from the SHOCK trial and registry included 2 models for prediction of in-hospital mortality, the first accounting for clinical variables and the second based on invasive hemodynamic data. Both models included age, end-organ hypoperfusion, and anoxic brain damage; the clinical model also included shock on admission, SBP, prior coronary artery bypass grafting, noninferior myocardial infarction, creatinine of ≥1.9 mg/dL, and the hemodynamic model added stroke work and LVEF less than 28%. The CardShock risk score incorporated common clinical variables for prediction of in-hospital mortality and found the following predictors: ACS as the etiology for CS, age, prior MI, prior coronary artery bypass grafting, confusion, reduced LVEF, and elevated serum lactate level. In a comparison with the SHOCK risk model the authors were able to show superiority in terms of c-statistics for prediction in both the CardShock cohort and in the IABP-SHOCK II cohort.[10]

Finally, cardiac power index may be useful not only as a means of estimating cardiac contractile reserve[14,15] but also as a strong predictor of mortality in AMI CS.[15] Low initial cardiac power index is considered a predictor of unfavorable outcomes in CS patients (0.6 W/m² in nonsurvivors vs 0.74 in survivors). This index accounts for the fact that in many CS patients, merely improving CO will not promote recovery from shock, as the inflammation-mediated decline of SVR remains prominent. The increase in mean arterial pressure in addition to improved CO serves as evidence of improvement of both the contractility component and recovery of SVR, and might be a useful tool to assess patients' prognosis and responsiveness to vasopressors.

## MANAGEMENT OF CARDIOGENIC SHOCK

The initial evaluation of patients presenting with CS should trigger an attempt to address all reversible causes according to the suspected etiology of the condition. For the rarer etiologies of CS other than ischemia, immediate intervention is necessary, as with pericardial tamponade or free wall rupture.[9] As for most CS patients, management of CS resulting from AMI includes the use of drugs such as inotropes and vasopressors, fluid management, and early revascularization. The introduction of early revascularization over the last decades has resulted in a decline in mortality compared with the pre-revascularization era.[9,53,54] Despite the sharp increase of percutaneous coronary intervention rates in CS patients and guideline recommendations for early revascularization in CS,[53,55] percutaneous coronary intervention rates remain underutilized, with only 50% to 70% of eligible patients receiving intervention.[4,56]

However, as summarized in **Fig. 3** reproduced from Thiele and colleagues,[4] commonly used

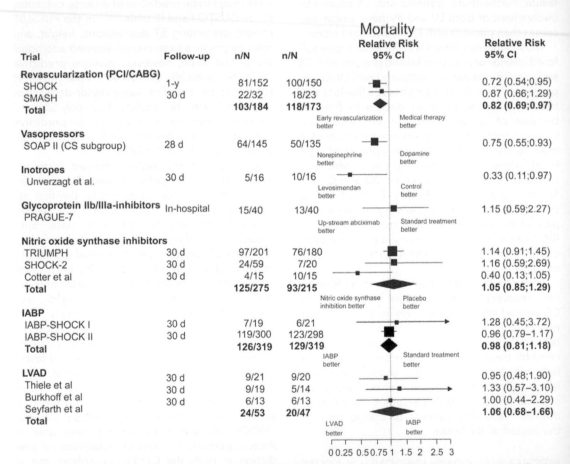

Fig. 3. Summary for the evidence from randomized, controlled trials studying different treatment modalities in cardiogenic shock patients. CABG, coronary artery bypass grafting; CI, confidence interval; IABP, intra-aortic balloon pump; IABP-SHOCK, intra-aortic balloon pump in shock; LVAD, left-ventricular assist device; PCI, percutaneous coronary intervention; SHOCK, SHould we emergently revascularize occluded coronaries for cardiogenic shocK; SMASH, Swiss multicenter trial of angioplasty for SHock; SOAP II, sepsis occurrence in acutely ill patients II; TRIUMPH, tilarginine acetate injection in a randomized international study in unstable MI patients with cardiogenic shock. (From Thiele H, Ohman EM, Desch S, et al. Management of cardiogenic shock. Eur Heart J 2015;36(20):1223–30; with permission.)

approaches have not shown benefit. Accordingly, guidelines for the management of CS are based on expert opinion.[57] As a result, practice varies significantly from institution to institution and even among physicians in the same institution.

Despite these advances in therapy, however, mortality rates of patients with refractory CS remain unacceptably high.[9] Major efforts are devoted in recent years toward introduction of new approaches, trying to (1) prevent the evolvement of massive cardiac injury after MI with intravenous β-blockers,[58] intramyocardial delivery of miR-29a,[59] intracoronary supersaturated oxygen,[60] and pressure-controlled intermittent coronary sinus occlusion[61] among many other approaches and (2) allowing better treatment once CS is present—as in the development of acute mechanical circulatory support (AMCS) devices.[62] Although these minimally invasive devices have the potential to transform the management and prognosis of many types of CS, ongoing studies are aimed at proving their hemodynamic effectiveness and impact on clinical outcomes. Effective use of AMCS

strategies can be done as a bridge to decision, recovery, long-term support devices (such as ventricular assist devices or total artificial hearts), or heart transplantation.[63] Historically, intra-aortic balloon pump was the only device of this class but failed to show significant mortality benefit in the large IABP-SHOCK II trial.[8] Different new generation devices are now in use, in which some are aimed at assisting the function of the LV, whereas others are designed to assist in cases of RV failure. The mechanism of action of each differs substantially, and a comprehensive understanding of the hemodynamics before its insertion and obviously once in use is warranted. A thorough review of this issue was published recently and may help in the consideration of the pros and cons of each device in different clinical scenarios (**Fig. 4**).[64]

Several key concepts to the management of CS and AMCS should be considered. First, survival of CS patients is time dependent. The introduction of the concept of "time to unload," rather than just "time to balloon," accentuates the need to act quickly and use AMCS earlier than is commonly practiced in the current

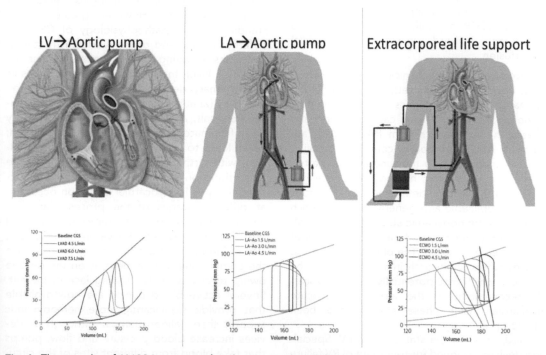

**Fig. 4.** Three modes of AMCS (*upper panel*) and corresponding PV loops (*lower panel*) in a cardiogenic shock state with progressively increasing rates of device flow. Although each mode can improve blood pressure and total blood flow, each mode has a different effect on LV because of the different sites from which blood is withdrawn. CGS, cardiogenic shock; LVAD, left ventricular assist device. (*From* Burkhoff D, Sayer G, Doshi D, et al. Hemodynamics of mechanical circulatory support. J Am Coll Cardiol 2015;66(23):2663–75; with permission.)

setting.[65] In fact, reserving the use of AMCS for patients already being treated with 2 or more inotropes might actually be too late, at a stage at which they already suffer irreversible organ dysfunction and metabolic derangements. Instead, using AMCS devices supplementary to aggressive fluid management and early revascularization could improve survival and allow for myocardial recovery, as the cardiac function is replaced by the device at a critical timing of myocardial ischemia, thereby interfering with the vicious cycle of myocardial deterioration.

Current understanding suggests that 3 aspects of treatment should be addressed to potentially improve chances of survival.[65]

1. Circulatory support—to treat tissue hypoperfusion and avoid accumulation of lactic acid and other metabolic products of anaerobic metabolism.
2. Ventricular unloading—normalizing (or even minimizing as much as possible) filling pressures, in addition to improving CO, has the potential to minimize the remodeling process and favorably impact prognosis; therefore, using and adjusting devices by their effect on PCWP or central venous pressure might be beneficial.
3. Myocardial perfusion—revascularization is essential, and allowing for higher DBP and lower LVEDP may shift the coronary pressure gradient toward increased myocardial perfusion.

Second, when a mechanical support device is used, optimization of its settings can be guided by change in hemodynamics and based on data gathered from right heart catheterization and invasive hemodynamics from PAC.[64] With advances in AMCS technology come an increasing role for understanding the fundamental pathophysiology underlying hemodynamic changes and using these to guide intervention. PV loops offer an applicable and generalizable approach to compare hemodynamic status before and after an intervention. Fig. 4 depicts 3 modes of AMCS used in practice. The physiology of these devices differs significantly in how they affect the ventricle, which may potentially impact myocardial recoverability in the setting of an acute myocardial insult; these effects have been detailed previously.[64]

Third, consider the status of the RV. Specialized devices designed for treatment of RV failure might be valuable in cases of isolated RV failure or combined with LV support in complex cases of biventricular failure.[47,66,67] The understanding of the interdependence between the 2 sides of the heart is crucial in many cases, and early identification and treatment of RV failure may help improve survival in many cases.

Finally, as new treatment algorithms in CS are developed that account for early intervention with AMCS,[65] future research is necessary to clarify safety and effectiveness. However, it must be recognized that appropriately powered randomized clinical trials of AMCS in CS are extremely difficult to conduct, in large part because of the need for informed consent in an urgent setting. Accordingly, we have advocated the conduct of smaller, well-conducted studies documenting the safety and effects on key physiologic parameters, including hemodynamics, LV function, and metabolic factors (eg, lactate).[68] Despite recognition that such parameters do not always correlate with clinical outcomes like mortality and progression to heart failure, it is clear that fundamental differences in hemodynamic effects of the different available devices are not fully appreciated in the clinical setting; such understanding has the potential to affect at least short-term clinical outcomes.

## SUMMARY

Treatment of CS remains a clinical challenge. Despite advances in technologies, there is a high mortality rate. However, greater understanding of the pathophysiology of CS from different causes and of the available treatment strategies is leading to new treatment concepts. At a high level, the pathophysiology consists of (1) a primary decrease in LV contractility; followed by (2) autonomic activation with vasoconstriction, salt, and water retention; followed by (3) inflammatory response with vasodilation; which leads to (4) progressive remodeling (dilation) with further worsening LV function. If the LV dysfunction is based on ischemia or infarction, changes in myocardial perfusion occurring at different stages of the process can play pivotal roles. No medical therapy has yet proved effective in improving survival in heart failure. Use of intra-aortic balloon therapy for CS, once the cornerstone of treatment, is on the decline owing to clinical trials showing lack of benefit. Several active blood pumps are now available that provide significantly more hemodynamic support than balloon pumps. Although all devices increase blood pressure and flow, pumps that take blood from different sites of the circulation (venous system, left atrium, LV) have different effects on pulmonary pressures and ventricular loading conditions. Furthermore, the responses to any one of these devices vary among patients because of differences in intrinsic RV and LV contractile reserves, pulmonary and systemic vascular properties, background medical therapies, and functionality of the baroreceptors. These factors can in part be quantified through the appropriate use of PAC, which has been inappropriately declined; prior studies showing no benefit of hemodynamic monitoring do not apply to CS, especially when mechanical circulatory support devices are being used. Furthermore, it is important that clinicians appreciate and understand the physiologic meaning of these measurements and take them into account when treating patients who have CS.

## REFERENCES

1. Thiele H, Allam B, Chatellier G, et al. Shock in acute myocardial infarction: the cape horn for trials? Eur Heart J 2010;31(15):1828–35.
2. Hasdai D. Cardiogenic shock, in cardiogenic shock. Springer; 2002. p. 3–6.
3. Menon V, Slater JN, White HD, et al. Acute myocardial infarction complicated by systemic hypoperfusion without hypotension: report of the SHOCK trial registry. Am J Med 2000;108(5):374–80.
4. Thiele H, Ohman EM, Desch S, et al. Management of cardiogenic shock. Eur Heart J 2015;36(20):1223–30.
5. Reynolds HR, Hochman JS. Cardiogenic shock current concepts and improving outcomes. Circulation 2008;117(5):686–97.
6. Goldberg RJ, Spencer FA, Gore JM, et al. Thirty-year trends (1975 to 2005) in the magnitude of, management of, and hospital death rates associated with cardiogenic shock in patients with acute myocardial infarction a population-based perspective. Circulation 2009;119(9):1211–9.
7. De Luca G, Parodi G, Sciagrà R, et al. Preprocedural TIMI flow and infarct size in STEMI undergoing primary angioplasty. J Thromb Thrombolysis 2014;38(1):81–6.
8. Thiele H, Zeymer U, Neumann FJ, et al. Intraaortic balloon support for myocardial infarction with cardiogenic shock. N Engl J Med 2012;367(14):1287–96.
9. Reyentovich A, Barghash MH, Hochman JS. Management of refractory cardiogenic shock. Nat Rev Cardiol 2016;13(8):481–92.
10. Harjola VP, Lassus J, Sionis A, et al. Clinical picture and risk prediction of short-term mortality in cardiogenic shock. Eur J Heart Fail 2015;17(5):501–9.
11. Tavazzi L, Maggioni AP, Lucci D, et al. Nationwide survey on acute heart failure in cardiology ward services in Italy. Eur Heart J 2006;27(10):1207–15.
12. Connors AF Jr, McCaffree DR, Gray BA. Evaluation of right-heart catheterization in the critically ill patient without acute myocardial infarction. N Engl J Med 1983;308(5):263–7.
13. Gorlin R. Practical cardiac hemodynamics. N Engl J Med 1977;296(4):203–5.
14. Fincke R, Hochman JS, Lowe AM, et al. Cardiac power is the strongest hemodynamic correlate of mortality in cardiogenic shock: a report from the SHOCK trial registry. J Am Coll Cardiol 2004;44(2):340–8.
15. Popovic B, Fay R, Cravoisy-Popovic A, et al. Cardiac power index, mean arterial pressure, and simplified acute physiology score II are strong predictors of survival and response to revascularization in cardiogenic shock. Shock 2014;42(1):22–6.
16. Wiener R, Welch H. TRends in the use of the pulmonary artery catheter in the United States, 1993-2004. JAMA 2007;298(4):423–9.
17. Binanay C, Califf RM, Hasselblad V, et al. Evaluation study of congestive heart failure and pulmonary artery catheterization effectiveness: the ESCAPE trial. JAMA 2005;294(13):1625–33.
18. Cohen MG, Kelly RV, Kong DF, et al. Pulmonary artery catheterization in acute coronary syndromes: insights from the GUSTO IIb and GUSTO III trials. Am J Med 2005;118(5):482–8.
19. Zion MM, Balkin J, Rosenmann D, et al. Use of pulmonary artery catheters in patients with acute myocardial infarction. Analysis of experience in 5,841 patients in the SPRINT registry. SPRINT study group. Chest 1990;98(6):1331–5.
20. Connors AF, Speroff T, Dawson NV, et al. The effectiveness of right heart catheterization in the initial care of critically III patients. JAMA 1996;276(11):889–97.
21. Murdoch SD, Cohen AT, Bellamy MC. Pulmonary artery catheterization and mortality in critically ill patients. Br J Anaesth 2000;85(4):611–5.
22. Staudinger T, Locker GJ, Laczika K, et al. Diagnostic validity of pulmonary artery catheterization for residents at an intensive care unit. J Trauma 1998;44(5):902–6.
23. Mimoz O, Rauss A, Rekik N, et al. Pulmonary artery catheterization in critically ill patients: a prospective analysis of outcome changes associated with catheter-prompted changes in therapy. Crit Care Med 1994;22(4):573–9.
24. Hadian M, Pinsky MR. Evidence-based review of the use of the pulmonary artery catheter: impact data and complications. Crit Care 2006;10(Suppl 3):S8.
25. Suess EM, Pinsky MR. Hemodynamic monitoring for the evaluation and treatment of shock: what is the current state of the art? Semin Respir Crit Care Med 2015;36(6):890–8.

26. Cooper LB, Mentz RJ, Stevens SR, et al. Hemodynamic predictors of heart failure morbidity and mortality: fluid or flow? J Card Fail 2016;22(3):182–9.

27. Uriel N, Sayer G, Addetia K, et al. Hemodynamic ramp tests in patients with left ventricular assist devices. JACC Heart Fail 2016;4(3):208–17.

28. Gnaegi A, Feihl F, Perret C. Intensive care physicians' insufficient knowledge of right-heart catheterization at the bedside: time to act? Crit Care Med 1997;25(2):213–20.

29. Harvey S, Harrison DA, Singer M, et al. Assessment of the clinical effectiveness of pulmonary artery catheters in management of patients in intensive care (PAC-Man): a randomised controlled trial. Lancet 2005;366(9484):472–7.

30. Picard MH, Davidoff R, Sleeper LA, et al. Echocardiographic predictors of survival and response to early revascularization in cardiogenic shock. Circulation 2003;107(2):279–84.

31. Lim N, Dubois MJ, De Backer D, et al. Do all nonsurvivors of cardiogenic shock die with a low cardiac index? Chest 2003;124(5):1885–91.

32. Robotham JL, Takata M, Berman M, et al. Ejection fraction revisited. Anesthesiology 1991;74(1):172–83.

33. Burkhoff D, Tyberg JV. Why does pulmonary venous pressure rise after onset of LV dysfunction: a theoretical analysis. Am J Physiol 1993;265(5):H1819–28.

34. Shpektor A. Cardiogenic shock: the role of inflammation. Acute Card Care 2010;12(4):115–8.

35. Gowda RM, Fox JT, Khan IA. Cardiogenic shock: basics and clinical considerations. Int J Cardiol 2008;123(3):221–8.

36. Kohsaka S, Menon V, Iwata K, et al. Microbiological profile of septic complication in patients with cardiogenic shock following acute myocardial infarction (from the SHOCK study). Am J Cardiol 2007;99(6):802–4.

37. Esposito E, Cuzzocrea S. Role of nitroso radicals as drug targets in circulatory shock. Br J Pharmacol 2009;157(4):494–508.

38. Pfeffer MA, Pfeffer JM, Fishbein MC, et al. Myocardial infarct size and ventricular function in rats. Circ Res 1979;44(4):503–12.

39. Widimsky P, Gregor P, Cervenka V, et al. Severe diffuse hypokinesis of the remote myocardium–the main cause of cardiogenic shock? An echocardiographic study of 75 patients with extremely large myocardial infarctions. Cor Vasa 1988;30(1):27–34.

40. Olivetti G, Quaini F, Sala R, et al. Acute myocardial infarction in humans is associated with activation of programmed myocyte cell death in the surviving portion of the heart. J Mol Cell Cardiol 1996;28(9):2005–16.

41. Stone GW, Selker HP, Thiele H, et al. Relationship between infarct size and outcomes following primary PCI: patient-level analysis from 10 randomized trials. J Am Coll Cardiol 2016;67(14):1674–83.

42. Jacobs AK, Leopold JA, Bates E, et al. Cardiogenic shock caused by right ventricular infarction: a report from the SHOCK registry. J Am Coll Cardiol 2003;41(8):1273–9.

43. Gayat E, Mebazaa A. Normal physiology and pathophysiology of the right ventricle. In: Mebazaa A, et al, editors. Acute heart failure. London: Springer London; 2008. p. 63–9.

44. Lee FA. Hemodynamics of the right ventricle in normal and disease states. Cardiol Clin 1992;10(1):59–67.

45. Goldstein JA, Tweddell JS, Barzilai B, et al. Importance of left ventricular function and systolic ventricular interaction to right ventricular performance during acute right heart ischemia. J Am Coll Cardiol 1992;19(3):704–11.

46. Ratliff NB, Hackel DB. Combined right and left ventricular infarction: pathogenesis and clinicopathologic correlations. Am J Cardiol 1980;45(2):217–21.

47. Anderson MB, Goldstein J, Milano C, et al. Benefits of a novel percutaneous ventricular assist device for right heart failure: the prospective RECOVER RIGHT study of the Impella RP device. J Heart Lung Transplant 2015;34(12):1549–60.

48. Dell'Italia LJ, Lembo NJ, Starling MR, et al. Hemodynamically important right ventricular infarction: follow-up evaluation of right ventricular systolic function at rest and during exercise with radionuclide ventriculography and respiratory gas exchange. Circulation 1987;75(5):996–1003.

49. Menon V, Webb JG, Hillis LD, et al. Outcome and profile of ventricular septal rupture with cardiogenic shock after myocardial infarction: a report from the SHOCK trial registry. J Am Coll Cardiol 2000;36(3 Suppl A):1110–6.

50. Hasdai D, Califf RM, Thompson TD, et al. Predictors of cardiogenic shock after thrombolytic therapy for acute myocardial infarction. J Am Coll Cardiol 2000;35(1):136–43.

51. Hasdai D, Topol EJ, Califf RM, et al. Cardiogenic shock complicating acute coronary syndromes. Lancet 2000;356(9231):749–56.

52. Katz JN, Stebbins AL, Alexander JH, et al. Predictors of 30-day mortality in patients with refractory cardiogenic shock following acute myocardial infarction despite a patent infarct artery. Am Heart J 2009;158(4):680–7.

53. De Luca L, Olivari Z, Farina A, et al. Temporal trends in the epidemiology, management, and outcome of patients with cardiogenic shock complicating acute coronary syndromes. Eur J Heart Fail 2015;17(11):1124–32.

54. Hochman JS, Sleeper LA, Webb JG, et al. Early revascularization and long-term survival in cardiogenic shock complicating acute myocardial infarction. JAMA 2006;295(21):2511–5.

55. Wayangankar SA, Bangalore S, McCoy LA, et al. Temporal trends and outcomes of patients undergoing percutaneous coronary interventions for cardiogenic shock in the setting of acute myocardial infarction: a report from the CathPCI registry. JACC Cardiovasc Interv 2016;9(4):341–51.

56. Jeger RV, Radovanovic D, Hunziker PR, et al. Ten-year trends in the incidence and treatment of cardiogenic shock. Ann Intern Med 2008;149(9):618–26.

57. Ponikowski P, Voors AA, Anker SD, et al. 2016 ESC guidelines for the diagnosis and treatment of acute and chronic heart failure. Eur J Heart Fail 2016; 18(8):891–975.

58. Pizarro G, Fernández-Friera L, Fuster V, et al. Long-term benefit of early pre-reperfusion metoprolol administration in patients with acute myocardial infarction: results from the METOCARD-CNIC trial (effect of metoprolol in cardioprotection during an acute myocardial infarction). J Am Coll Cardiol 2014;63(22):2356–62.

59. Ma Z, et al. Intramyocardial delivery of miR-29a improves cardiac function and prevents pathological remodelling following myocardial infarction. Heart Lung Circ 2016;25:S79.

60. Hanson ID, David SW, Dixon SR, et al. "Optimized" delivery of intracoronary supersaturated oxygen in acute anterior myocardial infarction: a feasibility and safety study. Catheter Cardiovasc Interv 2015; 86(Suppl 1):S51–7.

61. Egred M, et al. TCT-164 pressure-controlled intermittent coronary sinus occlusion reduces infarct size and results in functional recovery after STEMI; interim analysis of an ongoing trial. J Am Coll Cardiol 2016;68(18_S):B67.

62. Morine KJ, Kapur NK. Percutaneous mechanical circulatory support for cardiogenic shock. Curr Treat Options Cardiovasc Med 2016;18(1):1–14.

63. Shekar K, Gregory SD, Fraser JF. Mechanical circulatory support in the new era: an overview. Crit Care 2016;20:66.

64. Burkhoff D, Sayer G, Doshi D, et al. Hemodynamics of mechanical circulatory support. J Am Coll Cardiol 2015;66(23):2663–74.

65. Kapur NK, Esposito ML. Door to unload: a new paradigm for the management of cardiogenic shock. Curr Cardiovasc Risk Rep 2016;10(12):41.

66. Goldstein JA, Kern MJ. Percutaneous mechanical support for the failing right heart. Cardiol Clin 2012;30(2):303–10.

67. Cheung AW, White CW, Davis MK, et al. Short-term mechanical circulatory support for recovery from acute right ventricular failure: clinical outcomes. J Heart Lung Transpl 2014;33(8):794–9.

68. Burkhoff D. Device therapy: where next in cardiogenic shock owing to myocardial infarction? Nat Rev Cardiol 2015;12(7):383–4.

# SECTION II - Interventional Treatments to Improve/Reverse Heart Failure

# Transcatheter Aortic Valve Replacement and MitraClip to Reverse Heart Failure

 CrossMark

Sukhdeep Basra, MD, MPH, Molly Szerlip, MD, FSCAI*

## KEYWORDS

- Transcatheter aortic valve replacement • MitraClip • Heart failure • LV dysfunction • Outcomes

## KEY POINTS

- Transcatheter aortic valve replacement is safe and effective in severe heart failure and is associated with similar improvement in left ventricular ejection fraction (LVEF) as surgical aortic valve replacement.
- Baseline LVEF, mean gradient, and low flow are associated with improvement in LVEF and long-term outcomes in patients with severe heart failure.
- MitraClip implantation is safe and cost effective in patients with moderate to severe mitral regurgitation with severe heart failure.
- MitraClip is associated with reduction in mitral regurgitation and heart failure readmission, and improvement in quality of life.
- MitraClip is associated with reverse remodeling of left ventricle with improvement in left ventricular end-diastolic volume, left ventricular end-systolic volume, LVEF, left atrial volume, and pulmonary arterial systolic pressure.

## INTRODUCTION

Heart failure is known to affect about 2.2% of the population over the age of 20 years. The incidence and prevalence increases with age. An estimated 915,000 patients greater than 55 years of age were newly diagnosed with heart failure in 2012 and this was associated with $30.7 billion in health care costs in 2012.[1] Valvular heart disease, especially aortic stenosis (AS) and mitral regurgitation, are commonly seen in patients with heart failure and are frequently thought to be the cause of heart failure in a large proportion of these patients. Recently, catheter-based interventions, particularly transcatheter aortic valve replacement (TAVR) and percutaneous mitral valve repair (MitraClip) have been increasingly used in patients with heart failure to help improve their survival, quality of life, and left ventricular (LV) remodeling. We aim to systematically review the outcomes of these catheter-based interventions in patients with heart failure as well as review their role in reversing heart failure.

## TRANSCATHETER AORTIC VALVE REPLACEMENT IN PATIENTS WITH HEART FAILURE

TAVR has been associated with improved survival as compared with medical therapy in in-operable patients[2] with severe AS and has similar outcomes to surgical aortic valve replacement (SAVR) in patients with intermediate-risk and high-risk AS.[3,4] SAVR in patients with heart failure has been associated with improved outcomes as well as improved survival.[5] Similarly, TAVR has also been associated with improved outcomes and improvement in LV ejection fraction (LVEF) in patients with severe AS with heart failure.[6]

Department of Cardiology, The Heart Hospital Baylor Plano, 110 Allied Drive, Plano, TX 75093, USA
* Corresponding author.
E-mail address: molly.szerlip@bswhealth.org

Intervent Cardiol Clin 6 (2017) 373–386
http://dx.doi.org/10.1016/j.iccl.2017.03.007
2211-7458/17/© 2017 Elsevier Inc. All rights reserved.

## Outcomes of Transcatheter Aortic Valve Replacement in Patients with Heart Failure

The PARTNER trial (5-Year Outcomes of Transcatheter Aortic Valve Replacement or Surgical Aortic Valve Replacement for High Surgical Risk Patients With Aortic Stenosis) showed similar survival to SAVR and TAVR in high-risk patients with severe AS. Elmariah and colleagues[6] evaluated patients from the PARTNER high-risk cohort looking at the outcomes based on the presence of LV dysfunction (LVEF <50%; 657 patients: 332 TAVR, 304 SAVR; 203 of 657 patients with LV dysfunction). All-cause mortality was noted to be similar at 30 days and 1 year in patients with LV dysfunction undergoing TAVR or SAVR. The mean LVEF increased from 35.7 ± 8.5% to 48.6 ± 11.3% (P<.0001) at 1 year after TAVR and from 38.0 ± 8.0% to 50.1 ± 10.8% after SAVR (P<.0001; Fig. 1). Factors associated with improvement in LVEF of 10% or greater at 30 days included a higher baseline mean aortic valve gradient (odds ratio [OR], 1.04 per 1 mm Hg; 95% confidence interval [CI], 1.01–1.08), higher baseline LVEF (OR, 0.9; 95% CI, 0.86–0.95) and previous permanent pacemaker (OR, 0.34; 95% CI, 0.15–0.81). Failure to improve LVEF after 30 days was associated with increased mortality and repeat hospitalization after TAVR but not with SAVR[6] (Fig. 2, Table 1).

Patients with severe AS who were considered inoperable for SAVR by 2 independent cardiothoracic surgeons were randomized to treatment with either TAVR or medical therapy in the cohort B of the PARTNER trial. Passeri and colleagues[7] evaluated 342 patients (169 TAVR patients; 173 medical therapy patients) from the Partner B cohort of whom 46 patients (27.2%) had

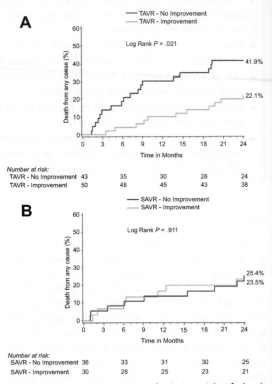

**Fig. 2.** Time-to-event curves depicting risk of death from any cause in patients with left ventricular (LV) dysfunction. Those who failed to improve by 30-days after transcatheter aortic valve replacement (TAVR) possessed an increased risk of death at 2 years (A), whereas lack of LV functional improvement after surgical aortic valve replacement (SAVR) did not influence survival (B). The event rates were calculated with the use of Kaplan–Meier methods and compared with the use of the log-rank test. Patients surviving fewer than 30 days were excluded from these analyses. (From Elmariah S, Palacios IF, McAndrew T, et al. Outcomes of transcatheter and surgical aortic valve replacement in high-risk patients with aortic stenosis and left ventricular dysfunction: results from the Placement of Aortic Transcatheter Valves (PARTNER) trial (cohort A). Circ Cardiovasc Interv 2013;6(6):604–14; with permission.)

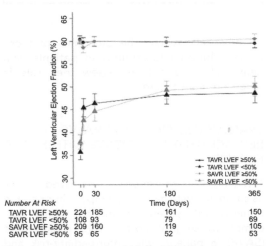

**Fig. 1.** Left ventricular (LV) functional recovery with time. LV ejection fraction (LVEF) remained stable in those with normal baseline function. In subjects with baseline LV dysfunction, LVEF improved quickly and equally after surgical aortic valve replacement (SAVR) and transcatheter aortic valve replacement (TAVR), with most LV functional improvement occurring within the first 30 days. Points represent mean values with error bars depicting standard deviations. (From Elmariah S, Palacios IF, McAndrew T, et al. Outcomes of transcatheter and surgical aortic valve replacement in high-risk patients with aortic stenosis and left ventricular dysfunction: results from the Placement of Aortic Transcatheter Valves (PARTNER) trial (cohort A). Circ Cardiovasc Interv 2013;6(6):604–14; with permission.)

**Table 1**
Clinical outcomes at 1 y by 30-d improvement in left ventricular ejection fraction in those with baseline left ventricular dysfunction (LVEF <50%)

| | Improvement | No Improvement | Hazard Ratio (95% CI) | P Value |
|---|---|---|---|---|
| **TAVR** | n = 50 | n = 43 | | |
| All-cause death | 10.0% (5) | 30.2% (13) | 0.28 (0.10–0.79) | .01 |
| Cardiac death | 2.1% (1) | 11.2% (4) | 0.18 (0.02–1.58) | .08 |
| Repeat hospitalization | 14.2% (7) | 42.4% (17) | 0.28 (0.11–0.67) | .002 |
| Death or repeat hospitalization | 20.0% (10) | 51.2% (22) | 0.30 (0.14–0.63) | .0008 |
| Stroke or TIA | 2.1% (1) | 7.6% (3) | 0.26 (0.03–2.48) | .20 |
| Stroke | 0.0% (0) | 5.3% (2) | N/A | .20 |
| TIA | 2.1% (1) | 2.3% (1) | 0.79 (0.05–12.69) | .87 |
| Death from any cause or major stroke | 10.0% (5) | 32.6% (14) | 0.26 (0.09–0.72) | .005 |
| Myocardial infarction | 0.0% (0) | 0.0% (0) | N/A | N/A |
| Dialysis lasting >30 d | 0.0% (0) | 0.0% (0) | N/A | N/A |
| **SAVR** | n = 30 | n = 36 | | |
| All-cause death | 16.7% (5) | 13.9% (5) | 1.19 (0.34–4.11) | .78 |
| Cardiac death | 3.6% (1) | 5.6% (2) | 0.59 (0.05–6.52) | .66 |
| Repeat hospitalization | 21.5% (6) | 8.9% (3) | 2.43 (0.61–9.73) | .19 |
| Death or repeat hospitalization | 33.3% (10) | 22.2% (8) | 1.53 (0.60–3.88) | .36 |
| Stroke or TIA | 0.0% (0) | 6.0% (2) | N/A | .19 |
| Stroke | 0.0% (0) | 6.0% (2) | N/A | .19 |
| TIA | 0.0% (0) | 0.0% (0) | N/A | N/A |
| Death from any cause or major stroke | 16.7% (5) | 19.4% (7) | 0.82 (0.26–2.60) | .74 |
| Myocardial infarction | 0.0% (0) | 0.0% (0) | N/A | N/A |
| Dialysis lasting >30 d | 0.0% (0) | 2.9% (1) | N/A | .36 |

Kaplan-Meier estimates (number of events) are shown.
*Abbreviations:* CI, confidence interval; LVEF, left ventricular ejection fraction; N/A, not applicable; SAVR, surgical aortic valve replacement; TAVR, transcatheter aortic valve replacement; TIA, transient ischemic attack.
*From* Elmariah S, Palacios IF, McAndrew T, et al. Outcomes of transcatheter and surgical aortic valve replacement in high-risk patients with aortic stenosis and left ventricular dysfunction: results from the Placement of Aortic Transcatheter Valves (PARTNER) trial (cohort A). Circ Cardiovasc Interv 2013;6(6):604–14; with permission.

LV dysfunction (LVEF <50%). LVEF improvement (≥10% improvement in LVEF at 30 days) occurred in 48.7% of the patients after TAVR and 30.4% of the patients treated with standard therapy (**Fig. 3**). Baseline LV dysfunction was not noted to affect survival after TAVR, but was noted to influence 1-year outcomes in patients on medical therapy (59.3% vs 45.8% in patients with normal LVEF; $P = .02$). Overall, TAVR was thought to improve outcomes and was associated with improved survival in patients with severe AS and heart failure.[7]

Although the impact of TAVR in patients with LV systolic dysfunction has been studied, there are lack of data with regard to the impact of diastolic dysfunction in patients undergoing TAVR. Kramer and colleagues[8] evaluated 500 patients undergoing TAVR for severe AS and 300 patients who were treated conservatively. A short deceleration time (<160 ms) was associated with worse survival as compared with patients with a long deceleration time (>220 ms; $P = .002$) and those with an intermediate deceleration time ($P = .05$). This was after adjustment for age, gender, stroke volume index, and comorbidities. Those patients with a short deceleration time before TAVR had the most improvements in deceleration time, E/A ratio, and systolic pulmonary arterial pressures (**Fig. 4**) after TAVR. More important, even among patients with a short deceleration time, TAVR was associated with improved survival when compared with conservative treatment (46 ± 7 vs 28 ± 12% at 3 years; $P = .05$), even after adjustment

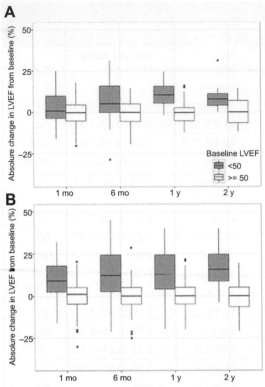

**Fig. 3.** Left ventricular functional recovery over time in subjects undergoing standard therapy (A) and transcatheter aortic valve replacement (B). LVEF, left ventricular ejection fraction. (From Passeri JJ, Elmariah S, Xu K, et al. Transcatheter aortic valve replacement and standard therapy in inoperable patients with aortic stenosis and low EF. Heart 2015;101(6):463–71; with permission.)

for age, gender, and stroke volume index ($P = .05$).[8]

## Left Ventricular Ejection Fraction Recovery After Transcatheter Aortic Valve Replacement: Determinants

Elhmidi and colleagues[9] evaluated 505 patients undergoing TAVR in a single center study and stratified the patients based on LV function (normal LV function [EF >50%, 64% of patients], moderate LV dysfunction [EF 35%–50%, 22% of patients], severe LV dysfunction [EF ≤35%, 14% of patients]). Patients with severe LV dysfunction were noted to have higher STS scores, higher logistic EuroSCORE, more coronary artery disease/previous coronary artery bypass surgery, higher NT-pro N-terminal pro-brain natriuretic peptide levels, lower mean transaortic valve gradients, and smaller aortic valve areas. The 6-month mortality was noted to be doubled in patients with severe LV dysfunction

as compared with those with normal LV function (27% vs 15%; $P \le .03$). In patients with an LVEF of 35% or less, 15% recovered to an LVEF of greater than 50% and 66% improved to an LVEF of 35% to 50%. Baseline LV function was the strongest independent predictor of improvement in LV function (OR, 85; 95% CI, 19–380; $P<.001$).

Patients with low-flow, low gradient AS are more difficult to treat. SAVR has not improved outcomes in these patients. Whether LV dysfunction is an independent predictor of poor outcomes or is associated with poor outcomes mediated by low flow needs to be investigated further. Low flow AS (defined as a stroke volume index $<35$ mL/m$^2$) can be present in both preserved EF and low EF. A retrospective analysis of 639 patients who underwent TAVR at 2 Canadian sites showed low flow to be present in 52.3% of the patients, and this was noted to be associated with a higher 30-day mortality (11.4% vs 5.9%; $P = .01$), 2-year all-cause mortality (35.3% vs 30.9%; $P = .005$), and 2-year cardiovascular mortality (25.7% vs 16.8%; $P = .01$). After multivariable adjustment, low-flow but not low-gradient or LV dysfunction was noted to be associated with worse outcomes in patients undergoing TAVR.[10]

Baron and associates evaluated the impact of ejection fraction and aortic valve gradient on outcomes in 11,292 patients treated with TAVR in the United States as part of the Transcatheter Valve Therapy registry. Patients were stratified based on levels of LV dysfunction (LVEF <30%, 30%–50%, and >50%) as well as aortic valve gradient (mean gradient <40 mm Hg or >40 mm Hg). At the 1-year follow-up, LV dysfunction as well as a low aortic gradient was associated with a higher rate of death and recurrent heart failure (**Fig. 5**). However, after adjustment for other factors, only low aortic valve gradient was associated with a higher mortality (hazard ratio, 1.21; 95% CI, 1.11–1.32; $P<.001$) and a higher rate of recurrent heart failure (hazard ratio, 1.52; 95% CI, 1.36–1.69; $P<.001$; **Figs. 6** and **7**). Importantly, at 30 days most patients noted improvement in quality of life scores (measured using Kansas City Cardiomyopathy Questionnaire Overall Summary questionnaires). Those patients with worse LV dysfunction improved the most (**Table 2**). This real-world study was important because it showed that patients with LV dysfunction undergoing TAVR had good long-term outcomes after TAVR and that patients with worse LV dysfunction had the most improvement in quality of life after TAVR.[11]

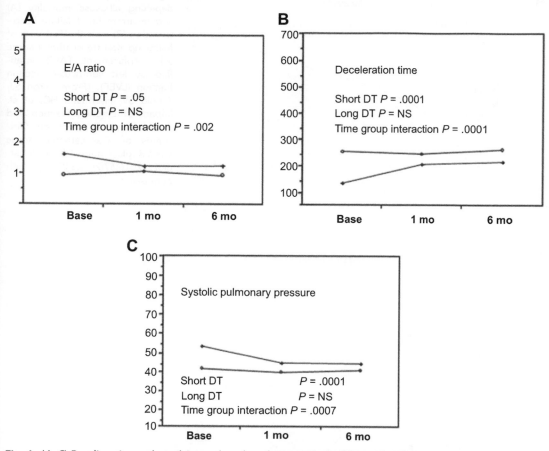

**Fig. 4.** (*A–C*) Baseline, 1-month, and 6-month early to late ventricular filling ratios (E/A ratios) (*A*), delay time (DT) (*B*), and systolic pulmonary artery pressure (SPAP) (*C*). Characteristics of the short DT at baseline (*blue line*) and long DT (*red line*) are shown. In patients with a baseline DT of 160 ms or greater, the E/A ratio, DT, and SPAP did not change between baseline, 1 month, and 6 months after transcatheter aortic valve replacement. However, patients with short DT at baseline showed a significant decrease in E/A ratio (*P* = .05), increase in DT (*P*<.0001), and decrease in SPAP (*P*<.0001). The groups × time interactions were significant for all comparisons, suggesting that, although patients with restrictive physiology at baseline are sicker and have inferior prognosis, they are also the patients who benefit most from a successful procedure. (*From* Kramer J, Biner S, Ghermezi M, et al. Impact of left ventricular filling parameters on outcome of patients undergoing trans-catheter aortic valve replacement. Eur Heart J Cardiovasc Imaging 2017;18(3):304–14; with permission.)

All of the trials to date have looked at patients with severe AS. The recently initiated TAVR-UNLOAD trial (Transcatheter Aortic Valve Replacement to UNload the Left Ventricle in Patients With ADvanced Heart Failure) aims to evaluate the safety and efficacy of TAVR in patients with moderate AS (defined as mean aortic valve gradient of >20 mm Hg and <40 mm Hg or aortic valve area >1.0 cm² and <1.5 cm² at rest or after dobutamine stress echocardiography) and heart failure on top of optimized medical management.[12] The primary endpoint is a hierarchical occurrence of all-cause death, disabling stroke, hospitalizations related to heart failure, symptomatic aortic valve disease or nondisabling stroke, and change in the Kansas City Cardiomyopathy Questionnaire at 1 year. The results of this trial may help us to better understand the role of TAVR in patients with severe heart failure.

## MITRACLIP IN PATIENTS WITH SEVERE HEART FAILURE

Mitral regurgitation affects 1% to 2% of the general population and is the second most common cause of valvular heart disease in the United States.[13] Mitral regurgitation remains a significant cause of heart failure either owing to a primary leaflet abnormality (degenerative/primary mitral regurgitation) or owing to underlying LV

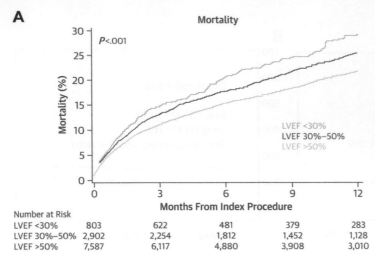

**A** Mortality

$P<.001$

Mortality (%)

LVEF <30%
LVEF 30%–50%
LVEF >50%

Months From Index Procedure

Number at Risk
| | | | | | |
|---|---|---|---|---|---|
| LVEF <30% | 803 | 622 | 481 | 379 | 283 |
| LVEF 30%–50% | 2,902 | 2,254 | 1,812 | 1,452 | 1,128 |
| LVEF >50% | 7,587 | 6,117 | 4,880 | 3,908 | 3,010 |

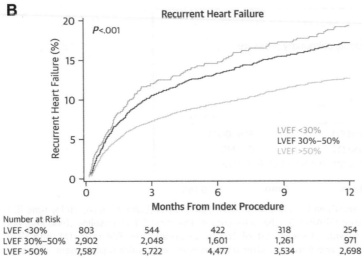

**B** Recurrent Heart Failure

$P<.001$

Recurrent Heart Failure (%)

LVEF <30%
LVEF 30%–50%
LVEF >50%

Months From Index Procedure

Number at Risk
| | | | | | |
|---|---|---|---|---|---|
| LVEF <30% | 803 | 544 | 422 | 318 | 254 |
| LVEF 30%–50% | 2,902 | 2,048 | 1,601 | 1,261 | 971 |
| LVEF >50% | 7,587 | 5,722 | 4,477 | 3,534 | 2,698 |

**Fig. 5.** Kaplan-Meier curves depicting all-cause mortality (*A*) and recurrent heart failure hospitalization (*B*) over the first year of follow-up after transcatheter aortic valve replacement (TAVR), stratified by left ventricular ejection fraction (LVEF). (*From* Baron SJ, Arnold SV, Herrmann HC, et al. Impact of Ejection Fraction and Aortic Valve Gradient on Outcomes of Transcatheter Aortic Valve Replacement. J Am Coll Cardiol 2016;67(20):2349–58; with permission.)

dysfunction or dilation (secondary or functional mitral regurgitation). The current American College of Cardiology/American Heart Association guidelines for the treatment of valvular heart diseases recommend the treatment of patients with severe symptomatic primary mitral regurgitation and an LVEF of greater than 30% or asymptomatic severe mitral regurgitation with an LVEF between 30% to 60% and an LV end-systolic diameter of 40 mm or greater (class I). Transcatheter mitral valve repair with the MitraClip percutaneous mitral valve edge to edge repair system (Abbott Vascular, Menlo Park, CA) has been recommended for patients with severe symptomatic chronic primary mitral regurgitation despite optimal medical therapy with prohibitive surgical risk and with favorable anatomy and reasonable life expectancy (class II).[14]

## MitraClip in Degenerative or Primary Mitral Regurgitation

The first large, randomized trial to look at percutaneous treatments for severe primary mitral regurgitation was the EVEREST trial (Endovascular Valve Edge-to-Edge REpair Study). The EVEREST I trial was a feasibility study of 107 patients (55 patients EVEREST 1 and 52 patients who were roll-ins for EVEREST II) with 3+ or 4+ functional or degenerative mitral regurgitation.[15] At the 1-year follow-up, 10 of the 107 patients (9%) had a major adverse event including a nonprocedural death, and 74% had acute procedural success and 64% were discharged with mitral regurgitation grade 1+ or lower. The primary efficacy endpoint of freedom from death, mitral valve surgery and mitral regurgitation of greater than 2+ was 95.9%, 94.0%, and 90.1% and freedom from surgery was 88.5%, 83.2%,

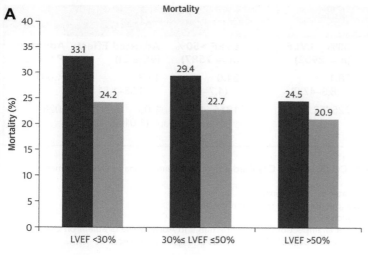

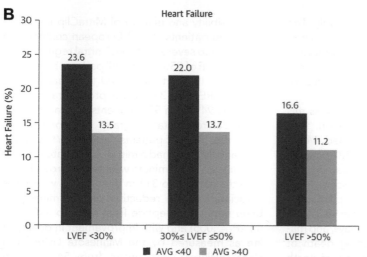

**Fig. 6.** One-year Kaplan-Meier estimates of all-cause mortality (*A*) and recurrent heart failure hospitalization (*B*) after transcatheter aortic valve replacement (TAVR), stratified by left ventricular ejection fraction (LVEF) and aortic valve gradient (AVG). (*From* Baron SJ, Arnold SV, Herrmann HC, et al. Impact of Ejection Fraction and Aortic Valve Gradient on Outcomes of Transcatheter Aortic Valve Replacement. J Am Coll Cardiol 2016;67(20):2349–58; with permission.)

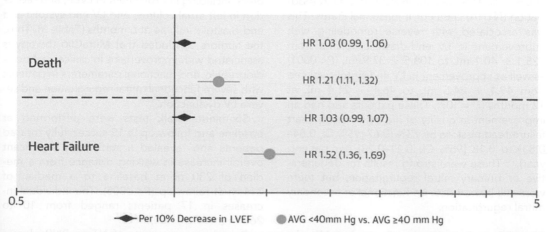

**Fig. 7.** Forest plot demonstrating the association of baseline left ventricular ejection fraction (LVEF) and aortic valve gradient (AVG) with all-cause mortality and recurrent heart failure after adjustment for potential confounders. (*From* Baron SJ, Arnold SV, Herrmann HC, et al. Impact of Ejection Fraction and Aortic Valve Gradient on Outcomes of Transcatheter Aortic Valve Replacement. J Am Coll Cardiol 2016;67(20):2349–58; with permission.)

**Table 2**
Health status outcomes at 30 days stratified by LVEF

| | LVEF <30% (n = 803) | 30% ≤ LVEF ≤50% (n = 2902) | LVEF >50% (n = 7587) | Adjusted Effect (95% CI) | Adjusted P Value |
|---|---|---|---|---|---|
| Change from baseline | 32.8 (11.5–54.5) | 28.1 (8.3–47.9) | 24.0 (4.7–43.8) | 1.03 (0.55–1.51)[b] | <.001 |
| Substantial health status improvement[a] | 201 (56.9) | 725 (52.3) | 1816 (48.2) | 1.06 (1.01–1.12)[c] | .028 |

Values are median (interquartile range) or n (%).
*Abbreviations:* CI, confidence interval; KCCQ-OS, Kansas City Cardiomyopathy Questionnaire Overall Summary score; LVEF, left ventricular ejection fraction.
[a] Change from baseline KCCQ-OS of greater than 20 points.
[b] Refers to absolute change in KCCQ-OS (per 10%-point reduction in LVEF).
[c] Adjusted odds ratio (per 10%-point reduction in LVEF).
*From* Baron SJ, Arnold SV, Herrmann HC, et al. Impact of Ejection Fraction and Aortic Valve Gradient on Outcomes of Transcatheter Aortic Valve Replacement. J Am Coll Cardiol 2016;67(20):2349–58; with permission.

and 76.3% at 1, 2, and 3 years, respectively. The authors concluded that the MitraClip system was safe and was able to achieve mitral regurgitation reduction to less than 2+ in the majority of patients with durable results and low rates of morbidity and mortality.

This led to a "real-world study" to assess this device in the same patient population. The REALISM study (Real World Expanded Multi-Center Study of MitraClip) looked at 127 patients with prohibitive risk degenerative mitral regurgitation (mean age, 82.4 years; STS score, 13.2 ± 7.3%) undergoing MitraClip implantation. MitraClip was successfully performed in 95.3% patients, duration of stay was 2.9 ± 3.1 days, and major adverse cardiac events, including death at 30 days, were 6.3%. At 1 year, the rate of death was 23.6%, with 82.9% of the surviving patients with mitral regurgitation of 2+ or less at 1 year and 86.9% of the patients in New York Heart Association (NYHA) class I or II functional status. This was associated with reverse remodeling with improvement in LV end-diastolic volume from 125.1 ± 40.1 mL to 108.5 ± 37.9 mL (P<.0001) as well as improvement in LV end systolic volume from 49.1 ± 24.5 mL to 46.1 ± 21.4 mL at 12 months (P = .07). These patients also had an improvement in quality of life by reducing heart failure readmissions by 73% (0.67 [95% CI, 0.54–0.83] to 0.18 [95% CI, 0.11–0.28] per patient-year).[16] These were strong results for degenerative or primary mitral regurgitation, but there were still limited data on functional or secondary mitral regurgitation.

## MitraClip in Functional or Secondary Mitral Regurgitation

To look at this technology in secondary mitral regurgitation, Franzen and colleagues[17] evaluated the feasibility and efficacy of MitraClip implantation in 50 patients from 7 European centers with moderate to severe functional mitral regurgitation and an LVEF of 25% or less. All patients had NYHA class III or IV heart failure and the mean logistic EuroSCORE was 34. Acute procedural success rate was 94% with 92% patients discharged with an mitral regurgitation grade of 2 or less. At 6 months, 72% of patients were in NYHA class I or II, and 87% still had a mitral regurgitation grade of 2 or less. The 6-minute walk test improved from a median of 230 to 311 m (P = .0005), which was associated with a reduction of N-terminal pro-brain natriuretic peptide from 4900 to 3300 pg/mL (P = .005) and with improvement in quality of life as measured by the Minnesota Living with Heart Failure Questionnaire from 54 ± 22 to 32 ± 20 (P = .0044). There was also significant improvement noted in echocardiographic parameters, including improvement in LVEF, and reduction in left atrial volume, and LV end-systolic and end-diastolic volume at 6 months (Table 3). Thus, the authors concluded that MitraClip therapy is associated with improvement in clinical, echocardiographic, and functional parameters in patients with severe functional mitral regurgitation and severe LV dysfunction.[17]

Six-minute walk tests were performed at baseline and follow-up in 19 successfully treated patients and revealed a statistically significant overall increase in walking distance from a median of 230 m at baseline to a median of 311 m at follow-up (P<.0005). The individual increases in 17 patients ranged from 10 to 263 m (median, 100).

Paired measurements of NT-proBNP plasma levels at baseline and follow-up were available from 18 patients. Overall, a significant decrease from a median of 4900 pg/mL (interquartile

**Table 3**
**Changes from baseline to 6 months in echocardiographic variables of successfully treated patients**

|  | n | Baseline (Mean ± SD) | 6 Months (Mean ± SD) | Δ (Mean ± SD) | P |
|---|---|---|---|---|---|
| Mitral valve orifice area (cm²) | 12 | 4.9 ± 1.6 | 3.2 ± 0.9 | −1.7 ± 1.4 | .002 |
| Mean transmitral gradient (mm Hg) | 19 | 1.7 ± 1.4 | 3.0 ± 2.6 | 1.3 ± 2.3 | .018 |
| LVEF (%) | 28 | 20 ± 4 | 25 ± 9 | 6 ± 9 | .003 |
| LV end-diastolic diameter (mm) | 30 | 71 ± 8 | 69 ± 8 | −2 ± 6 | .051 |
| LV end-systolic diameter (mm) | 30 | 62 ± 9 | 61 ± 8 | −1 ± 6 | .083 |
| LA diameter (mm) | 20 | 51 ± 7 | 45 ± 9 | −6 ± 9 | .023 |
| LV end-diastolic volume (mL) | 27 | 253 ± 73 | 237 ± 66 | −15 ± 35 | .010 |
| LV end-systolic volume (mL) | 26 | 196 ± 65 | 172 ± 55 | −24 ± 39 | .003 |

*Abbreviations:* Δ, difference; LA, left atrial; LV, left ventricular; LVEF, left ventricular ejection fraction; SD, standard deviation.

*From* Franzen O, van der Heyden J, Baldus S, et al. MitraClip® therapy in patients with end-stage systolic heart failure. Eur J Heart Fail 2011;13(5):569–76; with permission.

range, 3200–9500) at baseline to a median of 3300 pg/mL (interquartile range, 1500–5100; P<.005) at follow-up occurred, with individual relative decreases in 15 patients ranging from 27% to 282%.

Sixteen successfully treated patients completed the Minnesota Living with Heart Failure Questionnaire at baseline and at follow-up. Overall, a statistically significant score reduction from 54 ± 22 to 32 ± 20 (P<.0044) was noted, with individual score reductions in 13 patients ranging from -2 to -70. Changes were in echocardiographic parameters from baseline to 6 months after MitraClip implantation.

Schafer and colleagues[18] reported on the 12-month outcomes of 393 patients with moderate to severe functional mitral regurgitation who underwent MitraClip implantation in the ACCESS EU registry (a postapproval study of MitraClip). Patients were stratified by preprocedural LVEF (group A: 10%–20%; group B: >20%–30%; group C >30%–40%; group D >40%). Kaplan–Meier survival at 12 months was 81.8% (group A, 71%; group B, 79%; group C, 87%; group D, 86) with significant improvement in mitral regurgitation severity at 30 days and 12 months (P<.0001). There were similar improvements in NYHA class, 6-minute walk test, and Minnesota Living with Heart Failure Questionnaire at 12 months across all LVEF groups. Patients with an LVEF between 10% and 20% improved the most with 78.3% of patients in NYHA class I or II at 12 months as compared with 100% at baseline (Fig. 8). Similarly, the group with the LVEF between 10% and 20% had the most improvement in quality of life scores (51.5 vs 35.8; P = .02; Fig. 9).[18]

A metaanalysis of 9 studies with 875 patients with moderate to severe functional mitral regurgitation who underwent MitraClip implantation showed significant improvements in functional class and cardiac remodeling. Interestingly, patients with preexisting atrial fibrillation did not show similar improvements in LVEF, LV end-systolic volume, or LV end-diastolic volume after MitraClip implantation. This is similar to the poor prognostic effect of preexisting atrial fibrillation on outcomes after surgical mitral valve repair. In the overall cohort, after a median follow-up of 9 months, 78% of patients were in NYHA functional class I or II, with 11% of the patients still having moderate to severe residual mitral regurgitation. The 6-minute walk test improved by 100 m (range, 83–111) with significant reductions in LV volumes (>20 mL), left atrial volume (~40 mL) and systolic pulmonary arterial pressures (~12 mm Hg). They had a mild increase in LVEF (~4%). In-hospital mortality was low at 0.9%, 17% died at 12 months and 26% of the patients were rehospitalized for heart failure.[19]

The only randomized, controlled clinical trial to date on MitraClip in functional or secondary mitral regurgitation is currently enrolling at the time of the writing of this article. The COAPT trial (Cardiovascular Outcomes Assessment of MitraClip Therapy in Heart Failure Patients With Functional Mitral Regurgitation) aims to evaluate the effectiveness of MitraClip therapy in reducing heart failure hospitalizations in patients with functional mitral regurgitation and an LVEF between 20% and 50% and an LV end-systolic diameter of 70 mm or less. The trial randomizes patients with functional mitral regurgitation to MitraClip or standard medical

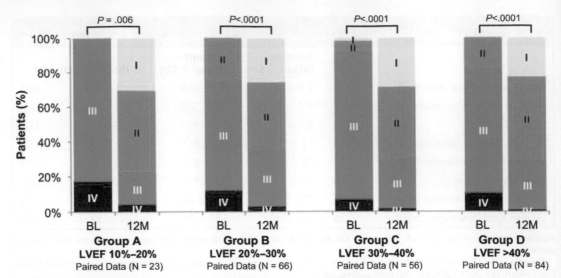

**Fig. 8.** Changes in New York Heart Association functional class from baseline to 12 months by left ventricular ejection fraction (LVEF) subgroups in patients with functional mitral regurgitation (paired data). BL, baseline; 12M, 12 months. (*From* Schäfer U, Maisano F, Butter C, et al. Impact of Preprocedural Left Ventricular Ejection Fraction on 1-Year Outcomes After MitraClip Implantation (from the ACCESS-EU Phase I, a Prospective, Multicenter, Nonrandomized Postapproval Study of the MitraClip Therapy in Europe). Am J Cardiol 2016;118(6):873–80; with permission.)

therapy. Total enrollment is 610 patients from 85 sites in the United States and Canada. The 30-day and 1-year outcomes of the 49 patients enrolled in the roll in period (34 US sites) were presented at TCT 2016 (mean STS score,

11 ± 7%; mean LVEF, 37 ± 11). Procedural success rate was 94% and mitral regurgitation was reduced to 2+ or less mitral regurgitation in 84% of patients. The 1-year mortality was 15.2%, heart failure rehospitalization was 28.3%

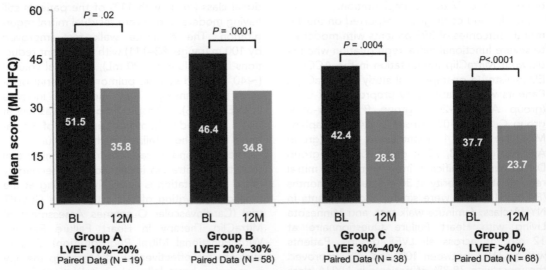

**Fig. 9.** Change in quality of life score from baseline to 12 months by left ventricular ejection fraction (LVEF) subgroups in patients with functional mitral regurgitation as measured using the Minnesota living with heart failure questionnaire (MLWHFQ; paired data). (*From* Schäfer U, Maisano F, Butter C, et al. Impact of Preprocedural Left Ventricular Ejection Fraction on 1-Year Outcomes After MitraClip Implantation (from the ACCESS-EU Phase I, a Prospective, Multicenter, Nonrandomized Postapproval Study of the MitraClip Therapy in Europe). Am J Cardiol 2016;118(6):873–80; with permission.)

and NYHA functional class improvement by 1 or more classes was 57.1%.[20] The results of this very important trial will help the understanding of the role of MitraClip implantation in patients with severe functional mitral regurgitation and are eagerly awaited.

The long-term safety and efficacy of the Mitra-Clip as compared with surgery was recently reported by Feldman and colleagues in the 5-year follow-up of the EVEREST II trial (Endovascular Valve Edge-to-Edge Repair Study). The trial included patients with both functional and degenerative mitral regurgitation and included 258 patients (178 MitraClip, 80 surgery). At 1 year, the MitraClip device arm was known to be less effective in reducing mitral regurgitation as compared with conventional surgery, but had superior safety and similar improvements in clinical and reverse remodeling parameters as compared with surgery. At 5 years, the composite outcome of freedom from death, surgery, and 3+ or 4+ mitral regurgitation was 44.2% in the device arm and 64.3% in the surgical arm (P = .01). This difference was driven mostly from increased rates of 3+ to 4+ mitral regurgitation in the device arm. After 6 months, the rates of repeat surgery for mitral regurgitation grade of 3+ or greater was similar between both groups and 5-year mortality was similar between both groups (MitraClip vs surgery 20.8% vs 26.8%; P = .4). Despite the lack of an annuloplasty ring and a higher residual mitral regurgitation, patients undergoing Mitra-Clip implantation had stable LV dimensions and similar improvements in heart failure symptoms at 5 years as compared with surgery, supporting the long-term durability and safety of MitraClip implantation.[21]

## MitraClip Effect on Remodeling

Grayburn and colleagues[22] evaluated the effect of MitraClip implantation on left atrial and LV volumes in 801 patients with degenerative and functional mitral regurgitation. The amount of reduction in left atrial and LV end-diastolic volumes after MitraClip implantation correlated with the degree of residual mitral regurgitation. There was greater remodeling with increasing degrees of mitral regurgitation reduction. The LV end-systolic volume after MitraClip was decreased in patients with functional mitral regurgitation but not in patients with degenerative mitral regurgitation. The authors concluded that, in patients with degenerative mitral regurgitation, reduction in the LV end-diastolic volume and left atrial volume but not in LV end-systolic volume is consistent with a decrease in volume overload in these patients. In patients

with functional mitral regurgitation, a reduction in both the LV end-diastolic and LV end-systolic volume as well as left atrial volume is consistent with reverse remodeling after MitraClip implantation when mitral regurgitation severity is reduced to either 1+ or 2+.

A large proportion of unoperated patients with severe mitral regurgitation continue to have recurrent heart failure hospitalizations and have a high overall mortality. Kapadia and colleagues[2] evaluated the prevalence and outcomes of unoperated patients with severe symptomatic mitral regurgitation with heart failure who presented to the Cleveland Clinic. Functional mitral regurgitation made up 90% of the heart failure patients and degenerative mitral regurgitation made up 6% of the patients. The 1-year and 5-year mortality rates were 20% and 50%, respectively, and the rates of hospitalization for heart failure in this population increased from 41% at 1 year to 90% at 5 years (Fig. 10). Based on echocardiograms, about 36% of these patients had anatomic characteristics favorable for MitraClip implantation. In light of the poor long-term outcomes of these patients if left untreated and the lack of survival benefit and high rate of recurrence of mitral regurgitation despite surgery in these patients, the authors suggested a large unmet need and potential opportunity for use of MitraClip. This could potentially reduce mitral regurgitation and heart failure hospitalizations in these patients.[23]

MitraClip has not only been shown to be effective, but also has been shown to be cost effective. Asgar and colleagues[24] suggested that treatment with MitraClip in patients with moderate to severe mitral regurgitation and heart failure is associated with superior survival and is cost effective when compared with medical therapy alone. At a mean follow-up of 22 months, all-cause mortality was 21% in the MitraClip cohort and 42% in the medical management cohort. MitraClip increased life expectancy by 1.87 to 3.6 years and quality-adjusted life-years from 1.13 to 2.76 years with an incremental cost-effectiveness ratio of $32,300 per quality-adjusted life-year gained.

In addition to being cost effective, MitraClip implantation is associated with improvement in cognitive and psychosocial functioning in heart failure patients. In 24 patients with heart failure and severe mitral regurgitation, MitraClip implantation was associated with improvement in long-term memory (P = .003) and executive function (planning ability; P<.001) as compared with a healthy group of patients without mitral regurgitation. Additionally, MitraClip

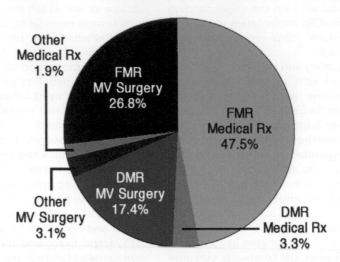

## A    Medically treated patients with severe MR

Other Medical Rx 1.9%

FMR MV Surgery 26.8%

FMR Medical Rx 47.5%

DMR MV Surgery 17.4%

Other MV Surgery 3.1%

DMR Medical Rx 3.3%

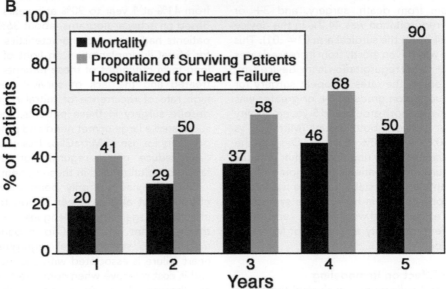

**B**

**Mortality**

**Proportion of Surviving Patients Hospitalized for Heart Failure**

% of Patients

Years

| Year | Mortality | Hospitalized |
|---|---|---|
| 1 | 20 | 41 |
| 2 | 29 | 50 |
| 3 | 37 | 58 |
| 4 | 46 | 68 |
| 5 | 50 | 90 |

Fig. 10. (A) Pie chart showing mechanism and management of 1095 patients with severe symptomatic mitral regurgitation. (B) Mortality and rates of hospitalization for heart failure in un-operated patients with severe mitral regurgitation. DMR, degenerative mitral regurgitation; FMR, functional mitral regurgitation; MV, mitral valve. (From Goel SS, Bajaj N, Aggarwal B, et al. Prevalence and Outcomes of Unoperated Patients With Severe Symptomatic Mitral Regurgitation and Heart Failure Comprehensive Analysis to Determine the Potential Role of MitraClip for This Unmet Need. J Am Coll Cardiol 2014;63(2):185–6; with permission.)

intervention also resulted in a significant improvement in depression (P = .002), anxiety (P = .003), and quality of life scores (physical P = .017; mental P = .013) over time.[25]

## SUMMARY

TAVR and MitraClip offer a unique, minimally invasive, percutaneous option to treat aortic stenosis and mitral regurgitation, respectively,

in patients with severe heart failure and are associated with improvement in LVEF, symptoms, quality of life, and reverse remodeling. These devices should be increasingly considered in patients with severe heart failure to help reduce the burden of heart failure hospitalizations as well as reverse heart failure, especially given their minimally invasive nature and consequent ability to treat a larger population of patients than open surgical options. Further studies are needed to evaluate the role of these devices in the heart failure population and to better understand the long-term benefit of these devices in patients with severe or end-stage heart failure.

## REFERENCES

1. Writing Group Members, Mozaffarian D, Benjamin EJ, et al. Executive summary: heart disease and stroke statistics–2016 update: a report from the American Heart Association. Circulation 2016;133(4):447–54.

2. Kapadia SR, Leon MB, Makkar RR, et al. 5-year outcomes of transcatheter aortic valve replacement compared with standard treatment for patients with inoperable aortic stenosis (PARTNER 1): a randomised controlled trial. Lancet 2015; 385(9986):2485–91.

3. Leon MB, Smith CR, Mack MJ, et al. Transcatheter or surgical aortic-valve replacement in intermediate-risk patients. N Engl J Med 2016;374(17):1609–20.

4. Mack MJ, Leon MB, Smith CR, et al. 5-year outcomes of transcatheter aortic valve replacement or surgical aortic valve replacement for high surgical risk patients with aortic stenosis (PARTNER 1): a randomised controlled trial. Lancet 2015;385(9986): 2477–84.

5. Pai RG, Varadarajan P, Razzouk A. Survival benefit of aortic valve replacement in patients with severe aortic stenosis with low ejection fraction and low gradient with normal ejection fraction. Ann Thorac Surg 2008;86(6):1781–9.

6. Elmariah S, Palacios IF, McAndrew T, et al. Outcomes of transcatheter and surgical aortic valve replacement in high-risk patients with aortic stenosis and left ventricular dysfunction: results from the placement of aortic transcatheter valves (PARTNER) trial (cohort A). Circ Cardiovasc Interv 2013;6(6):604–14.

7. Passeri JJ, Elmariah S, Xu K, et al. Transcatheter aortic valve replacement and standard therapy in inoperable patients with aortic stenosis and low EF. Heart 2015;101(6):463–71.

8. Kramer J, Biner S, Ghermezi M, et al. Impact of left ventricular filling parameters on outcome of patients undergoing trans-catheter aortic valve replacement. Eur Heart J Cardiovasc Imaging 2017;18(3):304–14.

9. Elhmidi Y, Bleiziffer S, Deutsch MA, et al. Transcatheter aortic valve implantation in patients with LV dysfunction: impact on mortality and predictors of LV function recovery. J Invasive Cardiol 2014; 26(3):132–8.

10. Le Ven F, Freeman M, Webb J, et al. Impact of low flow on the outcome of high-risk patients undergoing transcatheter aortic valve replacement. J Am Coll Cardiol 2013;62(9):782–8.

11. Baron SJ, Arnold SV, Herrmann HC, et al. Impact of ejection fraction and aortic valve gradient on outcomes of transcatheter aortic valve replacement. J Am Coll Cardiol 2016;67(20):2349–58.

12. Spitzer E, Van Mieghem NM, Pibarot P, et al. Rationale and design of the transcatheter aortic valve replacement to UNload the left ventricle in patients with ADvanced heart failure (TAVR UNLOAD) trial. Am Heart J 2016;182:80–8.

13. Fedak PW, McCarthy PM, Bonow RO. Evolving concepts and technologies in mitral valve repair. Circulation 2008;117(7):963–74.

14. Nishimura RA, Otto CM, Bonow RO, et al. 2014 AHA/ACC guideline for the management of patients with valvular heart disease: executive summary: a report of the American College of Cardiology/American heart association task force on practice guidelines. Circulation 2014;129(23): 2440–92.

15. Feldman T, Kar S, Rinaldi M, et al. Percutaneous mitral repair with the MitraClip system: safety and midterm durability in the initial EVEREST (Endovascular Valve Edge-to-Edge REpair Study) cohort. J Am Coll Cardiol 2009;54(8):686–94.

16. Lim DS, Reynolds MR, Feldman T, et al. Improved functional status and quality of life in prohibitive surgical risk patients with degenerative mitral regurgitation after transcatheter mitral valve repair. J Am Coll Cardiol 2014;64(2):182–92.

17. Franzen O, van der Heyden J, Baldus S, et al. MitraClip(R) therapy in patients with end-stage systolic heart failure. Eur J Heart Fail 2011;13(5): 569–76.

18. Schafer U, Maisano F, Butter C, et al. Impact of pre-procedural left ventricular ejection fraction on 1-year outcomes after MitraClip implantation (from the ACCESS-EU Phase I, a prospective, multi-center, nonrandomized postapproval study of the MitraClip therapy in Europe). Am J Cardiol 2016; 118(6):873–80.

19. D'ascenzo F, Moretti C, Marra WG, et al. Meta-analysis of the usefulness of MitraClip in patients with functional mitral regurgitation. Am J Cardiol 2015;116(2):325–31.

20. Stone G, Abraham W, Lindenfeld J, et al. Cardiovascular outcomes assessment of MitraClip therapy in heart failure patients with functional mitral regurgitation (The COAPT Trial): baseline characteristics and preliminary 30-day and 1-year outcomes of the roll-in cohort. J Am Coll Cardiol 2016;68(18):B255.

21. Feldman T, Kar S, Elmariah S, et al, EVEREST II investigators. Randomized comparison of percutaneous repair and surgery for mitral regurgitation: 5-year results of EVEREST II. J Am Coll Cardiol 2015;66(25):2844–54.

22. Grayburn PA, Foster E, Sangli C, et al. Relationship between the magnitude of reduction in mitral

regurgitation severity and left ventricular and left atrial reverse remodeling after MitraClip therapy. Circulation 2013;128(15):1667–74.

23. Goel SS, Bajaj N, Aggarwal B, et al. Prevalence and outcomes of unoperated patients with severe symptomatic mitral regurgitation and heart failure: comprehensive analysis to determine the potential role of MitraClip for this unmet need. J Am Coll Cardiol 2014;63(2):185–6.

24. Asgar AW, Khairy P, Guertin MC, et al. Clinical outcomes and economic impact of transcatheter mitral leaflet repair in heart failure patients. J Med Econ 2017;20(1):82–90.

25. Nikendei C, Schafer H, Weisbrod M, et al. The effects of mitral valve repair on memory performance, executive function, and psychological measures in patients with heart failure. Psychosom Med 2016;78(4):432–42.

# Mechanical Circulatory Support in Acute Decompensated Heart Failure and Shock

Nishtha Sodhi, MD, John M. Lasala, MD, PhD*

---

### KEYWORDS

- Interventional management • Cardiogenic shock • Decompensated heart failure
- Intraaortic balloon pump • TandemHeart • Extracorporeal membrane support

---

### KEY POINTS

- In the current era, failure of maximal medical therapy is no longer a justifiable endpoint given the array of available advanced mechanical options.
- Deciding which mechanical device is most suitable depends largely on the degree of support needed.
- These temporary support devices, if implemented in a timely fashion, can often bridge patients to decision, recovery, long-term support devices (ventricular assist devices [VADs] and total artificial heart), and/or heart transplant.

---

## INTRODUCTION

Approximately 6 million adults in the United States have congestive heart failure. Many of these patients, at some point in their care and evaluation, pass through a cardiac catheterization laboratory.[1] The emerging subspecialty of "interventional heart failure" has arisen due to this expanding patient population who require expertise in not only the pathophysiology but also the practical application and implementation of mechanical therapeutics to improve such hemodynamics, particularly once refractory to optimal medical management (Fig. 1).[2,3] An array of interventional therapeutics is available in the modern era, with uses depending on acute or chronic situations (Fig. 2). This article focuses on support in acute decompensated heart failure and cardiogenic shock, including intra-aortic balloon pumps (IABPs), continuous aortic flow augmentation, and extracorporeal membrane oxygenation (ECMO).

## INTRA-AORTIC BALLOON PUMP
### Introduction and Components

The IABP has grown to be the most widely used hemodynamic support device since its introduction in the 1960s.[4] This device uses the counterpulsation of a balloon in the descending aorta to improve cardiac output and increase coronary perfusion. The system comprises a dual-lumen 7.5F to 8.0F catheter with a polyethylene balloon and the control console. The inner catheter lumen accepts the guide wire during placement and transduces aortic pressure for monitoring. The gas lumen serves as the conduit for the rapid exchange of helium in and out of the balloon. Helium has low viscosity and is absorbed rapidly in blood if the balloon inadvertently ruptures.

### Hemodynamic Effects

The hemodynamic consequences of counterpulsation can be organized into those that occur during inflation and those during deflation

---

Disclosure Statement: None.

Cardiovascular Division, Washington University, 660 South Euclid Avenue, St Louis, MO 63110, USA

* Corresponding author.

E-mail address: jlasala@wustl.edu

Intervent Cardiol Clin 6 (2017) 387–405

http://dx.doi.org/10.1016/j.iccl.2017.03.008

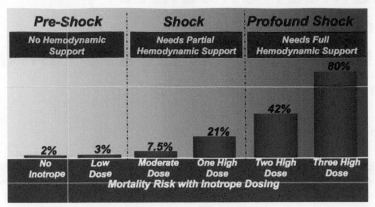

Fig. 1. The emerging subspecialty of "interventional heart failure" has arisen due to the expanding patient population who requires expertise in not only the pathophysiology but the practical application and implementation of mechanical therapeutics to improve such hemodynamics, particularly once refractory to optimal medical management, which forebodes incredible mortality. (*Adopted from* Samuels LE, Kaufman MS, Thomas MP, et al. Pharmacological criteria for ventricular assist device insertion following postcardiotomy shock: experience with the Abiomed BVS system. J Card Surg 1999;14(4):288–93.)

(Fig. 3). Inflation occurs at the onset of diastole and causes a displacement of blood that increases the diastolic pressure in the aorta. There is a resulting increase in systemic mean arterial pressure and cardiac output as well as an improvement in coronary perfusion. Balloon deflation is timed to occur immediately prior to systole, leading to an abrupt drop in aortic pressure just prior to ventricular ejection. This reduces the ventricular afterload and leads to

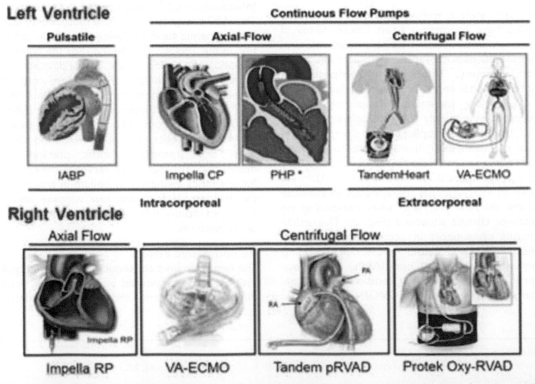

Fig. 2. The array of mechanical support options for LV failure and RV failure, respectively. (*Data from* Kapur NK, Esposito ML. Door to unload: a new paradigm for the management of cardiogenic shock. Curr Cardiovasc Risk Rep 2016;10:41.)

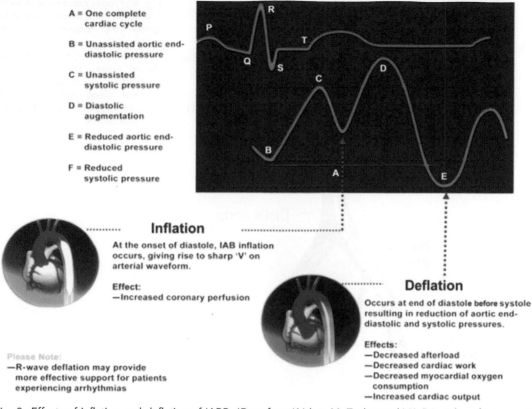

A = One complete cardiac cycle

B = Unassisted aortic end-diastolic pressure

C = Unassisted systolic pressure

D = Diastolic augmentation

E = Reduced aortic end-diastolic pressure

F = Reduced systolic pressure

**Inflation**

At the onset of diastole, IAB inflation occurs, giving rise to sharp 'V' on arterial waveform.

Effect:
—Increased coronary perfusion

**Deflation**

Occurs at end of diastole before systole resulting in reduction of aortic end-diastolic and systolic pressures.

Effects:
—Decreased afterload
—Decreased cardiac work
—Decreased myocardial oxygen consumption
—Increased cardiac output

Please Note:
—R-wave deflation may provide more effective support for patients experiencing arrhythmias

Fig. 3. Effects of inflation and deflation of IABP. (*Data from* Krishna M, Zacharowski K. Principles of intra-aortic balloon pump counterpulsation. Contin Educ Anaesth Crit Care Pain 2009;9(1): 24–28.)

decreased workload and improved cardiac output.

## Technical Considerations and Contraindications

Proper balloon volume sizing can maximize the hemodynamic benefit for patients. Increases in balloon volume (up to 50 mL) are accomplished by adding length to the balloon. Thus, sizing charts are based on patient height to avoid balloon obstruction of left subclavian and bilateral renal perfusion (Fig. 4). Balloon position should be performed under fluoroscopy to avoid this potential complication. If the placement cannot be performed under live fluoroscopy, then immediate verification via a chest plain film is warranted. The proper position of the distal tip is at 1 cm to 2 cm distal to left subclavian artery (second to third intercostal space), although one study suggests that placing the tip 2 cm above the carina may be a more reliable landmark.[5] Additionally, serial monitoring of the left radial pulse and urine output can signal malposition or movement of the IABP.

Contraindications to IABP placement include severe aortic insufficiency, aortic aneurysm, and peripheral vascular disease. The IABP may also be inserted without a sheath; however, this technique is contraindicated if there is significant scar tissue or if the patient is obese.

## Management

One of the most important functions of the console is to provide real-time information regarding the timing of balloon inflation and deflation. There are several modes to set balloon trigger, including ECG and pressure. ECG triggering is the most commonly used; however, it is susceptible to arrhythmias.

Recognition of mistimed balloon inflation and/or deflation is vital to ensuring proper hemodynamic support. The correct IABP waveform consists of inflation in diastole at the dicrotic notch, causing an augmentation of the diastolic pressure above the unassisted pressure (Fig. 5). Deflation should occur just before systole and cause a decrease in the end-diastolic pressure and peak systolic pressure. There are 4 scenarios to recognize: early inflation, late inflation, early deflation, and late deflation. When early inflation is occurring, the balloon is expanding prior to the dicrotic notch and can

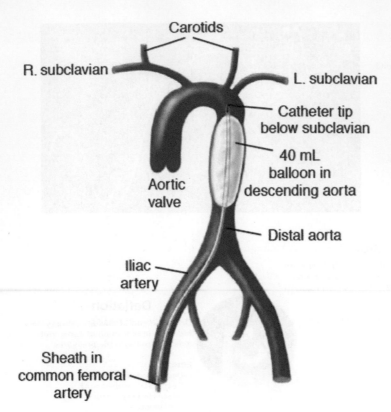

Fig. 4. Proper placement of IABP. The tip of the catheter should be below the subclavian, usually achieved by placing this at the tracheal bifurcation. Placement should ensure that there is no obstruction of left subclavian and bilateral renal perfusion. (*Data from* Ragosta M. Textbook of clinical hemodynamics. Philadelphia: Saunders/Elsevier; 2008.)

encroach onto the previous systolic phase (Fig. 6). The detrimental effects can include premature closure of the aortic valve with resulting increased filling pressures and afterload that results in increased myocardial oxygen demand. Late inflation occurs after the dicrotic notch and can lead to poor diastolic augmentation and with it poor coronary perfusion. In addition, there is ineffective afterload reduction and increased myocardial oxygen consumption demand. Early deflation leads to a sharp drop right in aortic pressure during the diastolic phase and limits pressure augmentation and coronary flow (Fig. 7). It can also lead to poor afterload reduction and increased myocardial oxygen demand. Finally, late deflation causes the balloon to impede on the subsequent systolic phase and the work of the heart against an inflated balloon leads to increased afterload and increased myocardial oxygen demand.

Potential complications of IABP use include limb ischemia, bleeding, thrombocytopenia,

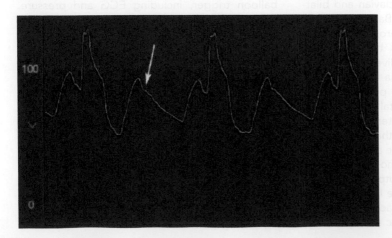

Fig. 5. Proper timing of inflation and deflation of an IABP. The balloon inflates after the dicrotic notch on the aortic pressure waveform (*arrow*). Deflation should be completed before aortic ejection begins on the next cardiac cycle, which is evident by a lower end-diastolic pressure of the augmented beat compared with the unaugmented beat. (*Data from* Ragosta M. Textbook of clinical hemodynamics. Philadelphia: Saunders/Elsevier; 2008.)

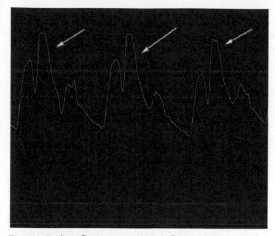

**Fig. 6.** Early inflation and late deflation. Balloon inflation is occurring prior to the dicrotic notch (*arrows*) and the end-diastolic pressure of the augmented beat is higher than that of the unaugmented beat consistent with late deflation. (*Data from* Ragosta M. Textbook of clinical hemodynamics. Philadelphia: Saunders/Elsevier; 2008.)

infection, and aortic dissection. Rupture of the balloon may also occur and is signaled by the presence of blood within the tubing or with a gas loss alarm. In this case, the device should be stopped immediately and removed.

Long-term IABP support can be safely accomplished via a subclavian approach that minimizes infection and allows patients to ambulate.[6] This approach can be considered for hemodynamic support for patients undergoing stabilization and subsequent work-up for transplant or left ventricular assist device (LVAD).

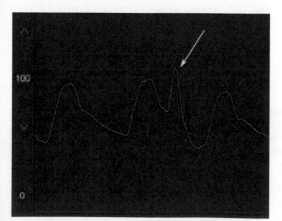

**Fig. 7.** Early deflation along with late inflation. Early deflation leads to a sharp drop in aortic pressure during diastole (*arrow*), thereby limiting coronary perfusion. (*Courtesy of* Ragosta M. Textbook of clinical hemodynamics. Philadelphia: Saunders/Elsevier; 2008.)

## Clinical Data and Guidelines for Intra-aortic Balloon Pump

In the Intra-aortic balloon counterpulsation in patients with acute myocardial infarction complicated by cardiogenic shock (IABP-SHOCK) I trial, there was no benefit in hemodynamics with IABP use in acute myocardial infarction (AMI) cardiogenic shock, likely due to poor native hemodynamics (**Fig. 8A**).[7] IABP-SHOCK II concluded no mortality benefit of IABP compared with medical therapy in the setting of AMI complicated by cardiogenic shock (**Fig. 8B**).[8] At 30 days, 39.7% of the patients in the IABP group and 41.3% of the patients in the control group had died. At 12-month follow-up of these patients, there was no survival benefit observed between the IABP arm and control arm.[8] In a meta-analysis, the IABP was found to increase the risk of bleeding and stroke in AMI cardiogenic shock patients.[9] Subsequently, the European Society of Cardiology downgraded the guidelines for the IABP to class III (harm), advising that the IABP should not be used routinely in cardiogenic shock patients.[10] The US population study by Stretch and colleagues analyzed the contemporary use of MCS devices from 2004 to 2011 and determined that IABP use prior to MCS was a predictor of mortality and increased costs (**Table 1**).[11,12] Thus, although it is readily available and used frequently, there is controversy regarding clinical benefits of IABP. Currently, IABP has received a class IIa indication for use during ST elevation myocardial infarction (STEMI) complicated by cardiogenic shock in the 2013 American College of Cardiology Foundation (ACCF)/American Heart Association (AHA) guidelines. The current ACCF/AHA and most recent Society for Cardiovascular Angiography and Interventions (SCAI) expert consensus document on percutaneous coronary intervention (PCI) without on-site cardiac surgery agree that the ability to provide IABP support during transport of unstable patients is a requirement for such centers.[13]

## LEFT ATRIAL TO AORTA ASSIST DEVICE: TANDEM HEART
### Introduction and Components

The TandemHeart (CardiacAssist, Pittsburgh, PA) is a support device that delivers blood from the left atrium (LA) to the arterial system (femoral artery) using an extracorporeal centrifugal pump. The TandemHeart system is composed of (1) an inflow cannula (21F) with transseptal placement into the LA, (2) an outflow cannula (15F or 17F) placed into the femoral artery, (3) centrifugal pump, and (4) control console (**Fig. 9**).

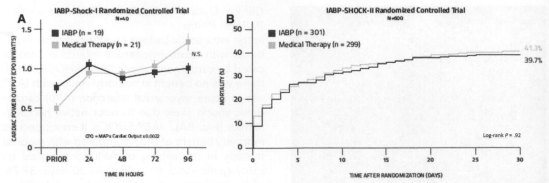

**Fig. 8.** (A) IABP-SHOCK I and (B) IABP-SHOCK II demonstrated no hemodynamic or mortality benefit with IABP use. (*Data from* Prondzinsky R, Unverzagt S, Russ M, et al. Hemodynamic effects of intra-aortic balloon counterpulsation in patients with acute myocardial infarction complicated by cardiogenic shock: the prospective, randomized IABP SHOCK trial. Shock 2012;37(4):378–84; and Thiele H, Zeymer U, Neumann FJ, et al. Intra-aortic balloon counterpulsation in acute myocardial infarction complicated by cardiogenic shock (IABP-SHOCK II): final 12 month results of a randomised, open-label trial. Lancet 2013;382(9905):1638–45.)

### Inflow and outflow cannulae

The inflow cannula is placed from the femoral vein into the LA via a transseptal puncture. The cannula is 21F and comes in either 62-cm or 72-cm lengths. Blood inflow comes through 14 side holes at the distal tip. The arterial outflow cannula is 17 cm in length and comes in either 15F or 17F. Both cannulae contain 3 radiopaque markings at the distal end, allowing accurate fluoroscopic placement.

### Centrifugal pump

The centrifugal pump is hydrodynamic and uses a fluid-bearing system created by constant saline infusion into the lower housing that minimizes friction. The pump itself has a maximum flow of 4 L/min to 5 L/min; however, flow is also dependent on inflow and outflow cannula size, with the variable in this system the outflow arterial cannula.

### Console

The controller is designed for ease of use with onscreen step-by-step set-up guidance as well as self-diagnostic algorithms and alarms. The console provides power to the system and has a battery backup that can provide up to 1 hour of operation.

### Hemodynamic Effects

The TandemHeart works in parallel, or in tandem, with the left ventricle (LV). The redirection of blood from the LA to the peripheral arterial system unloads the LV, thereby reducing workload, wall stress, and myocardial oxygen demand. Systemic circulation is perfused by both parallel pumps, generally with a greater contribution from the TandemHeart due to LV response to the pump, which may virtually cease due to changing loading conditions (decreased preload and increased afterload). The 19F arterial cannula allows up to 5 L/min of flow whereas the 15F cannula allows up to 3.5 L/min.

### Technical Considerations and Contraindications

As with other types of hemodynamic support devices, the size of the peripheral vasculature

| Table 1 | | | | |
| --- | --- | --- | --- | --- |
| Predictors of mortality in acute myocardial infarction cardiogenic shock | | | | |
| | **Odds Ratio** | **Lower 95% CI** | **Upper 95% CI** | ***P* Value** |
| CPR administration | 3.50 | 2.20 | 5.57 | <.001 |
| IABP use | 2.00 | 1.58 | 2.52 | <.001 |
| Intubation | 1.71 | 1.27 | 2.30 | <.001 |
| Vasopressor use | 1.39 | .75 | 2.58 | .30 |

Performed or administered up to 7 days before percutaneous ventricular assist device use. Data were collected from the Nationwide Inpatient Sample from the Healthcare Cost and Utilization Project between 2004 and 2011, and determined that IABP use prior to MCS was a predictor of mortality and increased costs.

*Data from* Stretch R, Sauer CM, Yuh DD, et al. National trends in the utilization of short-term mechanical circulatory support: incidence, outcomes, and cost analysis. J Am Coll Cardiol 2014;64(14):1407-15.

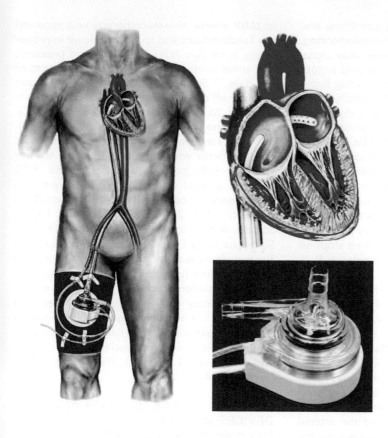

Fig. 9. TandemHeart. The Tandem-Heart system is composed of (1) an inflow cannula (21F) with transseptal placement into the LA, (2) an outflow cannula (15F or 17F) placed into the femoral artery, (3) centrifugal pump, and (4) control console. (*Data from* Naidu SS. Novel percutaneous cardiac assist devices. Circulation 2011;123:533–43.)

can limit the use of the TandemHeart. The venous cannula is 21F whereas the arterial cannula can be 15F or 17F. Serial assessment must be made of the access sites to assess for any possible complication or compromise of distal perfusion. Although frequent examination of limb color and temperature is needed, the distal pulse may not be palpable due to the nonpulsatile flow from the device. Placement of a sheath to provide antegrade flow to the distal limb may help prevent ischemia.

The placement of the TandemHeart venous cannula requires a transseptal puncture. For an experienced operator, a transseptal puncture is a relatively safe procedure. Approximately 1% of cases, however, develop complications 45, including cardiac wall perforation, aortic root puncture, pericardial effusion or tamponade, stroke, and death 46.

For those operators with less experience, methods to help delineate the atrial septal anatomy, such as intracardiac echo or transesophageal echo, may be more time consuming and costly but may minimize complications. The placement of a pigtail catheter to the aortic annulus marks the structure and helps avoid inadvertent puncture of the aortic root.

Adequate right ventricular (RV) function is required to maintain LA volume. Contraindications for the placement of the TandemHeart include any condition that prohibits anticoagulation. In addition, the presence of a ventricular septal defect or aortic insufficiency precludes placement.[13,14]

## Management

The flow provided by the TandemHeart is dependent on several factors, including the systemic and pulmonary resistance, cannula size and position, and fluid balance. Support is initiated at 5500 revolutions per minute (rpm) and subsequently raised by 250 rpm to 500 rpm until there is no long an increase in flow. This is the maximum flow for that particular set of parameters. Should more flow be desired, parameters, such as fluid balance, vascular resistance, and RV function, should be assessed and addressed. This highlights the need for continued hemodynamic monitoring as well as the utility of a Swan-Ganz catheter to help assess total cardiac output and filling pressures.

The TandemHeart console provides alarms categorized into 3 settings: low priority, medium priority, and high priority. The alarms are accompanied by the triggering conditions and associated causes that can guide troubleshooting.

Vibration in the system's tubing may signal inadequate filling of the LA and should trigger an evaluation for the root cause, including hypovolemia, pulmonary hypertension, cardiac tamponade, bleeding, RV failure, or arrhythmias. Kinks in the tubing, cannula migration, and thrombus in the circuit should also be assessed.

The importance of adequate anticoagulation has been discussed previously. Although protocols may vary among centers, activated clotting time (ACT) should be maintained between 180 seconds and 220 seconds. Additional heparin administration should be considered if the flow drops below 1 L/min or if the system is stopped for more than 5 minutes (not recommended).

Complications for this device are discussed previously but are summarized and include bleeding, limb ischemia, arrhythmias, tamponade, atrial perforation, and residual atrial septal defect.[13,14]

Weaning from the TandemHeart should be performed when deemed clinically appropriate by the managing team. Flow rate is decreased by 50% every hour but is not to be reduced below 1 L/min. If a patient remains stable, then the device may be turned off and the arterial cannula immediately clamped followed by the venous cannula. The device is then retracted from the LA into the right atrium and the heparin is stopped. Once the ACT reaches appropriate levels (per hospital protocol) the femoral cannulae may be removed.

### Clinical Data and Guidelines for TandemHeart

The Texas Heart experience analyzed 117 patients with severe cardiogenic shock refractory to IABP and/or pharmacotherapy who received the TandemHeart and found significant improvements in cardiac index, systolic blood pressure, and urine output over an average implant of 5.8 days.[15] Similar hemodynamics were found by Burkhoff and colleagues[16] in 33 patients randomized to TandemHeart or IABP (Fig. 10). Although no randomized trial of high-risk (HR)-PCI with TandemHeart exists, in a small series of 54 patients who were deemed high risk for surgery, 97% procedural success and 87% 6-month survival were found in those patients who underwent complex PCI with TandemHeart support.[17] The 2015 SCAI/ACC/Heart Failure Society of American (HFSA)/Society of Thoracic Surgeons (STS) Expert Consensus suggest that TandemHeart may be considered in (1) severe LV dysfunction (ejection fraction [EF] <35%) or recent decompensated heart failure with associated technically challenging or prolonged PCI (depending on vascular anatomy, local expertise, and availability) and (2) continued deterioration of cardiogenic shock patients despite IABP and/or Impella 2.5 or Impella CP (Abiomed, Danvers, MA).[13]

## LEFT VENTRICULAR TO AORTA ASSIST DEVICES: IMPELLA

### Introduction and Components

The Impella is a percutaneous ventricular support device that uses a microaxial pump to move blood continuously from the LV to the ascending aorta. There are 3 classes available that provide increasing levels of LV support: Impella 2.5 (2.5 L/min; 12F system), Impella CP (approximately 3.5 L/min; 14F system), and the Impella 5.0 (5.0 L/min; 21F system). All 3 have been approved in the United States to provide hemodynamic support for up to 6 hours.

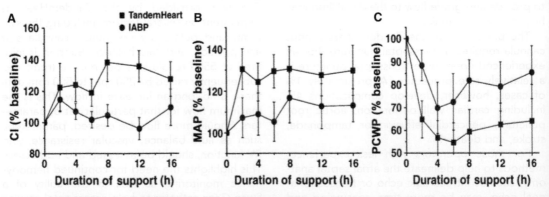

Fig. 10. Compared with the IABP, the patients who received the TandemHeart had a greater increase in cardiac index and mean arterial pressure (A, B) and decrease in pulmonary capillary wedge pressure (C) but no difference in severe adverse events of 30-day mortality. (Data from Burkhoff D, Cohen H, Brunckhorst C, et al. A randomized multicenter clinical study to evaluate the safety and efficacy of the TandemHeart percutaneous ventricular assist device versus conventional therapy with intraaortic balloon pumping for treatment of cardiogenic shock. Am Heart J 2006;152:469.e1–8.)

Additionally, based on data from trials, such as PROTECT I and PROTECT II,[9,18] the Impella 2.5 and, more recently, the Impella CP have been approved for use in hemodynamically stable patients undergoing elective or urgent HR-PCI.

The Impella support system is comprised of 3 major components: (1) catheter, (2) purge system, and (3) automated controller (Fig. 11). An impeller and its adjacent motor are located near the outlet area in the ascending aorta. As it rotates, negative pressure draws ventricular blood into the inlet area and through the cannula. The flow through the cannula is dependent on the rotation speed of the impeller for which there are 9 settings: P0 through P8. To protect the motor, the purge fluid (5% dextrose with heparin) forms a hydraulic pressure shield that prevents blood from migrating proximally past the impeller and into the motor housing.

## Hemodynamic Effects

There are 2 primary effects that the Impella imparts: (1) an unloading of the ventricle (lower end-diastolic volume and pressure) and (2) an increase in forward flow (higher mean arterial pressure). There is a reduction in LV end-diastolic pressure and volume that translates into decreased wall tension and myocardial oxygen demand.[13,14] Furthermore, there is evidence of improved coronary perfusion pressure and hyperemic flow velocity with a decrease in microvascular resistance with Impella 2.5.[13,14]

An important concept to recognize with Impella, as with other forms of LV support, is the device's reliance on a functional RV in providing LV filling (unless there is concurrent RV support). And although transient arrhythmias can be tolerated, more sustained tachycardias or asystole compromises the hemodynamic support.

## Technical Considerations and Contraindications

A common limitation to use of Impella support is the inadequacy of the peripheral vasculature in accommodating the large bore catheters. Although the Impella 2.5 (12F) and Impella CP (14F) can often be placed percutaneously via the femoral artery, the Impella 5.0 device requires a surgical cutdown of the femoral, axillary, or subclavian artery. There is a need for anticoagulation (goal ACT >250 s at placement, 160–180 s for maintenance), so the presence of a coagulopathy or recent hemorrhage may prohibit its use. The presence of a mechanical aortic valve or a LV mural thrombus precludes Impella use, as does significant aortic valve stenosis (valve area 0.6 cm$^2$ or less, except when performed with valvuloplasty) or insufficiency (2+ or greater by echo). These clinical parameters do not prohibit TandemHeart or ECMO utilization.

## Management

Appropriate postprocedural management of the Impella system is paramount. The Impella controller is an important tool that allows continuous automated oversight of device parameters and function. Although the device representative

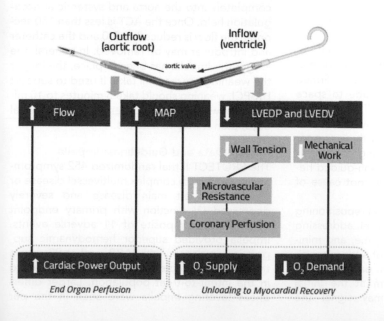

Fig. 11. Impella. The Impella support system comprises 3 major components: (1) catheter, (2) purge system, and (3) automated controller. (*Data from* Cardiogenic Shock Therapy with Impella Clinical Dossier.)

Outflow (aortic root)    Inflow (ventricle)

aortic valve

↑ Flow    ↑ MAP    ↓ LVEDP and LVEDV

↓ Wall Tension    ↓ Mechanical Work

↓ Microvascular Resistance

↑ Coronary Perfusion

↑ Cardiac Power Output    ↑ O$_2$ Supply    ↓ O$_2$ Demand

*End Organ Perfusion*    *Unloading to Myocardial Recovery*

is an invaluable resource for help with trouble-shooting, there are several scenarios with which operators should be familiar.

### Position monitoring

The automated Impella controller has 2 main displays that are useful in monitoring catheter position and function. The first is the home screen, which contains an alarm window that can display up to 3 alarms simultaneously with trouble-shooting suggestions. In addition, there is a central display area that displays an illustration of the determined Impella position with corresponding position indicator message. The placement screen displays 2 waveforms: placement signal waveform and motor current waveform. These waveforms signals can be used to determine the catheter position. If the catheter needs to be repositioned, then echocardiographic or fluoroscopic guidance is recommended.

A severely dysfunctional LV may be unable to generate a significant pressure difference across the aortic valve. This leads to dampening of the placement signal and motor current waveforms that limits their utility in determining catheter position. In this case, the operator must rely on patient hemodynamic parameter and imaging to monitor position.

During the initial placement of the Impella catheter, there is tendency for the catheter to dive forward into the ventricle. This can be avoided by taking precautionary steps, including placing the inlet area at approximately 3.5 cm below the aortic valve, removing the slack from the catheter over the aortic arch prior to starting the pump, tightening the Tuohy-Borst valve, and placing a leg immobilizer.

### Suction alarm

Suction may occur with the Impella due to improper positioning or inadequate LV volume. The Impella position should always be confirmed with imaging and adjustments made to space the inlet from the ventricular wall. Inadequate LV volume may be secondary to overall volume depletion but can be seen when there is poor RV function leading to poor filling of the left side. Echocardiographically or Swan-guided hemodynamics can help assess the root cause of a suction alarm.

When encountered with suction repositioning the catheter, decreasing the P-level, addressing disturbances in intravascular volume, and minimizing movement with the use of a leg immobilizer can be attempted. It is paramount to recognize that a suction alarm at the initial placement of the catheter may signal the presence of thrombus. If correct position has been confirmed, then the catheter may need to be removed and fully inspected while assuring that an appropriate ACT exists (>250 s). The presence of suction may lead to hemolysis.

### Hemolysis

Patients must be monitored for signs of possible hemolysis, such as new or worsening anemia and the presence of dark-colored urine. Laboratory testing may help confirm the presence of hemolysis, including bilirubin, lactate dehydrogenase, haptoglobin, and plasma-free hemoglobin. Hemolysis usually indicates improper position but may be due to 3 things: (1) inlet obstruction (position or volume), (2) obstruction within the cannula (eg, clot), and (3) outflow obstruction (AV or AO wall close to outlet). These scenarios can be visualized with transthoracic echo and Doppler assessment.

### Heparin-induced thrombocytopenia

If heparin-induced thrombocytopenia is suspected, then all heparin products should be stopped and confirmatory testing performed. The team must then make a risk-benefit decision as to continue without heparin in the system. Direct thrombin inhibitors may be used for systemic anticoagulation or in the purge solution (50).

### Weaning

Once a decision has been made to wean the patient from support, then the flow should be decreased 2 P-levels at a time as hemodynamically tolerated until reaching P-2. If a patient tolerates P-2, the catheter may be pulled completely into the aorta and systemic anticoagulation held. Once the ACT is less than 150 seconds, the flow is reduced to P-0 and the catheter and introducer may be removed. In general, the longer the Impella has been in place, the longer the weaning process will take. If used to support HR-PCI, weaning should take 5 minutes to 10 minutes; however, if it has been left in for several days, then it may take hours.

### Clinical Data and Guidelines: Impella

The PROTECT II trial randomized 452 symptomatic patients with complex multivessel disease or unprotected left main disease and severely depressed LV function with primary endpoint of a 30-day composite of 11 adverse events. Impella provided superior hemodynamic support in comparison with IABP, and at 90 days a trend toward decreased events was observed in the intent-to-treat population. Larger differences favoring Impella were seen in the per protocol population. A subsequent analysis redefining myocardial infarction as the development of new Q waves or creatine kinase–MB more than 8 times the upper limit of normal demonstrated lower rates of events, major cardiac adverse events, and cerebrovascular events in patients treated with Impella.[13,19–21]

The Catheter-based Ventricular Assist Device (cVAD) registry is an observational, multicenter, retrospective registry of patients supported with Impella 2.5, Impella CP, Impella 5.0, Impella LD, or Impella RP and reflects real-world use and suggests greater survival with pre-PCI Impella insertion compared with pre-PCI IABP and/or pharmacotherapy alone (Fig. 12).

Current guidelines for Impella use are summarized in Table 2.

## Impella RP

The RECOVER RIGHT study was conducted in 2014 to evaluate the safety and efficacy of the Impella RP. Findings included successful implantation in 90% of patients suffering from right heart failure and 73% successful survival to either 30 days or to hospital discharge.[22–24] The device is implanted into the femoral vein for inflow through the inferior vena cava to the outlet area in the pulmonary artery. Delivery is via a 0.08 wire preferentially placed in the left lower pulmonary artery.

The Impella RP is currently Food and Drug Administration approved for humanitarian device exemption for patients who develop acute right heart failure or decompensation after LVAD implantation, myocardial infarction, heart transplant, or open-heart surgery. Larger prospective study is ongoing.

## EXTRACORPOREAL MEMBRANE OXYGENATION

### Introduction and Components

ECMO is a form of mechanical cardiopulmonary support that can be provided for a prolonged period. There are 2 general modes of ECMO support: (1) venovenous (VV) and (2) venoarterial (VA) (Fig. 13). In VV-ECMO, blood is taken from the right atrium, then oxygenated, and $CO_2$ removed prior to being returned to the right atrium. This form of ECMO provides only respiratory support; patients are still dependent on their native hemodynamic condition. In contrast, VA-ECMO provides both respiratory and hemodynamic support. In this case, blood is pulled from the venous system (right atrium or inferior vena cava) and, after gas exchange, is delivered back to the arterial system at either central or peripheral cannulation sites.

There are a variety of configurations for an ECMO system; however, there are several fundamental components, including (1) drainage and perfusion cannulae, (2) centrifugal (most common) or roller pump, (3) membrane oxygenator and heat exchanger.

This discussion focuses on VA-ECMO and its role in hemodynamic support for patients with cardiogenic shock or requiring salvage during cardiac arrest. There several indications for VA-ECMO, all with the underlying notion that ultimately the patient is thought to have a reversible course of cardiac failure. This includes its

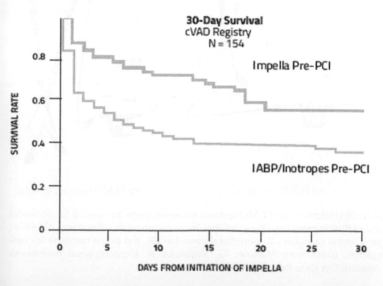

Fig. 12. The cVAD registry is an observational, multicenter, retrospective registry of patients supported with Impella 2.5, Impella CP, Impella 5.0, Impella LD, or Impella RP and reflects real-world use and suggests greater survival with pre-PCI Impella insertion compared with pre-PCI IABP and/or pharmacotherapy alone. (*Data from* O'Neill WW, Kleiman NS, Moses J, et al. A prospective, randomized clinical trial of hemodynamic support with Impella 2.5 versus intraaortic balloon pump in patients undergoing high-risk percutaneous coronary intervention: The PROTECT II study. Circulation 2012;126:1717–27.)

**30-Day Survival**
cVAD Registry
N = 154

Impella Pre-PCI

IABP/Inotropes Pre-PCI

SURVIVAL RATE

DAYS FROM INITIATION OF IMPELLA

**Table 2**
**Summary of guideline recommendations for Impella use**

| Clinical Society Guideline Populations[a] | Class | Latest Update | Impella Food and Drug Administration Approval |
|---|---|---|---|
| PCI in cardiogenic shock | I | 2013 | 2016 |
| Multiorgan failure, cardiogenic shock | I | 2013 | 2016 |
| PCI in low EF, complex CAD | IIb | 2011 | 2015 |
| Bridge to recovery or decision, cardiogenic shock | IIa | 2013 | 2016 |
| STEMI and cardiogenic shock | IIb | 2013 | 2016 |
| STEMI and urgent CABG | IIa | 2013 | 2016 |
| Acutely decompensated heart failure | IIa | 2012 | To be determined |
| Consensus document on hemodynamic support | N/A | 2015 | 2015/16 |

[a] ACCF, HFSA, Heart Rhythm Society, International Society for Heart & Lung Transplantation, SCAI, STS.
*Courtesy of* Cardiogenic Shock Therapy with Impella Clinical Dossier.

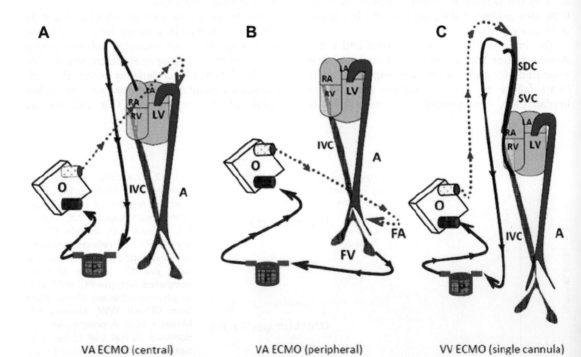

**VA ECMO (central)**          **VA ECMO (peripheral)**          **VV ECMO (single cannula)**

**Fig. 13.** ECMO: there are a variety of configurations for an ECMO system; however, there are several fundamental components, including (1) drainage and perfusion cannulae, (2) centrifugal (most common) or roller pump, (3) membrane oxygenator and heat exchanger. Central cannulae (*A*), peripheral cannulae (*B*), and single cannulae for respiratory support alone (*C*) are depicted. (*Data from* Martinez G, Vuylsteke A. Extracorporeal membrane oxygenation in adults. Contin Educ Anaesth Crit Care Pain 2012;12(2):57–61.)

common usage as a bridge to advanced heart failure therapies, such as LVAD and/or transplant.[25–27] Patients who fail to wean from cardiopulmonary bypass (CPB) after cardiac surgery can also be transitioned to VA-ECMO.[25–27]

## Hemodynamic Effects

There are 2 competing effects of ECMO on the LV. As blood is pulled from the venous system, there is a decrease in preload and consequently the end-diastolic volume and end-diastolic pressure in the LV, which reduces wall tension and work. In contrast, as blood returns to the arterial system there is an increase in afterload and work.[28]

## Technical Considerations and Contraindications

Contraindications to ECMO include the presence of an irreversible process, multiorgan failure, prolonged cardiopulmonary resuscitation (CPR) (>60 mins), aortic dissection, and severe aortic regurgitation. In addition, patients with active bleeding or with contraindication to anticoagulation are generally not candidates for ECMO support. Another factor to consider includes the presence of significant peripheral arterial disease.

Cannulae for VA ECMO can be placed either centrally or peripherally. Central access usually consists of the drainage cannula placed the in the right atrium and the perfusion cannula in the ascending aorta. This approach requires a sternotomy or thoracotomy and is most often an option for those surgical patients who fail to wean from CPB. Peripheral cannulation may require a cutdown but can often be performed percutaneously. The drainage cannula may access the venous circulation at the jugular or femoral vein. The perfusion cannula is most often placed in the femoral artery but may also use the axillary, subclavian, or in rare circumstances the carotid artery (although this site is more commonly used in infants). In femoral artery cannulation, especially in patients with peripheral vascular disease, there may be a need to place an additional cannula into the femoral artery directing blood flow anterograde down the ipsilateral limb to prevent ischemia (**Fig. 14**).[29]

## Management

The active management of ECMO can become complex and its discussion is outside of the scope of this article. This article aims to address several of the more practical aspects to management. A perfusionist is required to manage the

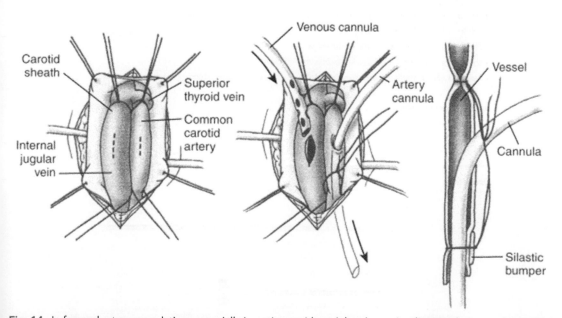

**Fig. 14.** In femoral artery cannulation, especially in patients with peripheral vascular disease, there may be a need to place an additional cannula into the femoral artery directing blood flow anterograde down the ipsilateral limb to prevent ischemia. (*Data from* Frischer JS, Stolar CJ. Extracorproeal membrane oxygenation. In: Holcomb GW, Murphy JP, Ostlie DJ. Ashcraft's Pediatric Surgery. 5th edition. Philadelphia: Elsevier; 2010. p. 74–86.)

ECMO circuits and should be present during any procedure in the cardiac catheterization laboratory. Anticoagulation is key in preventing the formation of thrombus in the system. Heparin is most commonly used with goal ACT of 180 to 250.

Common complications include bleeding, thrombosis, infection, and limb ischemia (58). Hemorrhage is often seen and most commonly involves the access site but may occur in any organ and can be devastating when the central nervous system is involved.[27,28] The risk of thrombosis can range from 8% to 17%.[27,28] Managing the balance between the risks for hemorrhage and thrombosis requires frequent monitoring. The risk of infection of any indwelling line must be recognized and appropriate aseptic procedures followed. Limb ischemia can be secondary to a direct effect of the cannula interrupting distal flow or from an embolic phenomenon. Supplemental antegrade flow via a cannula placed in the femoral artery, as discussed previously, may be help circumvent this problem. Other options include a cannula placed in the dorsalis pedis or posterior tibial arteries.[27,28]

## CLINICAL DATA AND GUIDELINES: EXTRACORPOREAL MEMBRANE OXYGENATION

There are no large randomized controlled trials on use of ECMO. The Extracorporeal Life Support Organization registry, however, demonstrated a 27% survival to hospital discharge.[13,30] More recently, a 49% survival was demonstrated with the use of either mechanical support or ECMO in cardiogenic shock.[13,31–33] Current expert guidelines recommend the use of ECMO when concomitant hypoxemia and RV failure are present.

## PERCUTANEOUS HEART PUMP

The SHIELD II trial is a prospective, randomized multicenter trial comparing HeartMate PHP (Thoratec, Pleasanton, CA) to the Impella 2.5 in patients undergoing HR-PCI. The PHP device is capable of generating 4 L/min to 5 L/min flow with the advantage of percutaneous insertion via a 14F introducer sheath. Once positioned across the aortic valve, the outer sheath of the PHP is retracted, thereby fully expanding the cannula to 24F (Fig. 15). The study is currently

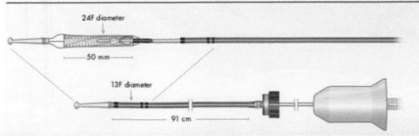

Fig. 15. The HeartMate PHP (Thoratec) is capable of generating 4 L/min to 5 L/min flow with the advantage of percutaneous insertion via a 14F introducer sheath. Once positioned across the aortic valve, the outer sheath of the PHP is retracted, thereby fully expanding the cannula to 24F. (*Courtesy of* Thoratec, Pleasanton, CA.)

**Table 3**
Options for mechanical device support in acute decompensated heart failure and cardiogenic shock

| Device | Pump Type | Vascular Access | Trigger | Maximum Support |
|---|---|---|---|---|
| IABP | Volume displacement pump | Femoral artery for 7F or 8F sheath | ECG or Pressure | Dependent on native circulation; 0.5 L/min |
| Impella | Axial continuous flow pump | Percutaneous—Impella 2.5 (12F) and Impella CP (14F) via femoral artery<br>Surgical cutdown of the femoral, axillary, or subclavian artery—Impella 5.0 (21F) | Continuous flow | Impella 2.5 (2.5 L/min) and Impella CP (approximately 3.5 L/min)<br>Impella 5.0 (5.0 L/min) |
| TandemHeart | Centrifugal continuous flow pump | 21F inflow cannula into femoral vein with transseptal placement into the LA<br>15F or 17F outflow cannula into femoral artery | Continuous flow | 15F—4.0 L/min<br>17F—5.0 L/min |
| VV-ECMO | Respiratory support alone | RA to oxygenator back to RA | Continuous oxygenation dependent on native circulation | Dependent on native circulation |
| VA-ECMO | Respiratory and hemodynamic support | Sternotomy or thoracotomy—central access—drainage cannula placed the in the right atrium and the perfusion cannula in the ascending aorta<br>Percutaneous—peripheral access—venous drainage cannula may access (jugular or femoral vein) and the arterial perfusion cannula (femoral, axillary, subclavian, carotid arteries) | Continuous oxygenation and hemodynamic flow and support | Complete CPB |

It is best to match device with severity of cardiogenic shock right from the initial clinical assessment rather than proceeding with a fixed predetermined algorithm of escalation of device therapy.

**Table 4**
**Hemodynamic impacts of the available pharmacologic and mechanical support options**

| | Inotropes | Intra-aortic Balloon Pump | Extracorporeal Membrane Oxygenation | TandemHeart | Impella | Surgical Ventricular Assist Device |
|---|---|---|---|---|---|---|
| **Advantages** | | | | | | |
| Flow (L/min) | <0.5 | 0.5 | 4 | 3.5 | 2.5–5.0 | 6.0 |
| Coronary perfusion | ↑ | ↑↑ | – | – | ↑↑ | ↑↑ |
| LV end-diastolic pressure | ↑ | ↓ | ↑↑↑↑ | ↓↓ | ↓↓↓ | ↓↓↓↓ |
| **Limitations** | | | | | | |
| Arrhythmia | +++ | – | – | – | – | – |
| Stoke | – | ++ | ++ | + | + | +++ |
| Limb ischemia | NA | + | +++ | ++ | + | NA |
| Bleeding | NA | ++ | ++++ | +++ | +/++ | ++++ |
| Cost | $ | $ | $$$ | $$$ | $$$ | $$$$$ |

enrolling and primary endpoint includes 90-day composite analysis of cardiac death, myocardial infarction, stroke, repeat revascularization (PCI or coronary artery bypass graft), bleeding (Bleeding Academic Research Consortium type 3 or 5), aortic insufficiency +2° over baseline, and severe hypotension (defined as systolic blood pressure <90 mm Hg while on a device support requiring inotropic/pressor medications to restore hemodynamics).[34]

## SUMMARY

In the current era, failure of maximal medical therapy is no longer a justifiable endpoint given the array of available advanced mechanical

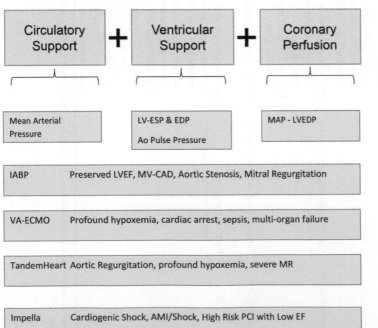

Fig. 16. Optimal patient selection for AMCS pumps. AMCS, acute mechanical circulatory support; EDP, end diastolic pressure; ESP, end systolic pressure; MAP, mean arterial pressure; MR, mitral regurgitation; MV-CAD, multivessel coronary artery disease. (*Data from* Kapur NK, Esposito ML. Door to unload: a new paradigm for the management of cardiogenic shock. Curr Cardiovasc Risk Rep 2016;10:41.)

options.[1,2,12,35–37] Deciding which device is most suitable depends largely on the degree of support needed (**Tables 3 and 4**). It is best to match device with severity of cardiogenic shock right from the initial clinical assessment rather than proceeding with a fixed predetermined algorithm of escalation of device therapy (**Fig. 16**). Certain hemodynamic parameters, such as cardiac index, pulmonary artery pulsatility index, pulmonary artery systolic pressure, and pulmonary capillary wedge pressure, can also be used to match mechanical support needed for the degree of LV and/or RV failure (**Figs. 17 and 18**).

These temporary support devices, if implemented in a timely fashion, can often bridge patients to decision, recovery, long-term support devices (VADs and total artificial heart), and/or heart transplant. They can even be sued as adjunct support for HR procedures targeting the underlying cardiogenic shock etiology (eg, HR-PCI) (see **Fig. 17**). Underlying successful device selection and ultimate outcome requires a multidisciplinary heart team approach, including heart failure specialists, interventional cardiologists, and cardiothoracic surgeons, along with patient preferences executed in a timely fashion. Door to support

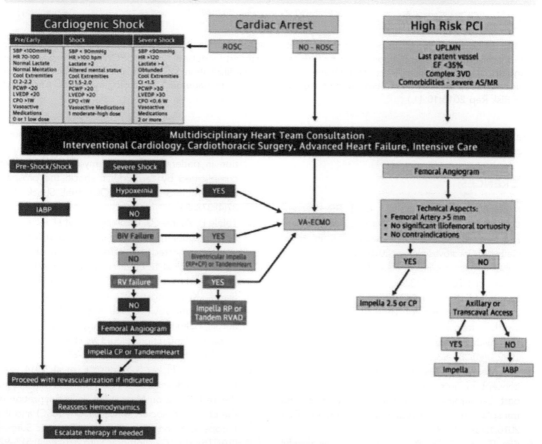

**CENTRAL ILLUSTRATION: Algorithm for Percutaneous MCS Device Selection in Patients with Cardiogenic Shock, Cardiac Arrest, and HR-PCI**

**Fig. 17.** Algorithm for percutaneous MCS device selection in patients with cardiogenic shock, cardiac arrest, and HR-PCI. 3VD, 3-vessel coronary artery disease; AS, aortic stenosis; BiV, biventricular; CI, cardiac index; CPO, cardiac power; HR, heart rate; LVEDP, LV end-diastolic pressure; MCS, mechanical circulatory support; MR, mitral regurgitation; PCWP, pulmonary capillary wedge pressure; ROSC, return of spontaneous circulation; RVAD, right VAD; SBP, systolic blood pressure; UPLMN, unprotected left main artery. (*Data from* Atkinson T, Ohman EM, O'Neill WW, et al. A practical approach to mechanical circulatory support in patients undergoing percutaneous coronary intervention. Interventional Scientific Council of the American College of Cardiology. JACC Cardiovasc Interv 2016;9(9):871–83.)

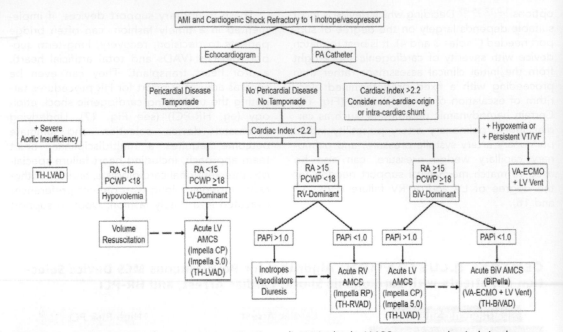

**Fig. 18.** Proposed algorithm for patient presenting in cardiogenic shock. AMCS, acute mechanical circulatory support; BiV, biventricular; PA, pulmonary artery; PAPi, pulmonary artery pulsatility index; PCWP, pulmonary capillary wedge pressure; TH, tandem heart; Vent, LV vent; VF, ventricular fibrillation; VT, ventricular tachycardia. (*Data from* Kapur NK, Esposito ML. Door to unload: a new paradigm for the management of cardiogenic shock. Curr Cardiovasc Risk Rep 2016;10:41.)

time is one of the most influential parameters in successful outcomes.

## REFERENCES

1. Kapur NK, Dimas V, Sorajja P, et al. The Interventional Heart Failure Initiative: a mission statement for the next generation of invasive cardiologists. Catheter Cardiovasc Interv 2015;86(2):353–5.

2. Kapur NK. Interventional Heart Failure. Cardiac Interventions Today 2013.

3. Samuels LE, Kaufman MS, Thomas MP, et al. Pharmacological criteria for ventricular assist device insertion following postcardiotomy shock: experience with the Abiomed BVS system. J Card Surg 1999;14(4):288–93.

4. Thompson KA, Philip KJ, Simsir S, et al. The new concept of 'interventional heart failure therapy': part 2–inotropes, valvular disease, pumps, and transplantation. J Cardiovasc Pharmacol Ther 2010;15(3):231–43.

5. Kim JT, Lee JR, Kim JK, et al. The carina as a useful radiographic landmark for positioning the intraaortic balloon pump. Anesth Analg 2007;105(3):735–8.

6. Estep JD, Cordero-Reyes AM, Bhimaraj A, et al. Percutaneous Placement of an Intra-Aortic Balloon Pump in the Left Axillary/Subclavian Position Provides Safe, Ambulatory Long-Term Support as Bridge to Heart Transplantation. JACC Heart Fail 2013;1(5):382–8.

7. Prondzinsky R, Unverzagt S, Russ M, et al. Hemodynamic effects of intra-aortic balloon counterpulsation in patients with acute myocardial infarction complicated by cardiogenic shock: the prospective, randomized IABP SHOCK trial. Shock 2012; 37(4):378–84.

8. Thiele H, Zeymer U, Neumann FJ, et al. Intra-aortic balloon counterpulsation in acute myocardial infarction complicated by cardiogenic shock (IABP-SHOCK II): final 12 month results of a randomised, open-label trial. Lancet 2013;382(9905):1638–45.

9. Sjauw KD, Engström AE, Vis MM, et al. A systematic review and meta-analysis of intra-aortic balloon pump therapy in ST-elevation myocardial infarction: should we change the guidelines? Eur Heart J 2009;30(4):459–68.

10. Kolh P, Windecker S, Alfonso F, et al. 2014 ESC/EACTS Guidelines on myocardial revascularization: the Task Force on Myocardial Revascularization of the European Society of Cardiology (ESC) and the European Association for Cardio-Thoracic Surgery (EACTS). Eur J Cardiothorac Surg 2014;46(4):517–92.

11. Stretch R, Sauer CM, Yuh DD, et al. National trends in the utilization of short-term mechanical circulatory support: incidence, outcomes, and cost analysis. J Am Coll Cardiol 2014;64(14):1407–15.

12. Atkinson T, Ohman EM, O'Neill WW, et al. A practical approach to mechanical circulatory support in patients undergoing percutaneous coronary

intervention. Interventional Scientific Council of the American College of Cardiology. JACC Cardiovasc Interv 2016;9(9):871–83.

13. Rihal CS, Naidu SS, Givertz MM, et al. 2015 SCAI/ACC/HFSA/STS Clinical Expert Consensus Statement on the Use of Percutaneous Mechanical Circulatory Support Devices in Cardiovascular Care. J Am Coll Cardiol 2015;65(19):2140–1.

14. Naidu SS. Novel percutaneous cardiac assist devices. Circulation 2011;123:533–43. originally published February 7, 2011.

15. Kar B, Gregoric ID, Basra SS, et al. The percutaneous ventricular assist device in severe refractory cardiogenic shock. J Am Coll Cardiol 2011;57:688–96.

16. Burkhoff D, Cohen H, Brunckhorst C, et al. A randomized multicenter clinical study to evaluate the safety and efficacy of the TandemHeart percutaneous ventricular assist device versus conventional therapy with intraaortic balloon pumping for treatment of cardiogenic shock. Am Heart J 2006;152:469.e1-8.

17. Alli OO, Singh IM, Holmes DR Jr, et al. Percutaneous left ventricular assist device with TandemHeart for high-risk percutaneous coronary intervention: The Mayo Clinic experience. Catheter Cardiovasc Interv 2012;80:728–34.

18. Krishna M, Zacharowski K. Principles of intra-aortic balloon pump counterpulsation. Contin Educ Anaesth Crit Care Pain 2009;9(1):24–8.

19. O'Neill WW, Kleiman NS, Moses J, et al. A prospective, randomized clinical trial of hemodynamic support with Impella 2.5 versus intraaortic balloon pump in patients undergoing high-risk percutaneous coronary intervention: The PROTECT II study. Circulation 2012;126:1717–27.

20. Dangas GD, Kini AS, Sharma SK, et al. Impact of hemodynamic support with Impella 2.5 versus intraaortic balloon pump on prognostically important clinical outcomes in patients undergoing high-risk percutaneous coronary intervention (from the PROTECT II randomized trial). Am J Cardiol 2014;113:222–8.

21. Cohen MG, Ghatak A, Kleiman NS, et al. Optimizing rotational atherectomy in high-risk percutaneous coronary interventions: Insights from the PROTECT Iotaiota study. Catheter Cardiovasc Interv 2014;83:1057–64.

22. Anderson MB, Goldstein J, Milano C, et al. Benefits of a novel percutaneous ventricular assist device for right heart failure: The prospective RECOVER RIGHT study of the Impella RP device. J Heart Lung Transplant 2015;34(12):1549–60.

23. Ragosta M. Textbook of clinical hemodynamics. Philadelphia: Saunders/Elsevier; 2008.

24. Martinez G, Vuylsteke A. Extracorporeal membrane oxygenation in adults. Contin Educ Anaesth Crit Care Pain 2012;12(2):57–61.

25. Rousse N, Juthier F, Pinçon C, et al. ECMO as a bridge to decision: Recovery, VAD, or heart transplantation? Int J Cardiol 2015;187:620–7.

26. Chung JC, Tsai PR, Chou NK, et al. Extracorporeal membrane oxygenation bridge to adult heart transplantation. Clin Transplant 2010;24(3):375–80.

27. Abrams D. Extracorporeal membrane oxygenation in cardiopulmonary disease in adults. J Am Coll Cardiol 2014;63(25 Pt A):2769–78.

28. Burkhoff D. Hemodynamics of mechanical circulatory support. J Am Coll Cardiol 2015;66(23):2663–74.

29. Gaffney AM, Wildhirt SM, Griffin MJ, et al. Extracorporeal life support. BMJ 2010;341:c5317.

30. Thiagarajan RR, Brogan TV, Scheurer MA, et al. Extracorporeal membrane oxygenation to support cardiopulmonary resuscitation in adults. Ann Thorac Surg 2009;87:778–85.

31. Takayama H, Truby L, Koekort M, et al. Clinical outcome of mechanical circulatory support for refractory cardiogenic shock in the current era. J Heart Lung Transplant 2013;32:106–11.

32. Frischer JS, Stolar CJ. Extracorproeal membrane oxygenation. In: Holcomb GW, Murphy JP, Ostlie DJ, editors. Ashcraft's Pediatric Surgery. 5th edition. Philadelphia: Elsevier; 2010. p. 74–86.

33. Kapur NK, Esposito ML. Door to unload: a new paradigm for the management of cardiogenic shock. Curr Cardiovasc Risk Rep 2016;10:41. http://dx.doi.org/10.1007/s12170-016-0524-3.

34. Supporting Patients Undergoing HIgh-Risk PCI Using a High-Flow PErcutaneous Left Ventricular Support Device (SHIELD II) (SHIELD II). Available at: https://clinicaltrials.gov/show/NCT02468778. Accessed September 1, 2016.

35. Shekar K, Gregory SD, Fraser JF, et al. Mechanical circulatory support in the new era: an overview. Crit Care 2016;20:66.

36. Burkhoff D, Naidu SS. The science behind percutaneous hemodynamic support: a review and comparison of support strategies. Catheter Cardiovasc Interv 2012;80(5):816–29.

37. Morley D, Litwak K, Ferber P, et al. Hemodynamic effects of partial ventricular support in chronic heart failure: results of simulation validated with in vivo data. J Thorac Cardiovasc Surg 2007;133(1):21–8.

# Multivessel Revascularization in Shock and High-Risk Percutaneous Coronary Intervention

Sandeep K. Krishnan, MD, Robert F. Riley, MD, MS,
Ravi S. Hira, MD, William L. Lombardi, MD*

## KEYWORDS

- Multivessel revascularization • Percutaneous coronary intervention • Coronary artery disease
- Cardiogenic shock • Revascularization

## KEY POINTS

- Current guidelines support multivessel percutaneous coronary intervention in the setting of cardiogenic shock.
- It remains to be determined if those benefits extend consistently to patients with stable coronary artery disease.
- Trials underway, including COMPLETE and OPEN-CTO—along with many others, may help to address these questions.
- It is clear that clinicians must remain vigilant to do what is best for each patient on a case-by-case basis after discussing all options.

## MULTIVESSEL CORONARY ARTERY DISEASE AND CARDIOGENIC SHOCK

Approximately 40% to 60% of patients undergoing percutaneous revascularization have multivessel coronary artery disease (CAD), defined as 70% or greater stenosis in 2 or more coronary arteries or involving the left main.[1] Coronary artery bypass grafting (CABG) continues to carry a class I recommendation for many of these patients from the latest American College of Cardiology/American Heart Association guidelines statement,[2] but as many as 30% to 40% of patients with multivessel disease (MVD) and class I indications for CABG undergo percutaneous coronary intervention (PCI) despite its class II recommendation in most patients with MVD.[3] The use of PCI in these patients may be partially explained by patient preference, anatomic factors, or comorbidities that preclude surgical candidacy.[4] Technical advancements in PCI and recent studies comparing PCI with CABG may justify multivessel PCI as a reasonable alternative for certain patients.[5–8] Moreover, in the setting of cardiogenic shock (CS), most guidelines tend to support the use of PCI as a therapeutic alternative to CABG in this setting.[2,9]

CS is a result of end-organ hypoperfusion owing to left ventricular (LV), right ventricular, or biventricular myocardial dysfunction resulting in systolic and/or diastolic myocardial pump failure.[10] Acute myocardial infarction accounts for approximately 75% of all patients with CS.[11,12] CS complicates 8.6% of ST-segment elevation myocardial infarctions (STEMI)[13] and 2.5% of non-STEMI,[14] is associated with a 60% to 70% mortality rate, and remains the leading cause of death in patients hospitalized with myocardial infarction in the era of reperfusion.[15] The only therapy found to improve outcomes in this

Division of Cardiology, University of Washington, School of Medicine, 1959 Northeast Pacific Street, Seattle, WA 98195, USA

* Corresponding author. Division of Cardiology, University of Washington Medical Center, 1959 Northeast Pacific Street, Seattle, WA 98103.
E-mail address: lombaw@cardiology.washington.edu

Intervent Cardiol Clin 6 (2017) 407–416
http://dx.doi.org/10.1016/j.iccl.2017.03.009
2211-7458/17/© 2017 Elsevier Inc. All rights reserved.

patient group remains revascularization, particularly complete revascularization.[9] However, given the potential negative outcomes associated with PCI, especially in the setting of shock (increased risk of stent thrombosis, ongoing ischemia, contrast-induced nephropathy, and longer radiation exposure[16]), multivessel revascularization during the initial presentation of CS continues to remain an infrequent practice despite its broad acceptance in the literature. Further, although the highest risk cases have the greatest incremental mortality benefit from treatment, they are simultaneously the least desirable to treat owing to the increased risk of adverse outcomes. This likely leads to errors of omission with patients being less likely to undergo cardiac catheterization in the setting of CS.

## CARDIOGENIC SHOCK

CS is defined by hemodynamic and clinical parameters. Hemodynamic parameters include persistent hypotension (systolic blood pressure <80–90 mm Hg or mean arterial pressure 30 mm Hg lower than baseline) for longer than 30 minutes, a cardiac index of less than 1.8 L/min/m$^2$ without support or less than 2.0 to 2.2 L/min/m$^2$ with support, and elevated filling pressures (LV end-diastolic pressure >18 mm Hg or right ventricular end-diastolic pressure >10–15 mm Hg). Clinically, signs and symptoms of hypoperfusion (ie, cool extremities, nausea, decreased urine output, and/or altered mental status) help to diagnose CS.[10] Decreased perfusion and end-organ dysfunction leads to lactic acidosis, catecholamine and neurohormonal release, along with activation of systemic inflammatory and coagulation cascades. This eventually results in a downward spiral (**Fig. 1**) with further myocardial depression and hypoperfusion.[17,18]

CS presents with a wide clinical spectrum ranging from "preshock" (significant risk of developing CS), "mild" CS (responsive to low-dose inotropes/vasopressors), "profound" CS (responsive to high-dose inotropes/vasopressors and intraaortic balloon pump [IABP]), and "severe refractory" CS (unresponsive to high-dose inotropes/vasopressors and IABP). The aim is to restore adequate perfusion and prevent end-organ dysfunction thus breaking the downward spiral of untreated CS. Given that many patients with CS present with acute coronary syndromes (ACS), these diagnoses and their pathologies are inextricably linked. Moreover, a large majority of these patients also have MVD as their etiology for CS.[19]

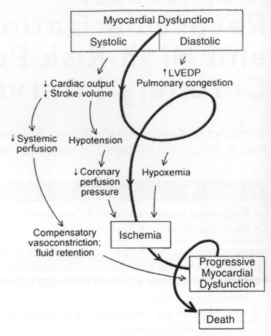

**Fig. 1.** The downward spiral in cardiogenic shock. LVEDP, left ventricular end-diastolic pressure. (*Reprinted from* Hollenberg SM, Kavinsky CJ, Parrillo JE. Cardiogenic shock. Ann Intern Med 1999;131:49; with permission.)

### Patients with Multivessel Disease Presenting with Acute Coronary Syndrome

Patients with MVD can be divided into 2 broad categories: those presenting with and those presenting without concurrent CS. Those patients with ACS, multivessel CAD, and also CS have a class I guideline recommendation from both American and European cardiac societies for CR (either surgical or percutaneous). Data supporting these recommendations were initially shown in the SHOCK trial (Should We Emergently Revascularize Occluded Coronaries for Cardiogenic Shock) and more recently in the IMPRESS in Severe Shock (IMPella vs IABP REduces mortality in STEMI patients treated with primary PCI in Severe cardiogenic SHOCK) trial. Those patients with ACS and multivessel CAD who do not present in CS are addressed by the PRAMI (Preventive Angioplasty in Acute Myocardial Infarction) and CvLPRIT (Complete vs Lesion-Only Primary PCI) data, currently with a class IIb recommendation in the guidelines for CR.[2,9]

The SHOCK trial, published in 1999, provided a modicum of clarity regarding the revascularization of patients presenting with CS. This study was a randomized trial comparing 2 treatment strategies—emergency revascularization and initial medical stabilization—at 30 centers. For patients assigned to revascularization, angioplasty or bypass surgery had to be performed as soon as possible and within 6 hours of randomization. For patients assigned to medical stabilization, intensive medical therapy was required. Intraaortic balloon counterpulsation (IABP) and thrombolytic therapy were recommended. Delayed revascularization at a minimum of 54 hours after randomization was recommended if clinically appropriate. The primary endpoint of the study was overall mortality 30 days after randomization. Secondary endpoints consisted of overall mortality 6 and 12 months after infarction. At 30 days, overall mortality did not differ significantly between the revascularization and medical therapy groups (46.7% and 56.0%, respectively; difference, −9.3%; 95% confidence interval [CI] for the difference, −20.5% to 1.9%; $P = .11$). However, the 6-month mortality was lower in the revascularization group than in the medical therapy group (50.3% vs 63.1%; $P = .027$).[20] This study highlighted the importance of revascularization in patients in CS with 85% of patients in the revascularization arm having MVD.[20] Despite these data, most patients with CS still do not undergo emergency revascularization, either because of lack of facilities at the hospitals where they present or because of doubt as to its efficacy.[21–24]

The IMPRESS trial was published as an exploratory assessment of mortality and other safety outcomes comparing percutaneous mechanical circulatory support with the Impella CP with IABP in mechanically ventilated patients with CS from acute myocardial infarction. Like the SHOCK trial, the primary study endpoint was 30-day overall mortality. The secondary endpoint was 6-month all-cause mortality. All patients underwent primary PCI. In MVD, the mode of revascularization (immediate or staged PCI of the nonculprit lesions) was left to the discretion of the operator. A total of 48 patients were randomly assigned to either Impella (n = 24) or IABP (n = 24). The mean age was 58 years, 79% were male, all patients were mechanically ventilated, 96% of the patients received catecholamines, and 92% had had a cardiac arrest before randomization. The authors found no difference at 30 days or 6 months between the 2 therapies. Further analysis showed no significant interaction in 30-day mortality between the IABP and patients treated with percutaneous mechanical circulatory support with respect to age, sex, return of spontaneous circulation times, lactate levels on admission,

moment of IABP or percutaneous mechanical circulatory support placement, systolic blood pressure before device placement, or traumatic injuries on admission. However, 96% of patients were post cardiac arrest (with a mean time of >20 minutes from start of cardiopulmonary resuscitation until the return of spontaneous circulation in both arms) and 23% were diagnosed with anoxic brain injury, indicating a poor prognosis before randomization. The majority of patients (46/48 subjects) were on catecholamines before MCS insertion and more than 80% of patients in both groups had devices placed after the intervention; these devices may have been placed beyond their potential therapeutic window. Finally, although 75% of subjects had multivessel CAD, less than 20% of these patients had PCI of nonculprit lesions, despite the current guidelines for CR in CS. Therefore, the IMPRESS trial can only be viewed as an exploratory analysis. It demonstrates the feasibility of a larger trial powered to study the aforementioned outcomes with a design that meets guideline-mediated standard of care.

The PRAMI and CvLPRIT trials also examined patients with MVD. The primary aim of the PRAMI trial was to determine whether performing PCI in nonculprit coronary arteries with obstructive CAD as part of the procedure to treat the infarct artery would reduce the combined incidence of death from cardiac causes, nonfatal myocardial infarction, or refractory angina. Four hundred sixty-five consecutive patients of any age with acute STEMI and multivessel coronary disease detected at the time of emergency PCI were enrolled at 5 coronary care centers. This trial excluded those patients in CS or with high-risk lesions (chronic total occlusions [CTO] or stenoses of the left main coronary artery). After the completion of PCI in the infarcted artery, eligible patients were randomly assigned to undergo no further PCI procedures or to undergo immediate preventive PCI in noninfarcted arteries with more than 50% stenoses (preventive PCI). The primary outcome was a composite of death from cardiac causes, nonfatal myocardial infarction, or refractory angina, and each of the components was also assessed individually. Secondary outcomes were death from noncardiac causes and repeat revascularization procedures (PCI or CABG).[25]

During a mean follow-up of 23 months, the primary outcome occurred in 21 patients assigned to preventive PCI and in 53 patients assigned to culprit-only PCI, which translated into rates of 9 events per 100 patients and 23 per 100, respectively (hazard ratio in the preventive PCI group, 0.35; 95% CI, 0.21–0.58; P<.001). Hazard ratios for the 3 components of the primary outcome were 0.34 (95% CI, 0.11–1.08) for death from cardiac causes, 0.32 (95% CI, 0.13–0.75) for nonfatal myocardial infarction, and 0.35 (95% CI, 0.18–0.69) for refractory angina—all significant. Thus, the authors concluded that in patients with STEMI and multivessel CAD undergoing infarct artery PCI, preventive PCI in nonculprit coronary arteries with stenoses of greater than 50% significantly reduced the risk of adverse cardiovascular events, as compared with PCI limited to the infarct artery.[25] Although this trial specifically excluded patients with concurrent CS, it did show an improvement in major adverse cardiovascular events (MACE) for subjects who underwent CR compared with culprit-only PCI.

Similarly, the CvLPRIT trial from 2015 is a UK multicenter, randomized, open-label study that set out to test the feasibility, safety, and potential benefit of undertaking in-hospital CR of angiographically significant nonculprit lesions in patients presenting with primary PCI for STEMI compared with PCI of the infarct-related artery alone. The hypothesis was that early treatment of significant nonculprit lesions during the index admission would reduce the global ischemic burden and protect against short- and medium-term recurrent ischemic events. CvLPRIT and PRAMI ask similar questions, but were initiated independently with slight differences in trial design. If patients fulfilled inclusion criteria after angiography, randomization was performed before culprit PCI in contrast with the PRAMI trial, in which patients were randomized after culprit lesion PCI was complete. In the PRAMI trial, if the patients were randomized to undergo PCI to nonculprit vessels it had to be performed immediately. In CvLPRIT, PCI of nonculprit vessels could be performed at any point during the index hospitalization. Patients were randomized to 1 of 2 groups after PCI: either CR (including all nonculprit lesions) or culprit-only treatment. Randomization was stratified by infarct location (anterior/nonanterior) and symptom onset (≤3 hours or >3 hours). There were 296 patients were randomized (146 to culprit-only and 150 to CR).

In the culprit-only PCI arm, 7 patients (5%) crossed over to receive CR. In the CR group, 11 patients (7%) received culprit-only PCI only, with 3 of these referred for CABG. On the basis of the operator decision, 64% of the CR group received noninfarct artery revascularization at the same procedural session as culprit lesion PCI. MACE was significantly lower in the

complete revascularization arm (10.0%) than in the culprit-only arm (21.2%; hazard ratio, 0.45; 95% CI, 0.24–0.84; P = .009). The individual components of the primary endpoint and cardiovascular mortality were all also lower, although none were statistically significant. There was no increase in stroke, major bleeding, or contrast-induced nephropathy in the CR group. CvLPRIT demonstrated that, in patients undergoing PCI for STEMI, CR during the index admission resulted in a significantly lower MACE rate at 12 months than when only the infarct-related artery was treated, with early separation of clinical event curves. Additionally, there was an incidence of predischarge HF, which prolonged hospitalization, with double the number (n = 7) in the culprit-only group compared with the CR group (n = 3).[26]

The ACUITY trial (Acute Catheterization and Urgent Intervention Triage Strategy) from 2012 provided further evidence that complete revascularization should be the goal in most cases of ACS. ACUITY was a multicenter, prospective, randomized trial of 13,819 patients with moderate- and high-risk non–ST-elevation ACS treated with an early invasive management strategy. Patients were randomly assigned before coronary angiography to heparin plus a glycoprotein IIb/IIIa inhibitor, bivalirudin plus a glycoprotein IIb/IIIa inhibitor, or bivalirudin monotherapy. Angiography was performed in all patients within 72 hours of randomization. Depending on coronary anatomy and the suitability of lesions for revascularization, patients were triaged to PCI, CABG, or medical management. In patients who were triaged to PCI, selection of stent type (bare metal or drug eluting) was at the operator's discretion. Regardless of stent type, dual antiplatelet therapy with aspirin and clopidogrel was recommended for at least 1 year.[27]

In these ACS patients, incomplete revascularization was variably defined if any lesion with diameter stenosis (DS) cutoffs ranging from 30% or more to 70% or more with a reference vessel diameter of 2.0 mm or greater remained after PCI. The primary outcome was 1-year composite rate of MACE (death, myocardial infarction, or ischemia-driven unplanned revascularization). The 1-year MACE rate was increased among patients with incomplete revascularization using all of the DS cutoffs. Incomplete revascularization (≥50% DS) was associated with higher 1-year rates of myocardial infarction (12.0% vs 8.2%; hazard ratio, 1.50; 95% CI, 1.18–1.89; P = .0007) and ischemia-driven unplanned revascularization (15.7% vs 10.2%; hazard ratio, 1.58; 95% CI, 1.28–1.96;

$P<.0001$). By multivariable analysis, incomplete revascularization ($\geq$50% DS) was an independent predictor of 1-year MACE (hazard ratio, 1.36; 95% CI, 1.12–1.64; $P = .002$).[27]

In the recently published KAMIR study (Korean Acute Myocardial Infarction Registry), data from 31,149 patients with STEMI and non-STEMI between 2006 and 2013 were retrieved and analyzed in this prospective, multicenter (53 centers participated), observational, registry-based study. One objective of the study was to compare the outcomes of patients presenting with ACS who underwent multivessel versus culprit-only revascularization. Primary outcomes were in-hospital mortality and all-cause death during follow-up. Secondary outcomes included cardiac death, recurrent myocardial infarction, any revascularization and MACE, consisting of all-cause death, recurrent myocardial infarction and any revascularization during follow-up. Multivessel revascularization was defined as PCI of a significant stenosis in a nonculprit vessel during admission. Procedural success was defined as Thrombolysis in Myocardial Infarction (TIMI) flow grade 3 in the infarct-related artery and less than 30% diameter residual stenosis in the treated segment at the end of the procedure. Adjusted incidences of in hospital mortality (2.4% vs 9.3%; $P<.001$) and all-cause death during follow-up (4.8% vs 13.1%; $P<.001$) were significantly lower in the multivessel versus culprit-only revascularization groups. Adjusted incidences of cardiac death (4.8% vs 9.7%; $P = .002$) and MACE (18.1% vs 20.3%; $P = .026$) were significantly lower in the multivessel versus culprit-only group. Limitations include anatomic and procedural factors, such as lesion difficulty (including culprit and nonculprit vessels), expected procedure time, and operator's expertise, all of which could have influenced the results.[28]

The EXPLORE trial (Evaluating Xience and Left Ventricular Function in Percutaneous Coronary Intervention on Occlusions After ST-Elevation Myocardial Infarction) evaluated whether patients with STEMI and concurrent CTO in a non–infarct-related artery benefit from additional PCI of CTO shortly after primary PCI. There were 304 patients with acute STEMI who underwent primary PCI and had concurrent CTO in 14 centers in Europe and Canada enrolled; 150 patients were randomly assigned to early PCI of the CTO, and 154 patients were assigned to conservative treatment without PCI of the CTO. Primary outcomes were LV ejection fraction and LV end-diastolic volume on cardiac magnetic resonance imaging after 4 months.

The adjudicated procedural success rate in the CTO PCI arm of the trial was 73%. At 4 months, mean LV ejection fraction did not differ between the 2 groups (44.1 ± 12.2% vs 44.8 ± 11.9%, respectively; $P = .60$). Mean LV end-diastolic volume also did not differ between groups at 4 months: LV end-diastolic volume was 215.6 ± 62.5 mL in the CTO PCI arm versus 212.8 ± 60.3 mL in the no CTO PCI arm ($P = .70$). Subgroup analysis revealed that patients with CTO located in the left anterior descending coronary artery who were randomized to the CTO PCI strategy had significantly higher LV ejection fraction compared with patients randomized to the no CTO PCI strategy (47.2 ± 12.3% vs 40.4 ± 11.9%; $P = .02$). There were no differences in terms of 4-month major adverse coronary events (5.4% vs 2.6%; $P = .25$). The authors concluded that CTO PCI within 1 week after the primary PCI for STEMI was safe and feasible with a high degree of success.[29] It is clear that the preponderance of data demonstrate that, in patients presenting with ACS and MVD, regardless of presence or absence of CS, complete revascularization is the preferred treatment modality.

## Patients with Multivessel Disease Presenting with Stable Coronary Artery Disease

Treatment of these patients remains a point of contention. In 3 landmark clinical trials in the 1970s, a total of 2234 patients with chronic stable angina were assigned randomly to undergo CABG or receive medical therapy. However, these trials excluded patients with an ejection fraction of less than 35%.[30–32] A metaanalysis of the trials demonstrated that only 7.2% of the patients who underwent randomization had an ejection fraction of 40% or less, and only 4.0% had primary symptoms of heart failure rather than angina.[33] Thus, before the STICH trial (Surgical Treatment for Ischemic Heart Failure), the role of CABG in the treatment of patients with CAD and heart failure had not been clearly established.

The STICH trial was designed to evaluate the role of cardiac surgery in the treatment of patients with CAD and LV systolic dysfunction. A major hypothesis of the trial was that CABG plus intensive medical therapy based on current guidelines, as compared with medical therapy alone, would reduce mortality. Eligible patients had CAD that was amenable to CABG and an ejection fraction of 35% or less. The primary outcome was all-cause mortality and secondary outcomes included the rate of death from cardiovascular causes and a composite outcome of death or hospitalization for cardiovascular causes.

The primary outcome occurred in 244 of the 602 patients (41%) assigned to medical therapy alone and in 218 of the 610 patients (36%) assigned to CABG (hazard ratio with CABG, 0.86; 95% CI, 0.72–1.04; $P = .12$) in the intention-to-treat analysis. However, an as-treated and per-protocol analysis done by the authors showed that CABG was superior to medical therapy in both cases.[34] LV dysfunction in patients with CAD is not always an irreversible process related to previous myocardial infarction and resultant transmyocardial scar formation, because LV function improves substantially in many patients and may even normalize after CABG.[35] Previous studies that have suggested an association between myocardial viability and outcome have been retrospective in nature. In a substudy of STICH, the authors report the outcome of patients who also underwent assessment of myocardial viability. Of 1212 patients enrolled in the original study, 601 who underwent assessment of myocardial viability were included in the viability subanalysis. The univariate analysis showed a significant association between myocardial viability and outcome. However, this association was not significant on multivariable analysis. The one caveat to this finding was that most of those patients that had viability testing underwent single photon emission computed tomography or dobutamine stress echocardiography to assess viability, neither of which are as accurate as the current gold standards to test viability—cardiac magnetic resonance imaging or PET.[36] STICH was the first of many studies to suggest that revascularization improves outcomes in patients with stable CAD.

The Synergy between Percutaneous Coronary Intervention with Taxus and Cardiac Surgery (SYNTAX) clinical trial is the largest study to date comparing stenting with surgery. The study randomized 1800 patients with left main and/or 3-vessel coronary disease to CABG or PCI using paclitaxel drug-eluting stents, with the intent of achieving complete revascularization.[7] Operators were allowed to be aggressive in treating chronically occluded vessels, long lesions, bifurcations, and unprotected left main disease. Minimally invasive CABG was not permitted. Reflecting this aggressive approach, in the PCI group 63% had a bifurcation or trifurcation treated, 39.5% had left main disease, 33% of patients had more than 100 mm of stents placed, and on average 3.6 ± 1.6 lesions were treated and 4.6 ± 2.3 stents were implanted per patient.

A higher proportion of CABG patients had complete revascularization, 63.2% versus 56.7% ($P<.01$). Although the study was designed as a noninferiority trial, at 12 months, death from any cause, stroke, myocardial infarction, or repeat revascularization was lower among CABG patients (12.4%) than the PCI group (17.8%, $P<.01$). This endpoint was almost entirely explained by revascularization, because the rate of death, stroke, or myocardial infarction was 7.7% for CABG versus 7.6% for PCI ($P = .98$). There were more than 3 times as many strokes in the CABG group (2.2% vs 0.6%; $P<.01$), although all-cause death and myocardial infarction were not statistically different. At 5 years of follow-up, the major adverse cardiac and cerebrovascular event rates remained higher in the PCI group; the rates of all-cause mortality and stroke, however, were not different between the groups.[37,38]

The 5-year SYNTAX trial results contain some insights into the importance of complete revascularization versus incomplete revascularization. All-cause death was significantly higher in all groups with incomplete revascularization with the exception of those patients with total occlusions. However, those with diabetes, unprotected left main disease, de novo triple vessel disease, and ejection fractions of less than 50% all did worse with incomplete revascularization. When looking specifically at those patients, many use the residual SYNTAX score (RSS) as a quantitative measure of incomplete revascularization. In the original SYNTAX trial, an RSS of greater than 8 was highly specific in its association with 5-year clinical outcomes (specificity, all-cause death, 88%; major adverse cardiac and cerebrovascular events, 90%).

Alidoosti and colleagues[39] performed a retrospective analysis of 760 patients (mean age = 59.14 ± 10.36 years, 70.4% males) who underwent successful PCI with incomplete revascularization between September 2008 and March 2010 to evaluate the clinical impact of the RSS after PCI in patients with multivessel CAD. The RSS was used to quantify the extent and complexity of residual coronary stenosis following PCI. Multivariable analysis was used to evaluate the impact of RSS on 1-year MACE, including death, myocardial infarction, and revascularization. The overall incidence of 1-year MACE was 4.74%. Using receiving operating characteristic curve analysis a cutoff of greater than 5 for baseline RSS had a significant association with occurrence of 12-month MACE (area under the curve = 0.769; $P<.001$; sensitivity = 75%, specificity = 72%). The unadjusted effect of an RSS of greater than 5 on 12 months MACE showed a hazard ratio of 7.34 (P<.001). After adjustment to clinical SYNTAX score as the sole confounder, an RSS of greater than 5 remained a strong associate with 12 months MACE and its effect outweighed that of before adjustment (hazard ratio, 8.03; P<.001).

Another potential method of quantifying completeness of revascularization is using the SYNTAX Revascularization Index (SRI). The baseline SYNTAX score (bSS), the RSS, and the delta SYNTAX score ($\Delta$SS) were determined from 888 angiograms of patients enrolled in the prospective SYNTAX trial. The SRI was then calculated for each patient using the following formula: SRI = ($\Delta$SS/bSS]) $\times$ 100. Outcomes were examined according to the proportion of revascularized myocardium (SRI = 100% [CR], 50%–<100%, and <50%). The mean bSS was 28.4 $\pm$ 11.5, and after PCI, the mean $\Delta$SS was 23.8 $\pm$ 10.9 and the mean RSS was 4.5 $\pm$ 6.9. The mean SRI was 85.3 $\pm$ 21.2% and was 100% in 385 patients (43.5%), less than 100% to 50% in 454 patients (51.1%), and less than 50% in 48 patients (5.4%). Five-year adverse outcomes, including death, were inversely proportional to the SRI. An SRI cutoff of less than 70% (present in 142 patients [16.0%] after PCI) had the best prognostic accuracy for prediction of death and, by multivariable analysis, was an independent predictor of 5-year mortality (hazard ratio, 4.13; 95% CI, 2.79–6.11; P<.0001). The authors concluded that "the SRI is a useful tool in assessing the degree of revascularization after PCI, with SRI $\geq$70% representing a 'reasonable' goal for patients with complex CAD."[40] As evidence, several studies evaluating complete revascularization versus incomplete revascularization have generally supported complete revascularization as a strategy for improving long-term outcomes.

One of the current hypotheses regarding the role of complete revascularization in improving outcomes is that complete revascularization works through resolving early myocardial stunning/hibernation. It is well-recognized that hibernation resulting from severe CAD can contribute to the development of heart failure. Multiple studies with different imaging techniques have shown that revascularization of hibernating myocardium results in improved LV function, and a metaanalysis suggests this is associated with improved clinical outcomes.[35] As well as preventing hibernation, non–infarct-related artery PCI may also improve myocardial salvage by increasing blood flow to watershed areas of infarction, which could translate into improved clinical outcomes.

PCI trials in high-risk patients also suggest a benefit for complete revascularization. The PROTECT II study (A prospective, randomized clinical trial of hemodynamic support with Impella 2.5 versus intra-aortic balloon pump in patients undergoing high-risk percutaneous coronary intervention) is a perfect example. Published in 2012, this multicenter, randomized trial enrolled patients 18 to 90 years of age scheduled to undergo a nonemergent PCI. It included patients with an unprotected left main or last patent coronary vessel with a LV ejection fraction of 35% or less; patients with 3-vessel disease and a LV ejection fraction of 30% or less were also eligible. In all, 452 symptomatic patients with complex 3-vessel disease or unprotected left main CAD and severely depressed LV function were randomized. Patients were randomized to IABP (n = 226) or Impella 2.5 (n = 226) support during nonemergent high-risk PCI at 112 centers in the United States, Canada, and Europe. The primary endpoint (30-day major adverse events) was not different between groups: 35.1% for Impella 2.5 versus 40.1% for IABP (P = .227) in the intent-to-treat population and 34.3% versus 42.2% (P = .092) in the per-protocol population. At 90 days, the per-protocol analysis revealed a decrease in major adverse events in the Impella 2.5–supported patients in comparison with IABP: 40.0% versus 51.0% (P = .023; although this was nonsignificant in the intention-to-treat analysis).[41]

In a substudy of PROTECT II, among patients with quantitative echocardiography (LV volumes and biplane ejection fraction), Daubert and colleagues[42] assessed the extent and predictors of reverse LV remodeling, defined as improved systolic function with an absolute increase in ejection fraction of 5% or greater and correlated these findings with clinical events. Quantitative echocardiography was performed in 184 patients at baseline and longest follow-up. The mean ejection fraction at baseline was 27.1%. Ninety-three patients (51%) demonstrated reverse LV remodeling with an absolute increase in ejection fraction of 13.2% (P<.001). End-systolic volume decreased from 137.7 to 106.6 mL (P = .002). No change in ejection fraction or end-systolic volume was seen among nonremodelers. Reverse LV remodeling occurred more frequently in patients with more extensive revascularization (odds ratio, 7.52; 95% CI, 1.31–43.25) and was associated with significantly fewer major adverse events (composite of death/myocardial infarction/stroke/transient ischemic attack): 9.7% versus 24.2% (P = .009). There was also a greater reduction in New York Heart Association functional class III/IV heart failure among reverse LV remodelers (from 66.7% to 24.0%) than nonremodelers (56.3% to 34.4%; $P = .045$).[42]

Although incomplete revascularization is common in many randomized studies (NY PCI registry, ARTS I [Arterial Revascularization Therapies Study], ARTS II, SYNTAX PCI, SYNTAX CABG), there is a propensity of data suggesting that complete revascularization should be performed in a staged fashion. Vlaar and colleagues[43] published a pairwise and network metaanalyses performed on 3 PCI strategies for multivessel CAD in STEMI patients: (1) culprit vessel only PCI strategy, defined as PCI confined to culprit vessel lesions only, (2) multivessel PCI strategy, defined as PCI of culprit vessel as well as 1 or more nonculprit vessel lesions during the index procedure, and (3) staged PCI strategy, defined as PCI confined to culprit vessel, after which 1 or more nonculprit vessel lesions are treated during staged procedures. Prospective and retrospective studies were included when research subjects were patients with STEMI and MVD undergoing PCI. The primary endpoint was all-cause mortality and 40,280 patients were included. Pairwise metaanalyses demonstrated that staged PCI was associated with lower short- and long-term all-cause mortality as compared with culprit PCI and multivessel PCI. Multivessel PCI was associated with highest mortality rates at both short- and long-term follow-up. In network analyses, staged PCI was also consistently associated with lower mortality. This metaanalysis supports the hypothesis that incomplete revascularization is suboptimal for patients and leads to poorer outcomes. The timing of nonculprit vessel PCI is important; staged procedures seem to yield the best results. It is of no surprise that as the difficulty of the lesions increase, the incidence of both surgical and percutaneous incomplete revascularization increases as well.[44]

Regardless of the criteria used, several limitations exist when trying to quantify the impact of complete revascularization on outcomes. First, there is no universally accepted definition of complete revascularization. Second, different patient populations, endpoint definitions, and levels of monitoring and other differences in study methodologies (including blinding) may explain the discordance between earlier studies. Third, the assessment of complete revascularization versus incomplete revascularization is based on what happened at the time of surgery (by operative report) or PCI (by angiographic review) and does not take into account immediate

and late graft attrition or subsequent in-stent restenosis or stent thrombosis. Importantly, in virtually every study comparing complete revascularization and incomplete revascularization, patients in the incomplete revascularization group have been sicker, and although multivariable analyses can adjust for this bias when overt, unmeasured residual confounders cannot be accounted for.

## SUMMARY

This comprehensive review of the literature has defined the incidence of multivessel coronary disease in routine angiography, defined CS, and discussed the incidence of CS in patients presenting with MVD and ACS. It has examined the various trials addressing the treatment of patients with MVD presenting with ACS and more stably. Additionally, there has been a discussion of the current literature examining complete revascularization versus incomplete revascularization as it relates to long-term outcomes. Current guidelines support multivessel PCI in the setting of CS but it remains to be determined if those benefits extend consistently to patients with stable CAD. Thankfully we have trials in the pipeline—COMPLETE (addressing STEMI patients) and OPEN-CTO (any patient with at least one CTO)—along with many others that may help to address these questions. What remains clear, however, is that clinicians must remain vigilant to do what is best for each patient on a case-by-case basis after discussing all options with the patient and his or her family.

## REFERENCES

1. Anderson HV, Shaw RE, Brindis RG, et al. A contemporary overview of percutaneous coronary interventions. The American College of Cardiology-National Cardiovascular Data Registry (ACC-NCDR). J Am Coll Cardiol 2002;39: 1096–103.

2. Levine GN, Bates ER, Blankenship JC, et al. 2011 ACCF/AHA/SCAI guideline for percutaneous coronary intervention: executive summary: a report of the American College of Cardiology Foundation/ American Heart Association Task Force on Practice Guidelines and the Society for Cardiovascular Angiography and Interventions. Circulation 2011; 124:2574–609.

3. Gogo PB Jr, Dauerman HL, Mulgund J, et al. Changes in patterns of coronary revascularization strategies for patients with acute coronary syndromes (from the CRUSADE Quality Improvement Initiative). Am J Cardiol 2007;99:1222–6.

4. Mokadam NA, Melford RE Jr, Maynard C, et al. Prevalence and procedural outcomes of percutaneous coronary intervention and coronary artery bypass grafting in patients with diabetes and multivessel coronary artery disease. J Card Surg 2011; 26:1–8.

5. Mack MJ, Banning AP, Serruys PW, et al. Bypass versus drug-eluting stents at three years in SYNTAX patients with diabetes mellitus or metabolic syndrome. Ann Thorac Surg 2011;92:2140–6.

6. Patel MR, Bailey SR, Bonow RO, et al. ACCF/SCAI/AATS/AHA/ASE/ASNC/HFSA/HRS/SCCM/SCCT/SCMR/STS 2012 appropriate use criteria for diagnostic catheterization: a report of the American College of Cardiology Foundation Appropriate Use Criteria Task Force, Society for Cardiovascular Angiography and Interventions, American Association for Thoracic Surgery, American Heart Association, American Society of Echocardiography, American Society of Nuclear Cardiology, Heart Failure Society of America, Heart Rhythm Society, Society of Critical Care Medicine, Society of Cardiovascular Computed Tomography, Society for Cardiovascular Magnetic Resonance, and Society of Thoracic Surgeons. J Am Coll Cardiol 2012;59:1995–2027.

7. Serruys PW, Morice MC, Kappetein AP, et al. Percutaneous coronary intervention versus coronary-artery bypass grafting for severe coronary artery disease. N Engl J Med 2009;360:961–72.

8. Park SJ, Kim YH, Park DW, et al. Randomized trial of stents versus bypass surgery for left main coronary artery disease. N Engl J Med 2011;364: 1718–27.

9. Task Force on Myocardial Revascularization of the European Society of Cardiology and the European Association for Cardio-Thoracic Surgery, Windecker S, Kolh P, Alfonso F, et al. 2014 ESC/EACTS Guidelines on myocardial revascularization: the Task Force on Myocardial Revascularization of the European Society of Cardiology (ESC) and the European Association for Cardio-Thoracic Surgery (EACTS)Developed with the special contribution of the European Association of Percutaneous Cardiovascular Interventions (EAPCI). Eur Heart J 2014;35:2541–619.

10. Kar B, Basra SS, Shah NR, et al. Percutaneous circulatory support in cardiogenic shock: interventional bridge to recovery. Circulation 2012;125: 1809–17.

11. Lindholm MG, Kober L, Boesgaard S, et al. Trandolapril Cardiac Evaluation study g. Cardiogenic shock complicating acute myocardial infarction; prognostic impact of early and late shock development. Eur Heart J 2003;24:258–65.

12. Katz JN, Stebbins AL, Alexander JH, et al. Predictors of 30-day mortality in patients with refractory cardiogenic shock following acute myocardial infarction despite a patent infarct artery. Am Heart J 2009;158:680–7.

13. Babaev A, Frederick PD, Pasta DJ, et al. Trends in management and outcomes of patients with acute myocardial infarction complicated by cardiogenic shock. JAMA 2005;294:448–54.

14. Hasdai D, Harrington RA, Hochman JS, et al. Platelet glycoprotein IIb/IIIa blockade and outcome of cardiogenic shock complicating acute coronary syndromes without persistent ST-segment elevation. J Am Coll Cardiol 2000;36: 685–92.

15. Holmes DR Jr, Bates ER, Kleiman NS, et al. Contemporary reperfusion therapy for cardiogenic shock: the GUSTO-I trial experience. The GUSTO-I Investigators. Global Utilization of Streptokinase and Tissue Plasminogen Activator for Occluded Coronary Arteries. J Am Coll Cardiol 1995;26: 668–74.

16. Widimsky P, Holmes DR Jr. How to treat patients with ST-elevation acute myocardial infarction and multi-vessel disease? Eur Heart J 2011;32:396–403.

17. Reynolds HR, Hochman JS. Cardiogenic shock: current concepts and improving outcomes. Circulation 2008;117:686–97.

18. Hollenberg SM, Kavinsky CJ, Parrillo JE. Cardiogenic shock. Ann Intern Med 1999;131:47–59.

19. Hira RS, Thamwiwat A, Kar B. TandemHeart placement for cardiogenic shock in acute severe mitral regurgitation and right ventricular failure. Catheter Cardiovasc Interv 2014;83:319–22.

20. Hochman JS, Sleeper LA, Webb JG, et al. Early revascularization in acute myocardial infarction complicated by cardiogenic shock. SHOCK Investigators. Should We Emergently Revascularize Occluded Coronaries for Cardiogenic Shock. N Engl J Med 1999;341:625–34.

21. Hochman JS, Boland J, Sleeper LA, et al. Current spectrum of cardiogenic shock and effect of early revascularization on mortality. Results of an International Registry. SHOCK Registry Investigators. Circulation 1995;91:873–81.

22. Tiefenbrunn AJ, Chandra NC, French WJ, et al. Clinical experience with primary percutaneous transluminal coronary angioplasty compared with alteplase (recombinant tissue-type plasminogen activator) in patients with acute myocardial infarction: a report from the Second National Registry of Myocardial Infarction (NRMI-2). J Am Coll Cardiol 1998;31:1240–5.

23. Berger PB, Holmes DR Jr, Stebbins AL, et al. Impact of an aggressive invasive catheterization and revascularization strategy on mortality in patients with cardiogenic shock in the Global Utilization of Streptokinase and Tissue Plasminogen Activator for Occluded Coronary Arteries (GUSTO-I) trial. An observational study. Circulation 1997;96:122–7.

24. Menon V, Hochman JS, Stebbins A, et al. Lack of progress in cardiogenic shock: lessons from the GUSTO trials. Eur Heart J 2000;21:1928–36.

25. Wald DS, Morris JK, Wald NJ, et al. Randomized trial of preventive angioplasty in myocardial infarction. N Engl J Med 2013;369:1115–23.

26. Gershlick AH, Khan JN, Kelly DJ, et al. Randomized trial of complete versus lesion-only revascularization in patients undergoing primary percutaneous coronary intervention for STEMI and multivessel disease: the CvLPRIT trial. J Am Coll Cardiol 2015;65:963–72.

27. Rosner GF, Kirtane AJ, Genereux P, et al. Impact of the presence and extent of incomplete angiographic revascularization after percutaneous coronary intervention in acute coronary syndromes: the Acute Catheterization and Urgent Intervention Triage Strategy (ACUITY) trial. Circulation 2012;125:2613–20.

28. Park JS, Cha KS, Lee DS, et al. Culprit or multivessel revascularisation in ST-elevation myocardial infarction with cardiogenic shock. Heart 2015;101:1225–32.

29. Henriques JP, Hoebers LP, Ramunddal T, et al. Percutaneous intervention for concurrent chronic total occlusions in patients With STEMI: the EXPLORE trial. J Am Coll Cardiol 2016;68:1622–32.

30. Coronary artery surgery study (CASS): a randomized trial of coronary artery bypass surgery. Survival data. Circulation 1983;68:939–50.

31. Eleven-year survival in the Veterans Administration randomized trial of coronary bypass surgery for stable angina. The Veterans Administration Coronary Artery Bypass Surgery Cooperative Study Group. N Engl J Med 1984;311:1333–9.

32. Varnauskas E. Twelve-year follow-up of survival in the randomized European Coronary Surgery Study. N Engl J Med 1988;319:332–7.

33. Yusuf S, Zucker D, Peduzzi P, et al. Effect of coronary artery bypass graft surgery on survival: overview of 10-year results from randomised trials by the Coronary Artery Bypass Graft Surgery Trialists Collaboration. Lancet 1994;344:563–70.

34. Velazquez EJ, Lee KL, Deja MA, et al. Coronary-artery bypass surgery in patients with left ventricular dysfunction. N Engl J Med 2011;364:1607–16.

35. Allman KC, Shaw LJ, Hachamovitch R, et al. Myocardial viability testing and impact of revascularization on prognosis in patients with coronary artery disease and left ventricular dysfunction: a meta-analysis. J Am Coll Cardiol 2002;39:1151–8.

36. Bonow RO, Maurer G, Lee KL, et al. Myocardial viability and survival in ischemic left ventricular dysfunction. N Engl J Med 2011;364:1617–25.

37. Mohr FW, Morice MC, Kappetein AP, et al. Coronary artery bypass graft surgery versus percutaneous coronary intervention in patients with three-vessel disease and left main coronary disease: 5-year follow-up of the randomised, clinical SYNTAX trial. Lancet 2013;381:629–38.

38. Kappetein AP, Feldman TE, Mack MJ, et al. Comparison of coronary bypass surgery with drug-eluting stenting for the treatment of left main and/or three-vessel disease: 3-year follow-up of the SYNTAX trial. Eur Heart J 2011;32:2125–34.

39. Alidoosti M, Saroukhani S, Lotfi-Tokaldany M, et al. Objectifying the level of incomplete revascularization by the residual SYNTAX score and evaluating its impact on the one-year outcome of percutaneous coronary intervention in patients with multivessel disease. Cardiovasc Revasc Med 2016;17:308–12.

40. Genereux P, Campos CM, Farooq V, et al. Validation of the SYNTAX revascularization index to quantify reasonable level of incomplete revascularization after percutaneous coronary intervention. Am J Cardiol 2015;116:174–86.

41. O'Neill WW, Kleiman NS, Moses J, et al. A prospective, randomized clinical trial of hemodynamic support with Impella 2.5 versus intra-aortic balloon pump in patients undergoing high-risk percutaneous coronary intervention: the PROTECT II study. Circulation 2012;126:1717–27.

42. Daubert MA, Massaro J, Liao L, et al. High-risk percutaneous coronary intervention is associated with reverse left ventricular remodeling and improved outcomes in patients with coronary artery disease and reduced ejection fraction. Am Heart J 2015;170(3):550–8.

43. Vlaar PJ, Mahmoud KD, Holmes DR Jr, et al. Culprit vessel only versus multivessel and staged percutaneous coronary intervention for multivessel disease in patients presenting with ST-segment elevation myocardial infarction: a pairwise and network meta-analysis. J Am Coll Cardiol 2011;58:692–703.

44. Sianos G, Morel MA, Kappetein AP, et al. The SYNTAX Score: an angiographic tool grading the complexity of coronary artery disease. EuroIntervention 2005;1:219–27.

# Cardiac Resynchronization Therapy for Heart Failure

Amole Ojo, MD, Sohaib Tariq, MD, Prakash Harikrishnan, MD,
Sei Iwai, MD, FHRS, Jason T. Jacobson, MD, FHRS*

---

## KEYWORDS

- Cardiac resynchronization therapy • Heart failure with reduced ejection fraction • Dyssynchrony
- Biventricular pacing

---

## KEY POINTS

- Cardiac resynchronization therapy (CRT) is indicated (Class I) for patients with ejection fraction no more than 35%, left bundle branch block (LBBB) with QRS duration ≥150 milliseconds and at least Class II New York Heart Association class symptoms despite optimal medical therapy.
- CRT can improve hemodynamic status, left ventricular structure and function, mitral regurgitation, and functional status.
- The benefit of CRT is less clear in patients with QRS duration of 120 to 150 milliseconds.
- There is no clear evidence that patients with non-LBBB conduction delay benefit from CRT.

---

## INTRODUCTION

Guideline-directed medical therapy, such as angiotensin-converting enzyme inhibitors, beta blockers, and spironolactone have improved symptoms and survival in patients with heart failure with reduced ejection fraction (HFrEF). Reduction in left ventricular ejection fraction (LVEF) is seen commonly in an aging population, and hospital admissions with heart failure (HF) contribute significantly to the economic burden in this population. Implanted devices, such as implantable cardioverter–defibrillators (ICDs) and pacemakers are also beneficial in such patients, especially the recommended use of ICDs for the primary prevention of sudden arrhythmic death in ischemic and nonischemic cardiomyopathy patients. In patients with HF and bundle branch block, cardiac resynchronization therapy (CRT), which involves simultaneous pacing of both right and left ventricles (biventricular pacing), is beneficial. Prognosis in HF patients is poor, but with wide use of these therapies in the last 2 decades, median life expectancy has improved. Worse prognosis is also seen

in patients with ventricular conduction delay. In a retrospective study of 241 HF patients by Shamim and colleagues,[1] after 36 months of follow-up, the mortality rate was 20% in the group with QRS less than 120 milliseconds, 36% in the group with QRS of 120 to 160 milliseconds, and 58.3% in the group with QRS greater than 160 milliseconds.

## SEQUELAE OF CONDUCTION ABNORMALITIES AND DYSSYNCHRONY IN HEART FAILURE

In patients with HF, assessment of conduction abnormalities via 12-lead electrocardiogram (ECG) is essential to determine eligibility for CRT. Interatrial conduction delay, prolonged PR interval, QRS duration greater than 120 milliseconds, right bundle branch block (RBBB), left bundle branch block (LBBB), and non-specific intraventricular conduction disturbances (IVCD) are commonly seen in HF patients.

Worsening HF symptoms and poor outcomes are associated with LBBB.[2] Inter- and intraventricular dyssynchrony is commonly seen in

---

Disclosure Statement: J.T. Jacobson – St. Jude Medical, consultant. S. Iwai – Biotronik, speaker.
Division of Cardiology, Westchester Medical Center, New York Medical College, 100 Woods Road, Valhalla, NY 10595, USA
* Corresponding author.
E-mail address: Jason.Jacobson@wmchealth.org

Intervent Cardiol Clin 6 (2017) 417–426
http://dx.doi.org/10.1016/j.iccl.2017.03.010
2211-7458/17/© 2017 Elsevier Inc. All rights reserved.

patients with HF and LBBB, regardless of the QRS duration. In intraventricular dyssynchrony, late activation of the lateral wall of the left ventricle (LV) occurs in comparison to the interventricular septum. Ventricular dyssynchrony can worsen HF by reducing the efficiency of contraction and causing ventricular remodeling leading to pump failure. Its impact is significant in patients with underlying LV dysfunction.

## FAVORABLE EFFECTS OF RESYNCHRONIZATION

Cardiac resynchronization therapy helps improve atrioventricular (AV) delay and corrects ventricular dyssynchrony, through which an improvement is seen in both left ventricular (LV) performance and mitral regurgitation. Due to coordinated contraction, a rise in systolic pressure and decrease in intracardiac filling pressures are seen. In the Cardiac Resynchronization—Heart Failure (CARE-HF) trial, LVEF increased by an absolute 3.7% at 3 months and 6.9% at 18 months from a baseline of 25% in the CRT group when compared with medical therapy.[3] Reduction in IVCD, mitral regurgitation, and end-systolic volume index was also seen.[3] In the Multicenter InSync Randomized Clinical Evaluation (MIRACLE) trial, significant improvement in LVEF (absolute 3.6% vs 0.4%) and reduction in mitral regurgitation was seen in patients with HFrEF treated with CRT compared with medical therapy.[4] Importantly, the improvement in ventricular contractility due to CRT does not appear to cause an increase in myocardial oxygen demand.[5] Improved contractility is seen at higher heart rates in patients with CRT compared with LV-only pacing, further enhancing exercise capacity.[6]

Biventricular (BiV) pacing reverses the harmful effects of LV remodeling. In the MIRACLE trial a reduction in LV mass was seen. CRT helps with reduction in intracardiac filling pressures, improvement in cardiac index, and toleration to aggressive up titration of medical therapy including beta blockers.[7,8] Improved diastolic function is also observed in patients treated with CRT, a result of the beneficial remodeling.[9] However, not every patient treated with CRT will respond in this way. The rate of nonresponse to CRT has been estimated to be around 20% to 30%.[10] Factors that predict response will be discussed later in this article. It is also of note that the placebo effect in the control group in some of the CRT studies is not insignificant. In the MIRACLE trial, for example, the clinical composite HF score of 39% of patients in the control group also improved.[11]

## PACING IN HEART FAILURE

Right ventricular (RV) pacing is a cause of ventricular dyssynchrony and is not recommended in patients with HFrEF, as it reduces the efficiency of cardiac pump function and exacerbates heart failure symptoms. The right ventricle contracts before the left ventricle, which leads to interventricular dyssynchrony. This results in an iatrogenic LBBB, with late activation of the lateral wall compared with septum, hence causing intraventricular dyssynchrony.

In the Dual Chamber and VVI Implantable Defibrillator (DAVID) Trial, the effect of dual-chamber (right atrial [RA] and RV) pacing in HFrEF patients (mean LVEF 27%) was associated with worse outcomes (ie, higher mortality and hospitalizations for HF) when compared with VVI pacing with a lower rate limit of 40 beats per minute (VVI-40).[12] RV pacing was significantly higher in dual-chamber pacing group (60%) compared with the VVI-40 group (1%).[12] RV pacing more than 40% of the time greatly increased the risk of poor outcomes.[12] Post-hoc analysis of data from the MOde Selection Trial (MOST) study also showed that ventricular pacing is associated with increased hospitalizations of HF patients even with baseline QRS duration less than 120 milliseconds.[13] The DAVID II trial compared atrial pacing with back-up ventricular pacing (VVI-40), and no difference was seen in event-free survival and quality of life between both groups,[14] adding further evidence for the deleterious effects of RV pacing.

## OPTIMAL HEART FAILURE PATIENT SELECTION FOR RESYNCHRONIZATION

There is strong evidence of beneficial effects of CRT in patients with New York Heart Association (NYHA) Class III HF by improving symptoms, exercise capacity, and LF function. LVEF no more than ≤35% and QRS duration of at least 120 to 150 milliseconds were the inclusion criteria in most of the trials. The CARE-HF and Comparison of Medical Therapy, Pacing and Defibrillation in Heart Failure (COMPANION) trials showed significant reduction in all-cause mortality and hospitalizations for HF.[3,15] In the MIRACLE trial, improvement in NYHA class was seen as early as 1 month.[11] A meta-analysis included 14 randomized controlled trials with 4420 patients. All patients had LV systolic dysfunction (mean LVEF range 21%–30%), prolonged QRS duration (mean range, 155–209 milliseconds), and most had NYHA Class III and IV symptoms despite being on optimal medical therapy.[16] Reduction in hospitalizations by 37% and all-cause mortality by 22% was seen with CRT.[16] It also improved LVEF, quality of life, and functional class.[16]

CRT is also beneficial in HFrEF patients with mild HF symptoms, including NYHA Class I and II. The Multicenter Automatic Defibrillator Implantation Trial with Cardiac Resynchronization Therapy (MADIT-CRT) trial included 1820 patients with an LVEF of no more than 30%, QRS of at least 130 milliseconds, and NYHA Class I (ischemic cardiomyopathy) or II (ischemic and nonischemic cardiomyopathy) HF symptoms.[17] Patients were randomly assigned to CRT plus ICD or ICD alone. A 41% reduction in HF events was seen in the CRT group of patients, primarily with QRS duration of 150 milliseconds or more. Reduction in LV volume and improvement in LVEF was also seen. A subanalysis of the MADIT-CRT data showed that patients with LBBB receiving CRT-D had a significant reduction in HF progression and risk of ventricular arrhythmias when compared with patients with non-LBBB QRS pattern (right bundle branch block or intraventricular conduction disturbances).[1] A meta-analysis of 5 randomized controlled trials included 4213 patients of whom 91% had NYHA Class II HF.[18] CRT significantly reduced mortality and the risk of HF events. CRT also induced a significant reverse LV remodeling (defined as improvement in the LVEF and reduction in the LV end-systolic volume index).

## CARDIAC RESYNCHRONIZATION THERAPY IN HEART FAILURE WITH SPECIFIC CONDITIONS

### Cardiac Resynchronization Therapy in Atrial Fibrillation

The prevalence of atrial fibrillation (AF) in HF depends on the severity and ranges from less than 10% in patients with NYHA Functional Class I HF to approximately 50% in those with NYHA Class IV HF.[19] Among patients with persistent AF, CRT is generally considered in 3 clinical settings that may overlap: in the setting of systolic HF, atrioventricular (AV) block secondary to conduction system disease, and following AV node ablation. By using CRT, patients with AF who require pacemaker for AV block due to conduction system disease and those who require pacemaker following AV node ablation for the purpose of rate control can avoid the detrimental effects of dyssynchrony induced by RV pacing. The benefits of CRT were seen in the Left Ventricular-Based Cardiac Stimulation Post AV Nodal Ablation Evaluation (PAVE) trial, which included AF patients who underwent AV node ablation to treat medically refractory rapid ventricular rates[20] and in the Biventricular versus Right Ventricular Pacing in Heart Failure Patients with Atrioventricular Block (BLOCK HF) trial (which

included patients with indications for pacing for AV block, LVEF ≤50% with NYHA Class I, II or III HF), over 50% of whom had AF at baseline.[21]

In order to receive maximal benefits from CRT, a high rate of BiV pacing is required,[22] which may be difficult in patients with AF with intact AV conduction. The reported BiV pacing rates by the CRT devices may be misleading, as these include fusion and pseudofusion between intrinsic conduction and device pacing. In order to accurately determine the BiV pacing rates in these AF patients with intact AV conduction, Holter monitoring is often required.[23] VVIR pacing modality can be used in persistent AF patients, while DDDR or VDDR pacing modality can be used in those with paroxysmal AF. In 1 observational study, among 1285 patients treated with CRT, 243 were in AF. In patients with AF, AV node ablation in addition to CRT was found to significantly improve survival compared with CRT alone.[24] In order for patients with AF to achieve maximum CRT benefits, therefore, clinicians should target complete (100%) BiV pacing.

CRT has not been shown to reduce the incidence of new or recurrent AF even though it has a favorable impact on risk factors for AF such as LV systolic dysfunction, atrial size, degree of mitral regurgitation, and neurohormonal activation.[25] Hence, CRT is not currently indicated to reduce AF burden.[26]

### Cardiac Resynchronization Therapy in Patients Who are Pacemaker-Dependent

Patients who are pacemaker-dependent for different reasons are at risk for both interventricular and intraventricular dyssynchrony. RV pacing causes the right ventricle to contract before the left ventricle, which causes the septum to contract before the lateral wall.[27] CRT therefore offers a way of avoiding the negative effects of RV pacing in patients with reduced LVEF. It is unclear what the EF threshold for CRT should be, but it should be remembered that BLOCK-HF enrolled patients with EF 50% or less.[21]

### Cardiac Resynchronization Therapy in Patients with Mitral Regurgitation

Patients with mitral regurgitation (MR) should receive CRT according to the standard CRT indications, as previously discussed. CRT frequently improves secondary MR in patients with ventricular dyssynchrony.[4] Improvement in MR was noted in the CARE-HF and MIRACLE randomized trials of CRT.[3,11] However, ischemic MR has not been associated with significant improvement with CRT.[28] Lack of response to CRT among patients with ischemic MR may be due to an inability to pace infarcted areas. Hence, careful patient selection is required for CRT, especially in the setting of ischemic MR.

### Cardiac Resynchronization Therapy in Patients with Right Ventricular Dysfunction

Baseline RV function should not be used to determine CRT eligibility. A post-hoc analysis from 688 patients in the CARE-HF trial demonstrated that CRT has little effect on RV function and that RV dysfunction is not an important determinant of relative benefits of CRT.[29] The effect of CRT was similar across tertiles of RV function (identified by tricuspid plane systolic excursion). However, the analysis showed that RV dysfunction is a predictor of mortality.

## OPTIMIZATION OF CARDIAC RESYNCHRONIZATION THERAPY

Many factors must be considered in order to optimize the benefits of CRT. The LV pacing location is a major determinant of hemodynamic response in CRT.[30] The preferred location is in the posterolateral wall, as it is often the last segment to contract in a dyssynchronous LV. A post-hoc analysis of MADIT CRT[31] showed that apical LV lead location is associated with unfavorable outcomes, as opposed to placement in the basal portion of the venous branch. Observational studies have shown that the presence, location, and burden of LV scar have an impact on response to CRT.[32–34] The study by Roubicek and colleagues[35] showed that the electrical LV lead position as assessed by the ratio of the electrical delay (from the beginning of the QRS complex to the local LV electrogram) to the QRS duration (QLV ratio) is a strong predictor of HF hospitalization cardiac mortality in LBBB/IVCD patients who received CRT. In their study, patients with a QLV ratio of no more than 0.70 had worse outcomes.[35]

In a small study, Bernheim and colleagues[36] showed that right atrial (RA) pacing has adverse effects in patients treated with CRT. RA pacing leads to delayed activation of the left atrium (LA), which reduces LA contribution to the LV preload. Bernheim and colleagues showed avoidance of RA pacing was associated with greater improvement in ventricular dyssynchrony and in myocardial performance.

In standard dual-chamber pacing, the AV delay is often programmed to approximate the physiologic AV interval or longer to allow native AV conduction, thereby minimizing ventricular pacing. This is opposed to CRT, where ventricular pacing is desired. Hence, a shorter AV delay is often used to prevent native AV conduction.[37]

However, the best method for AV delay optimization is still not known. A small study by Meluzin and colleagues[38] proposed defining optimal AV delay by Doppler echocardiography; the end of the A wave should coincide with the onset of systolic MR flow. The need for routine AV delay optimization in CRT patients remains controversial.[26] The SMART-AV delay trial did not show any significant difference in primary outcome among these 3 AV delay strategies: empiric, device algorithm-based, and echo-guided.[39] Accordingly, routine AV delay optimization in CRT patients was not recommended in the 2012 EHRA/HRS expert consensus statement on cardiac resynchronization therapy in HF.[26] However, there is possible utility in selected patients who do not respond to CRT. Ventriculo-ventricular (VV) delay optimization should also be restricted to CRT nonresponders.[26] van Gelder and colleagues[40] showed that most CRT patients appear to benefit from LV pre-excitation or simultaneous activation.

In a data analysis from CRT devices in 36,935 patients, a higher percentage of BiV pacing was associated with improved survival.[22] The largest magnitude of reduction in mortality was observed in patients with greater than 98.5% BiV pacing. A post-hoc analysis of MADIT-CRT study showed that within the CRT-D group, for every 1% point increase in BiV pacing above 90%, the risk of HF/death and death alone significantly decreased by 6% and 10%, respectively.[41] Frequent premature ventricular complexes (PVCs) can reduce the BiV pacing percentage, thereby reducing the benefits of CRT. Hence, measures should be taken to aggressively reduce the PVC burden in those so afflicted.

## TIMING OF RESPONSE TO RESYNCHRONIZATION

Symptomatic benefit from CRT (such as increased 6-minute walk distance and improvement in NYHA class) occurs early and is persistent.[3,11,15,42] In CARE-HF and COMPANION, symptomatic benefit from CRT was not assessed before 3 months,[3,15] while most of the symptomatic improvement was seen in the MIRACLE trial at 1 month.[11] Mortality benefit and improvement in the LVEF were evident in many studies by 4 months.[3,11,15]

## PREDICTORS OF RESPONSE TO RESYNCHRONIZATION

End-stage HF patients, including those who are inotrope dependent, appear to have a poor response rate. Hence, CRT should be used carefully in patients with American College of Cardiology (ACC)/American Heart Association (AHA) Stage D, refractory NYHA Class IV symptoms. A meta-analysis by Sipahi and colleagues,[43] which included the CARE-HF, COMPANION, Resynchronization reverses remodeling in systolic left ventricular dysfunction trial (REVERSE), MADIT-CRT, and Resynchronization–Defibrillation for Ambulatory Heart Failure (RAFT) trials, found that CRT reduced adverse clinical events in patients with a baseline QRS interval of at least 150 milliseconds, but CRT did not reduce events in patients with a QRS less than 150 milliseconds. Two retrospective studies have suggested that the delta QRS duration (QRS shortening associated with biventricular pacing) is a better predictor of CRT benefit than the baseline QRS duration.[44,45] The efficacy of CRT in patients without underlying LBBB is not established.

Cardiac magnetic resonance tissue characteristics have been found to be predictive of CRT effect. In ischemic cardiomyopathy (ICM), response is associated with findings of less than 15% of total infarcted myocardium and the absence of significant postero-lateral scar.[46–48]

Preimplant quantification of mechanical synchrony (mainly performed by echocardiography) has failed to show significant predictive value for CRT benefit.[49,50] However, in expert hands, a comprehensive assessment that integrates multiple mechanical dyssynchrony parameters might help to identify CRT responders. Many studies have shown that women tend to respond to CRT more frequently than men.[51]

After device implantation for CRT, objective criteria such as cardiopulmonary testing or 6-minute walk in addition to LV volumes and function in combination with symptoms assessment should be used to assess response. If a patient is deemed as a nonresponder, effort should be made to identify reversible causes and treat as needed. The assessment should include physical examination, review of medications, assessment of lead location, and device interrogation (which should include assessment for atrial and ventricular arrhythmias and presence and frequency of continuous BiV pacing). An echo-guided or device-guided AV optimization can be considered, although its benefit seems marginal from several studies.[26]

## DEFIBRILLATOR BENEFITS

Sustained ventricular tachycardia (VT) and ventricular fibrillation (VF) are common in patients with HF with reduced LVEF and may lead to sudden cardiac death (SCD). Given that SCD is frequently the first presentation of a ventricular arrhythmia, there is a clear role for primary prevention ICDs in selected patients. Hence, patients who are candidates for CRT and at the same time meet any of the indications for ICD should get a combination device with an ICD (CRT-D).[52] In the COMPANION trial, 1520 patients were randomized to optimal medical therapy, CRT with a pacemaker alone (CRT-P) or CRT-D and were followed for a median time of more than 12 months. CRT-P reduced the risk of death from any cause by 24% (adjusted $P = .06$), while CRT-D reduced the risk by 36% (adjusted $P = .004$). Among patients with nonischemic cardiomyopathy (NICM), the CRT-D but not the CRT-P arm experienced a significant improvement in all-cause mortality.[15]

The Defibrillator Implantation in Patients with Nonischemic Systolic Heart Failure (DANISH) trial randomized 1116 patients with NICM to an ICD with modern (enrollment 2008–2015) medical therapy or medical therapy alone, which in over half of subjects included CRT pacing. There was no significant difference in the primary outcome of mortality from any cause. However, there was a significant reduction in the secondary outcome of SCD in the ICD group compared with the no ICD group. Subgroup analysis showed a significant reduction in total mortality for patients with ICD and age no more than 58 years.[53] Due to the low overall mortality rate in the DANISH trial, it may have been underpowered to show a mortality benefit of ICD therapy on top of guideline-directed optimal medical therapy and a high frequency of CRT pacing. More so, elderly patients tend to have greater comorbidities, which could contribute to other causes of death. It is, however, premature at this time to withhold potentially life-saving ICD therapy from all NICM patients. It is the authors' opinion that all patients who qualify for CRT including NICM patients, who are also candidates for ICD, should be offered CRT-D.

## COMPLICATIONS OF CARDIAC RESYNCHRONIZATION THERAPY DEVICE

Complications related to CRT device implantation occur in 13.8% of patients peri-procedurally and 10% of patients post-procedurally among all patients undergoing implant attempts,[54] indicating a higher complication rate than standard dual-chamber RA/RV pacing. In the COMPANION trial, moderate or severe procedure-related adverse events were seen in 8% of patients with CRT-D and 10% of patients with CRT-P.[15] The CRT device implantation procedure is not successful in about 7% of patients in whom implantation is attempted, the main reason being failure to implant the LV lead into a coronary sinus tributary.[16,54] Lead dislodgement is the most common postprocedural complication (5.8%) seen in patients in whom the CRT implant was successful.[54] LV lead is the most common lead to dislodge and in 1 study had to be repositioned in 4% of patients within 30 days of implantation.[17] Other complications include extracardiac stimulation, coronary sinus or venous dissection or perforation, hemothorax, pneumothorax, pocket hematoma, pocket erosion, infection, and arrhythmias.[3,15–17,54]

In the MADIT-CRT study, among 1089 patients in the CRT-D group, 0.5% developed coronary venous dissection with pericardial effusion during implantation; 1.7% developed pneumothorax; 1.1% developed infection, and 3.3% developed pocket hematoma requiring evacuation in the first 30 days after CRT-D implantation.[17] In a meta-analysis of 54 studies of CRT-P, the device malfunction rate was 5%, and the infection rate was 1.8% at 6 months; the rate of lead problems was 6.6% at 11 months. In a meta-analysis of 36 studies of CRT-D, the device malfunction rate was 5%; the infection rate was 1.1%, and the rate of lead problems was 7.2% at 12 months.[16]

Procedure-related mortality has been reported to be about 0.3% to 0.5% after CRT device implantation.[16,54] Age greater than 80 has been found to be an independent predictor of in-hospital mortality after CRT device implantation.[55]

## COST-EFFECTIVENESS OF CARDIAC RESYNCHRONIZATION THERAPY DEVICE IN HEART FAILURE

The CRT devices reduce the cost associated with recurrent hospitalizations for HF and so have proven to be cost-effective in HF patients, despite their high cost. In the COMPANION trial, the cost of follow-up hospitalization at 2 years was reduced by 29% by CRT-D and 37% by CRT-P compared with medical therapy alone. Over a period of 7 years, the incremental cost-effectiveness ratio per quality adjusted life-years (QALY) was $19,600 for CRT-P and $43,000 for CRT-D, which were well below the accepted cost-effectiveness ratio of $50,000 to 100,000 per QALY for therapeutic procedures.[56] These data also show that CRT-P is more cost-effective than CRT-D. Cost analysis data from other trials including CARE-HF and MADIT-CRT trials also show that CRT devices are cost-effective in HF patients.[57,58]

## CURRENT INDICATIONS OF CARDIAC RESYNCHRONIZATION THERAPY IN HEART FAILURE

As per the ACC/AHA 2013 guidelines for the management of HF, CRT is indicated for the following subgroup of Stage C HF patients with LVEF of no more than 35% who are already on optimal medical therapy.[59]

### Class I
Class I is defined as sinus rhythm, LBBB with a QRS duration of at least 150 milliseconds, and NYHA class II, III, or ambulatory IV symptoms.

### Class IIa
Class IIa can be defined as

1. Sinus rhythm, a non-LBBB pattern with a QRS duration of at least 150 milliseconds, and NYHA Class III, or ambulatory class IV symptoms
2. Sinus rhythm, LBBB with a QRS duration of 120 to 149 milliseconds, and NYHA Class II, III, or ambulatory IV symptoms
3. AF with slow ventricular rate requiring ventricular pacing or otherwise meets CRT criteria and atrioventricular nodal ablation or pharmacologic rate control will allow near 100% ventricular pacing with CRT
4. Anticipated requirement for significant (>40%) ventricular pacing

### Class IIb
Class IIb can be defined as

1. The usefulness of implantation of an ICD is of uncertain benefit to prolong meaningful survival in patients with a high risk of nonsudden death as predicted by frequent hospitalizations, advanced frailty, or comorbidities such as systemic malignancy or severe renal dysfunction
2. Sinus rhythm, a non-LBBB pattern with QRS duration of 120 to 149 milliseconds, and NYHA Class III, or ambulatory class IV.
3. Sinus rhythm, a non-LBBB pattern with a QRS duration of at least 150 milliseconds and NYHA Class II symptoms.
4. LVEF of 30% or less, ischemic etiology of HF, sinus rhythm, LBBB with a QRS duration of at least 150 milliseconds, and NYHA Class I symptoms

### Class III: Contraindications for Cardiac Resynchronization Therapy
Contraindications include

1. NYHA Class I or II symptoms and non-LBBB pattern with QRS duration less than 150 milliseconds

2. Patients whose comorbidities or frailty limit survival with good functional capacity to less than 1 year

The recent European Society of Cardiology (ESC) guidelines for HF[60] published in 2016 upgraded the indications for CRT in HF patients based on recently published trials. After the BLOCK-HF trial,[21] ESC guidelines have given CRT a class I indication for HFrEF patients, regardless of the NYHA class, who have an indication for pacing such as a high-degree AV block. CRT is contraindicated in patients with QRS duration less than 130 milliseconds based on the Cardiac Resynchronization Therapy in Patients with Heart Failure and Narrow QRS trial (RETHINQ),[50] Echo-CRT trial,[61] and IPD meta-analysis.[62]

## FUTURE DIRECTIONS OF CARDIAC RESYNCHRONIZATION THERAPY IN HEART FAILURE

Despite the fact that several randomized controlled trials have been conducted to assess the efficacy and safety of CRT in HF, these trials included only a few thousand patients, and about one-third of the patients did not derive any symptomatic benefit from CRT and were termed nonresponders. Further studies are needed to refine patient selection characteristics to maximize the benefits of CRT. Theoretically, multisite or multipoint LV pacing may be beneficial in some of these nonresponders who have severe LV dyssynchrony. The utility of CRT in patients who have severe LV dyssynchrony on echocardiography but without HF is not known. In patients in whom the LV lead could not be implanted into the coronary sinus, there are too few data on the feasibility, safety, and efficacy of surgical epicardial or endocardial LV lead implantation. Large randomized controlled trials are needed to address these issues with respect to CRT.

## SUMMARY

Conduction abnormalities and ventricular dyssynchrony are relatively common in patients with HF. Ventricular dyssynchrony causes adverse LV remodeling leading to worsening heart failure. Cardiac resynchronization helps in favorable remodeling of the LV and improving the cardiac hemodynamics, which may also improve MR in some patients. CRT device implantation has been shown to improve mortality and reduce HF hospitalizations in a subset of patients with HFrEF. The patients who benefit the most from CRT are HFrEF patients with severe LV dyssynchrony in the form of LBBB,

QRS duration of greater than 150 milliseconds, and NYHA Class III/IV symptoms. Appropriate patient selection, as directed by the existing guidelines and prompt recognition of procedure-related complications are important in order to maximize the efficacy of CRT and to minimize the adverse events related to device implantation.

## REFERENCES

1. Shamim W, Francis DP, Yousufuddin M, et al. Intraventricular conduction delay: a prognostic marker in chronic heart failure. Int J Cardiol 1999;70:171–8.
2. Baldasseroni S, Opasich C, Gorini M, et al. Left bundle-branch block is associated with increased 1-year sudden and total mortality rate in 5517 outpatients with congestive heart failure: a report from the Italian network on congestive heart failure. Am Heart J 2002;143:398.
3. Cleland JG, Daubert JC, Erdmann E, et al. The effect of cardiac resynchronization on morbidity and mortality in heart failure. N Engl J Med 2005;352:1539.
4. St John Sutton MG, Plappert T, Abraham WT, et al. Effect of cardiac resynchronization therapy on left ventricular size and function in chronic heart failure. Circulation 2003;107:1985.
5. Ukkonen H, Beanlands RS, Burwash IG, et al. Effect of cardiac resynchronization on myocardial efficiency and regional oxidative metabolism. Circulation 2003;107:28.
6. Vollmann D, Lüthje L, Schott P, et al. Biventricular pacing improves the blunted force-frequency relation present during univentricular pacing in patients with heart failure and conduction delay. Circulation 2006;113:953.
7. Leclercq C, Cazeau S, Le Breton H, et al. Acute hemodynamic effects of biventricular DDD pacing in patients with end-stage heart failure. J Am Coll Cardiol 1998;32:1825.
8. Aranda JM Jr, Woo GW, Conti JB, et al. Use of cardiac resynchronization therapy to optimize betablocker therapy in patients with heart failure and prolonged QRS duration. Am J Cardiol 2005;95:889.
9. Waggoner AD, Faddis MN, Gleva MJ, et al. Improvements in left ventricular diastolic function after cardiac resynchronization therapy are coupled to response in systolic performance. J Am Coll Cardiol 2005;46:2244.
10. Saxon LA, Ellenbogen KA. Resynchronization therapy for the treatment of heart failure. Circulation 2003;108(9):1044–8.
11. Abraham WT, Fisher WG, Smith AL, et al. Cardiac resynchronization in chronic heart failure. N Engl J Med 2002;346:1845.

12. Wilkoff BL, Cook JR, Epstein AE, et al. Dual-chamber pacing or ventricular backup pacing in patients with an implantable defibrillator: the Dual Chamber and VVI Implantable Defibrillator (DAVID) Trial. JAMA 2002;288:3115.

13. Sweeney MO, Hellkamp AS, Ellenbogen KA, et al. Adverse effect of ventricular pacing on heart failure and atrial fibrillation among patients with normal baseline QRS duration in a clinical trial of pacemaker therapy for sinus node dysfunction. Circulation 2003;107:2932.

14. Wilkoff BL, Kudenchuk PJ, Buxton AE, et al. The DAVID (Dual Chamber and VVI Implantable Defibrillator) II trial. J Am Coll Cardiol 2009;53:872.

15. Bristow MR, Saxon LA, Boehmer J, et al. Cardiac-resynchronization therapy with or without an implantable defibrillator in advanced chronic heart failure. N Engl J Med 2004;350:2140–50.

16. McAlister FA, Ezekowitz J, Hooton N, et al. Cardiac resynchronization therapy for patients with left ventricular systolic dysfunction: a systematic review. JAMA 2007;297:2502.

17. Moss AJ, Hall WJ, Cannom DS, et al. Cardiac-resynchronization therapy for the prevention of heart-failure events. N Engl J Med 2009;361:1329.

18. Santangeli P, Di Biase L, Pelargonio G, et al. Cardiac resynchronization therapy in patients with mild heart failure: a systematic review and meta-analysis. J Interv Card Electrophysiol 2011;32:125.

19. Maisel WH, Stevenson LW. Atrial fibrillation in heart failure: epidemiology, pathophysiology, and rationale for therapy. Am J Cardiol 2003;91(6A):2D–8D.

20. Doshi RN, Daoud EG, Fellows C, et al. Left ventricular-based cardiac stimulation post AV nodal ablation evaluation (the PAVE study). J Cardiovasc Electrophysiol 2005;16(11):1160–5.

21. Curtis AB, Worley SJ, Adamson PB, et al. Biventricular pacing for atrioventricular block and systolic dysfunction. N Engl J Med 2013;368(17):1585–93.

22. Hayes DL, Boehmer JP, Day JD, et al. Cardiac resynchronization therapy and the relationship of percent biventricular pacing to symptoms and survival. Heart Rhythm 2011;8(9):1469–75.

23. Kamath GS, Cotiga D, Koneru JN, et al. The utility of 12-lead Holter monitoring in patients with permanent atrial fibrillation for the identification of nonresponders after cardiac resynchronization therapy. J Am Coll Cardiol 2009;53(12):1050–5.

24. Gasparini M, Auricchio A, Metra M, et al. Long-term survival in patients undergoing cardiac resynchronization therapy: the importance of performing atrio-ventricular junction ablation in patients with permanent atrial fibrillation. Eur Heart J 2008;29(13):1644–52.

25. Saxon LA. Does cardiac resynchronization therapy reduce the incidence of atrial fibrillation, and does atrial fibrillation compromise the cardiac resynchronization therapy effect? Heart Rhythm 2007;4(3 Suppl):S31–3.

26. Daubert JC, Saxon L, Adamson PB, et al. 2012 EHRA/HRS expert consensus statement on cardiac resynchronization therapy in heart failure: implant and follow-up recommendations and management. Heart Rhythm 2012;9(9):1524–76.

27. Tops LF, Schalij MJ, Holman ER, et al. Right ventricular pacing can induce ventricular dyssynchrony in patients with atrial fibrillation after atrioventricular node ablation. J Am Coll Cardiol 2006;48(8):1642–8.

28. van Bommel RJ, Marsan NA, Delgado V, et al. Cardiac resynchronization therapy as a therapeutic option in patients with moderate-severe functional mitral regurgitation and high operative risk. Circulation 2011;124(8):912–9.

29. Damy T, Ghio S, Rigby AS, et al. Interplay between right ventricular function and cardiac resynchronization therapy: an analysis of the CARE-HF trial (Cardiac Resynchronization-Heart Failure). J Am Coll Cardiol 2013;61(21):2153–60.

30. Derval N, Steendijk P, Gula LJ, et al. Optimizing hemodynamics in heart failure patients by systematic screening of left ventricular pacing sites: the lateral left ventricular wall and the coronary sinus are rarely the best sites. J Am Coll Cardiol 2010;55(6):566–75.

31. Singh JP, Klein HU, Huang DT, et al. Left ventricular lead position and clinical outcome in the multicenter automatic defibrillator implantation trial-cardiac resynchronization therapy (MADIT-CRT) trial. Circulation 2011;123(11):1159–66.

32. Bleeker GB, Kaandorp TA, Lamb HJ, et al. Effect of posterolateral scar tissue on clinical and echocardiographic improvement after cardiac resynchronization therapy. Circulation 2006;113(7):969–76.

33. Adelstein EC, Saba S. Scar burden by myocardial perfusion imaging predicts echocardiographic response to cardiac resynchronization therapy in ischemic cardiomyopathy. Am Heart J 2007;153(1):105–12.

34. Sweeney MO, van Bommel RJ, Schalij MJ, et al. Analysis of ventricular activation using surface electrocardiography to predict left ventricular reverse volumetric remodeling during cardiac resynchronization therapy. Circulation 2010;121(5):626–34.

35. Roubicek T, Wichterle D, Kucera P, et al. Left ventricular lead electrical delay is a predictor of mortality in patients with cardiac resynchronization therapy. Circ Arrhythm Electrophysiol 2015;8(5):1113–21.

36. Bernheim A, Ammann P, Sticherling C, et al. Right atrial pacing impairs cardiac function during resynchronization therapy: acute effects of DDD pacing compared to VDD pacing. J Am Coll Cardiol 2005;45(9):1482–7.

37. Steinberg BA, Wehrenberg S, Jackson KP. Atrioventricular and ventricular-to-ventricular programming in patients with cardiac resynchronization therapy: results from ALTITUDE. J Interv Card Electrophysiol 2015;44(3):279–87.

38. Meluzin J, Novak M, Mullerova J, et al. A fast and simple echocardiographic method of determination of the optimal atrioventricular delay in patients after biventricular stimulation. Pacing Clin Electrophysiol 2004;27(1):58–64.

39. Ellenbogen KA, Gold MR, Meyer TE, et al. Primary results from the SmartDelay determined AV optimization: a comparison to other AV delay methods used in cardiac resynchronization therapy (SMART-AV) trial: a randomized trial comparing empirical, echocardiography-guided, and algorithmic atrioventricular delay programming in cardiac resynchronization therapy. Circulation 2010;122(25):2660–8.

40. van Gelder BM, Bracke FA, Meijer A, et al. Effect of optimizing the VV interval on left ventricular contractility in cardiac resynchronization therapy. Am J Cardiol 2004;93(12):1500–3.

41. Ruwald AC, Kutyifa V, Ruwald MH, et al. The association between biventricular pacing and cardiac resynchronization therapy-defibrillator efficacy when compared with implantable cardioverter defibrillator on outcomes and reverse remodeling. Eur Heart J 2015;36(7):440–8.

42. Steendijk P, Tulner SA, Bax JJ, et al. Hemodynamic effects of long-term cardiac resynchronization therapy: analysis by pressure-volume loops. Circulation 2006;113(10):1295–304.

43. Sipahi I, Carrigan TP, Rowland DY, et al. Impact of QRS duration on clinical event reduction with cardiac resynchronization therapy: meta-analysis of randomized controlled trials. Arch Intern Med 2011;171(16):1454–62.

44. Molhoek SG, VAN Erven L, Bootsma M, et al. QRS duration and shortening to predict clinical response to cardiac resynchronization therapy in patients with end-stage heart failure. Pacing Clin Electrophysiol 2004;27(3):308–13.

45. Lecoq G, Leclercq C, Leray E, et al. Clinical and electrocardiographic predictors of a positive response to cardiac resynchronization therapy in advanced heart failure. Eur Heart J 2005;26(11):1094–100.

46. White JA, Yee R, Yuan X, et al. Delayed enhancement magnetic resonance imaging predicts response to cardiac resynchronization therapy in patients with intraventricular dyssynchrony. J Am Coll Cardiol 2006;48(10):1953–60.

47. Chalil S, Stegemann B, Muyhaldeen SA, et al. Effect of posterolateral left ventricular scar on mortality and morbidity following cardiac resynchronization therapy. Pacing Clin Electrophysiol 2007;30(10):1201–9.

48. Chalil S, Foley PW, Muyhaldeen SA, et al. Late gadolinium enhancement-cardiovascular magnetic resonance as a predictor of response to cardiac resynchronization therapy in patients with ischaemic cardiomyopathy. Europace 2007;9(11):1031–7.

49. Chung ES, Leon AR, Tavazzi L, et al. Results of the predictors of response to CRT (PROSPECT) trial. Circulation 2008;117(20):2608–16.

50. Beshai JF, Grimm RA, Nagueh SF, et al. Cardiac-resynchronization therapy in heart failure with narrow QRS complexes. N Engl J Med 2007;357(24):2461–71.

51. Goldenberg I, Moss AJ, Hall WJ, et al. Predictors of response to cardiac resynchronization therapy in the multicenter automatic defibrillator implantation trial with cardiac resynchronization therapy (MADIT-CRT). Circulation 2011;124(14):1527–36.

52. Kuhlkamp V, InSync 7272 ICD World Wide Investigators. Initial experience with an implantable cardioverter-defibrillator incorporating cardiac resynchronization therapy. J Am Coll Cardiol 2002;39(5):790–7.

53. Kober L, Thune JJ, Nielsen JC, et al. Defibrillator implantation in patients with nonischemic systolic heart failure. N Engl J Med 2016;375(13):1221–30.

54. León AR, Abraham WT, Curtis AB, et al. Safety of transvenous cardiac resynchronization system implantation in patients with chronic heart failure: combined results of over 2,000 patients from a multicenter study program. J Am Coll Cardiol 2005;46(12):2348–56.

55. Swindle JP, Rich MW, McCann P, et al. Implantable cardiac device procedures in older patients: use and in-hospital outcomes. Arch Intern Med 2010;170(7):631–7.

56. Feldman AM, de Lissovoy G, Bristow MR, et al. Cost effectiveness of cardiac resynchronization therapy in the comparison of medical therapy, pacing, and defibrillation in heart failure (COMPANION) trial. J Am Coll Cardiol 2005;46(12):2322–4.

57. Calvert MJ, Freemantle N, Yao G, et al. Cost-effectiveness of cardiac resynchronization therapy: results from the CARE-HF trial. Eur Heart J 2005;26(24):2681–8.

58. Noyes K, Veazie P, Hall WJ, et al. Cost-effectiveness of cardiac resynchronization therapy in the MADIT-CRT trial. J Cardiovasc Electrophysiol 2013;24(1):66–74.

59. Yancy CW, Jessup M, Bozkurt B, et al. 2013 ACCF/AHA guideline for the management of heart failure: a report of the American College of Cardiology Foundation/American Heart Association Task Force on practice guidelines. Circulation 2013;128(16):e240–327.

60. Ponikowski P, Voors AA, Anker SD, et al. 2016 ESC Guidelines for the diagnosis and treatment of acute and chronic heart failure: the task force for the

diagnosis and treatment of acute and chronic heart failure of the European Society of Cardiology (ESC) Developed with the special contribution of the Heart Failure Association (HFA) of the ESC. Eur Heart J 2016;37(27):2129–200.

61. Steffel J, Robertson M, Singh JP, et al. The effect of QRS duration on cardiac resynchronization therapy in patients with a narrow QRS complex: a subgroup analysis of the EchoCRT trial. Eur Heart J 2015;36: 1983–9.

62. Cleland JG, Abraham WT, Linde C, et al. An individual patient meta-analysis of five randomized trials assessing the effects of cardiac resynchronization therapy on morbidity and mortality in patients with symptomatic heart failure. Eur Heart J 2013;34: 3547–56.

# Adult Congenital Interventions in Heart Failure

Hussam S. Suradi, MD, FSCAI[a,b,c,]*,
Ziyad M. Hijazi, MD, MPH, MSCAI[d]

**KEYWORDS**

- Adult congenital heart disease • Heart failure • Congenital interventions

**KEY POINTS**

- The advances in medical and surgical therapies for children with congenital heart disease (CHD) have resulted in a growing population of patients reaching adulthood, with survival rates exceeding 85%.
- Many of these patients, especially if they are managed inappropriately, face the prospect of future complications, including heart failure and premature death.
- Transcatheter interventions have evolved over the past decades to become the primary treatment for many forms of CHD.
- In this article, we discuss the role of transcatheter interventions in the treatment of heart failure in adults with CHD.

## INTRODUCTION

Congenital heart disease (CHD) is present in 0.8% to 1.0% of live births, and the vast majority of these patients are diagnosed and treated in infancy or childhood. The advances in medical and surgical therapies for children with CHD have resulted in a growing population of patients reaching adulthood, with survival rates exceeding 85%[1]. As a result, there are now an estimated 1.2 million patients included in this group in the United States.[2] This has created a well-established field on its own, the adult with CHD (ACHD), that serves as a fundamental component of any center providing care for these patients.[3] Further, board certification is now offered in this unique subspecialty.

ACHDs form 3 distinct groups: those with lesions that have not been previously diagnosed (new diagnoses); those who were treated appropriately (corrected), however, they require lifelong follow-up; and those who have had palliative procedures and also require lifelong follow-up. The first group is a rapidly diminishing group, as most forms of CHD are routinely diagnosed and treated in infancy or childhood. The most common diagnosis in this group is secundum atrial septal defect (ASD). The second group is rapidly expanding, as the children with corrected CHD reach adolescence and adulthood. Examples of patients in this group include patients following tetralogy of Fallot repair and arterial switch operation. The third group fortunately is also diminishing and

Disclosure Statement: H.S. Suradi: Nothing to disclose. Z.M. Hijazi: Consultant for Occlutech & Venus Medtech.
[a] Interventional Cardiology, Structural Heart & Valve Center, St. Mary Medical Center, 1500 South Lake Park Avenue, Suite 100, Hobart, IN 46342, USA; [b] Department of Cardiology, Community Hospital, Munster, IN 46321, USA; [c] Rush Center for Structural Heart Disease, Rush University Medical Center, Chicago, IL 60612, USA; [d] Sidra Cardiac Program, Department of Pediatrics, Sidra Medical & Research Center, Weill Cornell Medicine, PO Box 26999, Doha, Qatar
* Corresponding author. Interventional Cardiology, Structural Heart & Valve Center, St. Mary Medical Center, 1500 South Lake Park Avenue, Suite 100, Hobart, IN 46342.
E-mail address: Hussam_suradi@rush.edu

Intervent Cardiol Clin 6 (2017) 427–443
http://dx.doi.org/10.1016/j.iccl.2017.03.011
2211-7458/17/© 2017 Elsevier Inc. All rights reserved.

includes patients who had palliative procedures for single ventricle and are not candidates for the Fontan pathway.

In ACHD, heart failure is the ultimate expression of the sequelae and complications that patients with ACHD often face even after successful repair of their primary defect. Exercise intolerance is the main feature of heart failure, affecting more than a third of patients in the Euro Heart Survey, a large registry of patients with ACHD across Europe.[4] Patients with cyanotic lesions tend to be with the highest prevalence of exercise intolerance. Within the cyanotic population, those with significant pulmonary arterial hypertension (Eisenmenger syndrome) tend to be most severely limited. Patients with the right ventricle in the systemic position, either as a result of congenitally corrected transposition of the great arteries or after atrial switch operation (Mustard or Senning procedure) for transposition of the great arteries also tend to become severely limited in their exercise capacity, especially after the third decade of life. Patients with univentricular circulation and a Fontan-type operation are also typically limited in their exercise capacity, especially in the presence of ventricular dysfunction, atrioventricular valve regurgitation, or a failing Fontan circulation. Even patients with simple lesions, such as ASD, often present with reduced exercise capacity, even though often at a later stage.

Myocardial dysfunction is common in ACHD and can be caused by multiple factors. Hemodynamic overload of 1 or both ventricles due to obstructive or regurgitant lesions, shunting, and pulmonary or systemic hypertension is common in ACHD. This long-standing overload can eventually lead to severe ventricular dysfunction. Right ventricular systolic dysfunction is common in patients with significant volume overload, such as those with large ASDs or patients with tetralogy of Fallot and severe pulmonary regurgitation. Ventricular dysfunction also can result from repeated cardiac surgeries, anomalous coronary circulation, and abnormal myocardial perfusion. Ventricular-ventricular interaction is not uncommon in ACHD, with right-sided lesions often affecting the left ventricle and vice versa, such as in Ebstein anomaly. Acquired coronary and noncoronary heart disease superimposed to the congenitally abnormal heart also may cause deterioration of myocardial dysfunction, such as coronary atherosclerosis, infective endocarditis, systemic hypertension, myocarditis, and substance abuse. Coronary artery disease always should be suspected in ACHD when ventricular dysfunction is encountered and should be managed accordingly. Medications, permanent pacing, and arrhythmias are other important causes of heart failure in this population. Therefore, identification of the mechanisms responsible for heart failure is essential in the management of patients with ACHD because these can become targets for therapies (Box 1).

Over the past decades, interventional pediatric and adult cardiologists have become increasingly experienced with transcatheter interventional therapy for CHD. The rapid development of successful transcatheter procedures has led to interventional procedures becoming the primary treatment for many forms of CHD. These same techniques are currently being applied to ACHDs with excellent results. In this article, we focus in a defect-specific approach on the role of catheter-based interventions in the treatment of ACHDs.

## PREPROCEDURAL ASSESSMENT

All patients with CHD should undergo a comprehensive, multidisciplinary evaluation with close collaboration between the clinical cardiologist, interventionalist, and surgeon. Details of the procedure and the benefits and risks of any anticipated intervention should be discussed with the patient. Alternative options, including surgical treatment, should be discussed and a meeting with a surgeon should be offered if the patient desires. A thorough review of the patient's complete history and physical examination, including all previous pertinent noninvasive studies, cardiac

---

**Box 1**
**Potential mechanisms of heart failure in adults with congenital heart disease**

Valve disease

Outflow obstruction

Shunting

Volume/pressure overload

Residual lesions

Coronary anomalies

Coronary artery disease

Prior surgery

Arrhythmias

Pericardial disease

Pacing

Medications

Chronotropic incompetence

catheterizations, and reviewing operative notes from previous surgeries is essential. Patients may be severely ill or have various comorbidities, and recognition of these conditions and appropriate anticipation of potential complications is vitally important before cardiac catheterization. Laboratory studies should be ordered as indicated by the clinical findings and blood typing should be obtained for patients at significant complication risk and in whom intervention potentially may be needed. It also is important to review all relevant imaging modalities pertinent to the procedure. Airway management and the use of conscious sedation versus general anesthesia should be planned in advance of the catheterization procedure.

## DEFECT-SPECIFIC CONDITIONS
### Shunt Lesions
#### Atrial septal defects
The ASD is the most common form of CHD to escape detection in childhood. They comprise between 20% and 40% of all newly diagnosed CHD in adults. Under normal physiologic conditions, flow through an ASD occurs from left-to-right to a variable degree depending on the defect size, ventricular compliance, and the pulmonary vascular resistance. Excessive flow through the defect will eventually result in a chronic right heart volume loading state, eventually leading to long-term complications in the second or third decade of life. These include premature death, atrial arrhythmias, reduced exercise tolerance, right ventricular diastolic and systolic failure, left ventricular diastolic failure, and pulmonary arterial hypertension.[5,6] Therefore, early closure of hemodynamically significant defects is recommended. There are 4 different types of ASDs that have different anatomic and clinical features: ostium secundum, ostium primum, coronary sinus defects, and sinus venosus ASDs. Secundum ASD is the most common (75% of cases) and is usually located at the level of the fossa ovalis. The primum ASD (15%–20% of cases) is located in the inferior part of the atrial septum, near the crux of the heart, and is associated with atrioventricular septal defects. The sinus venosus type (5%–10% of cases) is located in the superior or inferior part of the septum, near the superior or inferior vena cavae entry to the right atrium. The superior part is usually associated with partial anomalous pulmonary venous drainage. The uncommon coronary sinus septal defect (<1%) allows shunting across the ostium of the coronary sinus.

The most common accepted indications for closure are evidence of a significant left-to-right shunt with Qp/Qs ratio greater than 1.5:1.0 or the presence of right heart enlargement as seen by transthoracic echocardiography. None of these defects, with the exception of secundum ASD, is amenable for device closure due to anatomic limitations. In patients with either severe irreversible pulmonary hypertension or severe left ventricular dysfunction, ASD closure is an absolute contraindication, as it is physiologically needed to act as a "pop-off valve" for either the right or left ventricle, respectively. ASD balloon test occlusion with observation of resultant hemodynamics may aid in observing the acute hemodynamic effects of closure, although studies assessing the longer-term predictive nature of such testing have not been performed. Complex strategies using concomitant pulmonary vasodilator therapies or customized "fenestrated" closure devices have been reported in patients with large-volume left-to-right shunting and moderate to severe pulmonary hypertension.

Even though there are no randomized trials comparing percutaneous versus surgical closure of ASDs, percutaneous closure of secundum ASD is currently the standard of care with a success rate exceeding 98% of patients who have suitable margins and defect size. An atrial septum rim greater than 5 mm around most of the defect is required for the safe use of any closure device, although more deficient anterior superior aortic rim is typical and does not preclude percutaneous closure. Depending on the experience of the operator, the procedure may be done under conscious sedation by using intracardiac echocardiography (ICE) or under general anesthesia with the use of transesophageal echocardiography to define the anatomy of the defect and to guide device deployment. It is advisable to perform balloon sizing of the defect to aid in selecting the appropriate device size (Fig. 1). The choice of device depends on its availability, the exact anatomy of the defect, and operator preference. In the United States, 2 devices are approved by the Food and Drug Administration for this indication: the Amplatzer Septal Occluder device (St Jude Medical, Plymouth, MN) and the Gore Helex Septal Occluder (Gore Medical, Flagstaff, AZ). Both devices are variations of "umbrella" devices that hold both sides of the atrial septum. Multiple other devices are available internationally, the most commonly used is the Occlutech Figulla Flex II device (Occlutech GmbH, Jena, Germany), a double-desk device similar in design to the Amplatzer septal occluder.

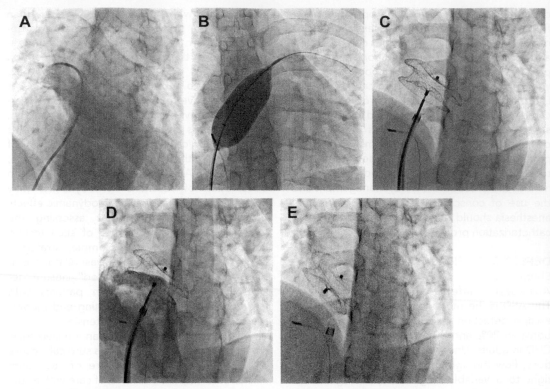

**Fig. 1.** Cine fluoroscopic steps during Amplatzer septal occluder (ASO) device deployment and evaluation post deployment. (*A*) Right upper pulmonary vein angiogram in the 4-chamber view profiling the atrial septum with a central secundum ASD. (*B*) Balloon sizing of the ASD to measure the "stop-flow diameter." (*C*) ASO deployment. (*D*) Right atrial angiogram after the device has been deployed but not released showing good device position, (*E*) ASO device has been released.

## Ventricular septal defect

Ventricular septal defects (VSDs) comprise as many as 10% of CHD in adults and are classified as inflow, muscular, or perimembranous depending on location in the septum. Significant VSD can develop left ventricular volume overload, ventricular failure, and pulmonary hypertension, typically at a younger age than patients with ASDs. Therefore, most patients with large shunts are usually diagnosed and treated in childhood. VSD closure in the adult is recommended for significant left-to-right shunt greater than 1.5:1.0, evidence of left ventricular volume overload, symptoms of heart failure, when accompanied by progressive aortic regurgitation or post episode of endocarditis. There are 2 main reasons to perform cardiac catheterization for VSDs: (1) to define the magnitude and level of the shunt, and (2) to exclude significant pulmonary vascular disease. Based on these data, decision for closure is determined.

Device closure of VSDs has become more common and can be performed safely and effectively. The defect is crossed with the use of a hydrophilic wire from the left ventricular side, the

guide wire is snared from the right side of the heart and exteriorized forming an arteriovenous vascular loop, and subsequent device deployment across the defect proceeds without interference to adjacent intracardiac structures (**Fig. 2**). Since the introduction of the Amplatzer devices to close VSDs in 1998 (St Jude Medical), the outcomes of percutaneous VSD closure have significantly improved and results have been promising, as these were specifically designed for closure of VSDs. The wide variability in VSD location, size, and morphology led to the development of different designs of the Amplatzer VSD devices (**Fig. 3**). The Amplatzer muscular VSD device has 2 symmetric disks that exceed the diameter of the connecting waist by 8 mm. The Amplatzer membranous VSD occluder is an asymmetrical device that was specifically designed for perimembranous VSDs to account for the surrounding cardiac structures. In 2002, Hijazi and colleagues[7] reported the first successful attempt in humans, whereby 6 patients underwent complete VSD closure without any significant complications. However, later studies raised the concern of complete heart block when

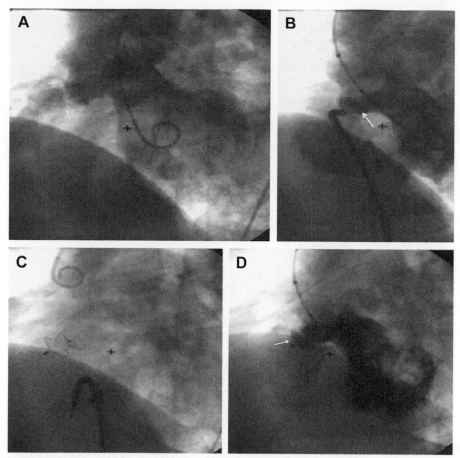

**Fig. 2.** Perimembranous VSD closure in a 39-year-old male patient using Amplatzer membranous VSD device. (*A*) Left ventricular angiogram in long axial oblique (LAO 60, Cranial 20) demonstrating a membranous VSD (*arrow*). (*B*) Repeat left ventricular angiogram after deployment of the left ventricular desk (*arrow*) of a 12-mm device showing good desk position. (*C*) The device has been released. (*D*) Repeat left ventricular angiogram after device release demonstrating good device position and minimal foaming through the device (*Arrow* indicates the membranous VSD occluder device).

using this original device due to impingement of the device on the atrioventricular node and the His-Purkinje fibers, which run through that portion of the septum. The European registry reported a complete heart block rate of 5%[8]; however, some centers have cited a rate as high as 22%.[9] This has led to the introduction of the Amplatzer membranous VSD occluder II, with the hope that the new design will have a lower rate of impact on the conduction system and subsequent heart block. Initial experiences have shown it to be encouraging, having no incidence of heart block reported.[10] Other Amplatzer devices (eg, Amplatzer duct occluder II) and non-Amplatzer devices (eg, Nit-Occlud) have been used as well to close perimembranous VSDs. Additionally, periventricular "hybrid" surgical approaches have been performed, in which a surgical incision exposes the right ventricular free wall followed by device closure in the usual fashion.

*Patent ductus arteriosus*
The overwhelming majority of patent ductus arterioses (PDA) are diagnosed and treated during childhood by using a variety of catheter-based techniques. Our standard practice for PDA closure in the pediatric population is for hemodynamically significant shunt with evidence of left heart enlargement or when there is a continuous murmur. Silent PDAs without an audible murmur are considered benign and do not warrant closure. In adults, however, PDA is a relatively uncommon finding, usually discovered incidentally while investigating symptoms such as dyspnea or palpitations, evaluation of a murmur, or following an episode of endarteritis. Similar to the pediatric population,

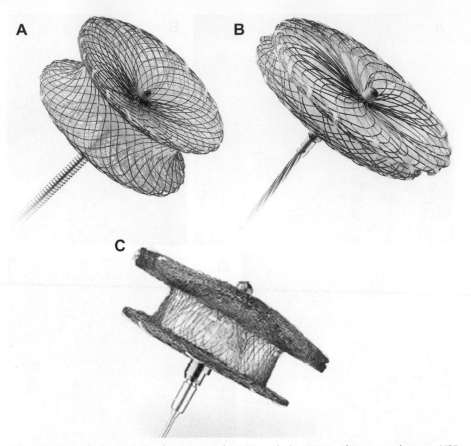

Fig. 3. Amplatzer VSD occluders. (*A*) Amplatzer muscular VSD occluder. (*B*) Amplatzer membranous VSD occluder I. (*C*) Amplatzer membranous VSD occluder II. (*Courtesy of* St Jude Medical, St Paul, MN; with permission.)

large PDAs with significant left-to-right shunt should be closed to reduce occurrence of the sequelae of ventricular failure or pulmonary arterial hypertension.

Catheter-based closure of PDAs in adults can be more challenging and complex as compared with closure in the pediatric population, as PDAs tend to be increasingly calcified and more tortuous. Nevertheless, transcatheter closure remains more desirable compared with surgery because of the potential for recurrent laryngeal nerve damage during surgery for calcified PDAs. With the availability of different devices developed specifically for PDA closure, more than 99% of PDAs are amenable to transcatheter closure. Devices currently available include the Amplatzer Duct Occluders (ADO I and II) (St Jude Medical) (Fig. 4), Nit-occlud PDA Occlusion system (pfm medical, Cologne, Germany), Occlutech PDA device, and detachable coils. The Amplatzer Atrial Septal and Muscular Ventricular Septal Defect Occluders also have been used to close larger PDAs. The ADO comes in a variety of sizes that allows it to be used

effectively in PDAs up to 11 mm and it can be used in all PDA types (Fig. 5).

## Coronary artery fistula

Coronary artery fistulae are connections between the coronary arteries and the cardiac chambers or great vessels. Most fistulae originate from the right coronary artery, with the left anterior descending artery being the next most frequently involved. The major termination sites are the right cardiac chambers and pulmonary arteries. Less frequently, fistulae drain into the superior vena cava, coronary sinus, or left cardiac chambers. Most fistulae are small and clinically silent. However, larger fistulae can lead to significant left-to-right shunting with right-sided volume overload and effective coronary arterial steal leading to ischemia.

Most coronary fistulae are amenable to percutaneous closure via either retrograde or antegrade approach, using a variety of coils, plugs, or duct occluders (Fig. 6). The aim of catheter closure is to occlude the fistulous artery as distally as possible, avoiding any possibility of

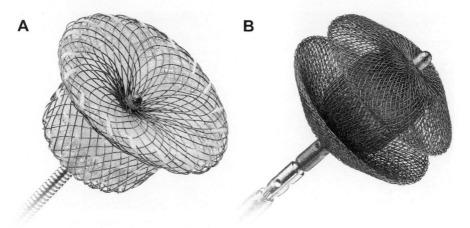

**Fig. 4.** ADO (*A*) I and (*B*) II. (*Courtesy of* St Jude Medical, Plymouth, MN; with permission.)

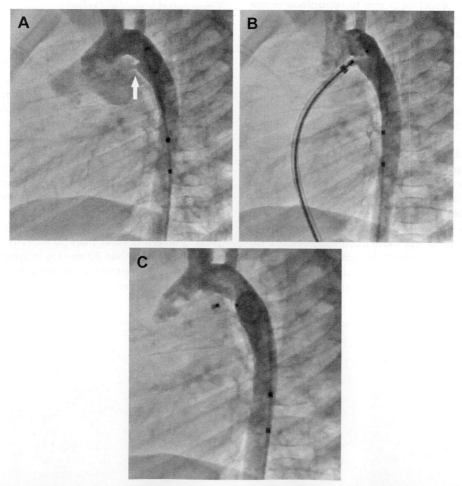

**Fig. 5.** Cine angiographic images during PDA closure using an ADO device. (*A*) Aortic angiogram demonstrating small PDA (*arrow*). (*B*) Repeat angiogram before device release demonstrating good device position. (*C*) Final angiogram after device release demonstrating good device position and no residual shunt.

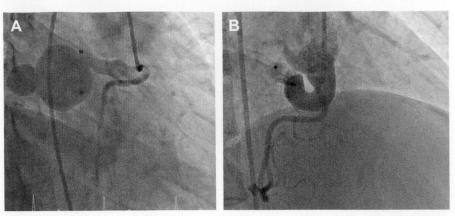

Fig. 6. (*A*) Selective right coronary angiogram demonstrating a large right coronary artery fistula draining to the right atrium. (*B*) Successful occlusion of fistula using Amplatzer muscular occluder.

occluding branches to the normal myocardium. Risks of fistula closure with these devices include myocardial infarction (due to inadvertent closure of viable branches or due to retrograde propagation of thrombus occluding viable branches) and migration of coils or discs to extracoronary vascular structures or within the coronary artery branches.[11] Long-term effects of intravascular fistula occlusion are yet to be demonstrated.

### Aortopulmonary collaterals

Aortopulmonary collaterals may be observed in patients with congenital malformations associated with decreased pulmonary flow, including pulmonary atresia, as well as variations of single-ventricle physiology or after Glenn shunt or Fontan palliation. These collaterals can arise from any systemic artery and connect directly to the pulmonary arteries (**Fig. 7**). The resulting left-to-right shunting may cause pulmonary vascular disease, systemic ventricular volume loading, and ultimate heart failure. Embolization is typically performed with coils; however, larger collaterals can be occluded using Amplatzer vascular plugs with similar success.

### Congenital Valvular Defects
#### Pulmonary valve stenosis

Valvar pulmonary stenosis is a common congenital lesion in pediatrics that may escape detection in childhood and present in adulthood with significant stenosis. It is typically caused by commissural fusion resulting in diminished valve orifice and increased right ventricular afterload. Symptoms may vary from mild exertional dyspnea to signs and symptoms of right heart failure, depending on the severity of obstruction and the degree of myocardial compensation. Balloon pulmonary valvuloplasty has evolved to be the procedure of choice for the treatment of pulmonary valve stenosis. Indications for intervention on isolated pulmonic stenosis include peak gradient greater than 50 mm Hg or mean gradient greater than 30 mm Hg in symptomatic patients. In asymptomatic patients, intervention may be considered with peak gradient greater

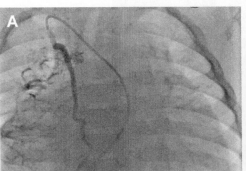
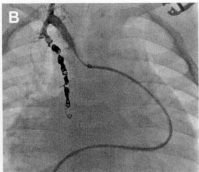

Fig. 7. (*A*) Selective injection into the right internal mammary artery showing collaterals to the right lung. (*B*) Coil occlusion of the right internal mammary artery. (*Courtesy of* Dr Damien Kenny, MD, Crumin, Dublin, Ireland.)

than 60 mm Hg or mean gradient greater than 40 mm Hg.[12] However, from our experience and that of others, we have found even low gradients of peak of 35 mm Hg to cause symptoms. Therefore, coupled with the safety of the procedure, we have been intervening on valves with gradients as low as 35 mm Hg with very good resolution of symptoms. Before balloon valvuloplasty, it is very important to carefully assess the pulmonary valve morphology and degree of calcification. The determinant of favorable result is the presence of commissural fusion. Dysplastic valves may be present in a small percentage of patients and are characterized by thickened, nodular, and redundant valve leaflets with minimal or no commissural fusion and lack of poststenotic dilatation of the pulmonary artery. Some investigators consider dysplastic valves as a relative contraindication for balloon dilatation; however, in our experience and that of others, balloon valvuloplasty remains the initial treatment of choice. It is generally recommended that the optimal balloon size selection should not exceed 125% of pulmonary valve annulus size to achieve favorable results and to avoid the risk of significant regurgitation. Balloon pulmonary valvuloplasty has uniformly excellent results in all age groups, with results comparable to surgical valvotomy, has low recurrence risk and can be easily repeated if necessary. The double-balloon technique, which uses 2 smaller balloons from each femoral vein, also has been applied to pulmonary valve stenosis with equally excellent results.[13]

## Percutaneous pulmonary valve implantation

Transcatheter pulmonary valve replacement (tPVR) is one of the most exciting recent developments in the treatment of structural heart disease and has evolved as an attractive alternative to surgery in patients with dysfunctional right ventricle–pulmonary artery conduits or bioprosthetic valves. The most common indication of pulmonary valve implantation is residual right ventricular outflow tract (RVOT) lesion after repair of CHD that can be stenotic, regurgitant, or mixed. The common congenital heart lesions falling in this group are pulmonary atresia, tetralogy of Fallot, Truncus arteriosus, Rastelli-type repair of transposition, and after Ross operation. The advent of tPVR with Melody (Medtronic Inc, Minneapolis, MN) and Sapien (Edwards Lifesciences, Irvine, CA) valves have dramatically altered the management of these patients. Patients with tetralogy of Fallot who have had valved conduits or bioprosthetic valves placed,

and patients who underwent the Ross procedure, in which the pulmonary valve is autotransplanted to replace the diseased aortic valve and a valved-conduit is used between the right ventricle and pulmonary artery, represent the 2 largest patient populations that are receiving these valves. Even though tPVR is not currently a standard indication in adults with native RVOT dysfunction, many centers have performed percutaneous pulmonic valve implantation in a select group of adults who have a native outflow tract (post transannular patch repair of tetralogy of Fallot) that is of an appropriate size or one that can be altered to a suitable size by insertion of multiple stents.[14]

Appropriate patient selection for pulmonary valve replacement is crucial, and the guidelines for both surgical and transcatheter pulmonary valve replacement have continued to evolve over the past decade.[15–19] In general, it is recommended to use a composite measure of clinical data (symptoms, exercise capacity, presence of arrhythmias), electrocardiogram and echo data, and MRI-based data elements, such as right ventricular end diastolic volume index ($\geq$150 mL/m$^2$), right ventricular end-systolic volume index (>80 mL/m$^2$), pulmonary regurgitant fraction ($\geq$40%), and right ventricular function (ejection fraction <40%).[20,21] Pulmonary valve replacement ideally should be performed before right ventricular function declines. In addition to clinical indications, several anatomic criteria need to be fulfilled to qualify for tPVR. The ideal anatomy for tPVR is a uniform diameter from RVOT to pulmonary artery with adequate main pulmonary artery length to avoid stenting into the pulmonary artery bifurcation. With the current iterations of the Melody valve, the RVOT, pulmonary valve annulus, and proximal main pulmonary artery must be 22 mm or less to prevent leaflet malcoaptation. Using the 22-mm Ensemble delivery system, the outer diameter of the Melody valve is approximately 24 mm, and therefore any inner diameter of a conduit larger than this would be insufficient to securely anchor the valve. Nevertheless, there is limited experience with mounting the Melody valve on a 24-mm balloon delivered through a 24-French sheath.[22] On the other hand, the SAPIEN valve can be deployed in RVOT sizes up to 29 mm in diameter.

During cardiac catheterization, routine hemodynamic data are obtained. Gradients are obtained in the RVOT/conduit, at the level of the pulmonary valve, and the pulmonary arteries. The pulmonary artery and branch morphology should be delineated by pulmonary arteriograms to define the architecture. After hemodynamic assessment, evaluation of the coronary arteries must be made with balloon inflation in the right ventricle outflow tract to assess the proximity of the coronary arteries to the outflow tract. When the conduit is placed on the anterior surface of the heart, coronary branches may pass directly beneath it, and may be potentially compressed by placement of the stented valve and distension of the conduit.[23] If no evidence of coronary compression is noted, prestenting of the RVOT using bare/covered metal stents is performed to create an appropriate landing zone for the transcatheter valve. Prestenting the landing site has significantly improved the survival of the implant, minimizing stent fracture, which affected 23% of the initially reported cases of the Melody valve. The appropriate valve is then introduced and deployed (Fig. 8 for implantation steps).

## Aortic stenosis

Congenital aortic stenosis is quite different from the more common calcific or senile aortic stenosis. The inherent abnormality in the valve morphology, most commonly bicuspid leaflets, can be associated with a variety of subvalvular, supravalvular, aortic root, and arch abnormalities. In general, congenitally stenotic aortic valves do not cause heart failure early in the disease process, and as such, are usually intervened on well before this would manifest itself in deteriorating ventricular function and associated symptoms of congestive heart failure. Unlike senile aortic stenosis, balloon aortic valvuloplasty (BAV) remains an excellent alternative to surgical valvotomy or valve replacement in young adults with congenital valvar aortic stenosis. The pathology involved in the latter includes more commissural fusion and less leaflet rigidity compared with the calcified senile aortic valves. The bicuspid aortic valve typically becomes thickened and calcified by the fourth decade of life, becoming less suitable to balloon dilatation. The retrograde approach is used most commonly for aortic valvuloplasty. It is important that the noncompliant balloon size does not exceed the aortic annulus size measured by aortography to prevent aortic regurgitation

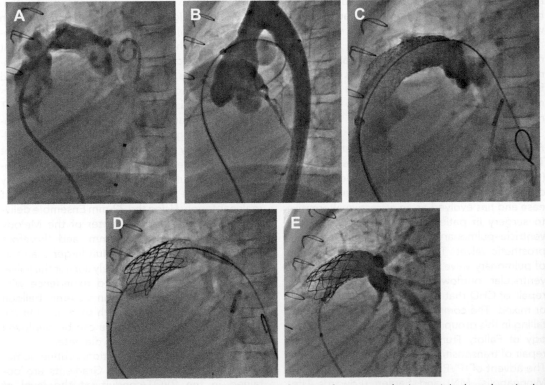

Fig. 8. Melody valve implantation steps. (A) Pulmonary homograft angiography in straight lateral projection demonstrating severe pulmonic regurgitation and stenosis. (B) Conduit balloon sizing with simultaneous aortic root angiography demonstrating left coronary artery with an acceptable distance from the conduit. (C) Angiography post stent deployment demonstrating no conduit stenosis with free pulmonary regurgitation. (D) Melody valve deployment. (E) Final angiography demonstrating no significant pulmonary regurgitation.

from occurring. In the presence of severe peripheral arterial disease, BAV via antegrade approach with transseptal puncture can be performed.

Congenital cardiovascular practice guidelines for patients with aortic stenosis have been established on the basis of valvular peak-to-peak gradients rather than echocardiographically estimated valve areas, in large part because of concerns regarding difficulties in accurately measuring systemic cardiac output and the uncommon presence of low output in pediatric patients. Data are few regarding timing and indications for intervention for adults with congenital aortic stenosis, although current practice guidelines suggest that for symptomatic young adults without severe calcification and less than moderate regurgitation, peak-to-peak gradient of 50 mm Hg (or asymptomatic young adults with ST-T changes and peak-to-peak gradient of 60 mm Hg) is an indication for BAV.[24]

Experience with transcatheter aortic valve replacement (TAVR) in patients with bicuspid aortic valve disease remains limited, as pivotal trials excluded bicuspid valves due to concern of paravalvular regurgitation. This is thought to be related to the larger annulus size, and larger sinus of Valsalva and ascending aortic dimension encountered with bicuspid aortic valves. However, a recent meta-analysis found no significant difference in the risk of post-TAVR paravalvular regurgitation in patients with bicuspid aortic valve compared with other patients (25.7% vs 19.9%).[25] Furthermore, the enhanced paravalvular sealing effect of the third-generation SAPIEN 3 valve has shown promising results in bicuspid aortic valve stenosis in a multicenter study with no patients having more than mild paravalvular regurgitation.[26] TAVR may eventually become an option for the adult patient with bicuspid aortic valve stenosis, but at this point, this treatment strategy is not yet well established for this patient population.

## Obstructive Vascular Lesions
### Coarctation of aorta
Coarctation of the aorta (CoA) is the sixth most common congenital lesion accounting for 4% to 6% of live births with CHD.[27,28] Aortic coarctation is typically located just distal to the origin of the left subclavian artery, although various degrees of obstruction also can occur throughout the aortic arch. Despite these anatomic variations, the effect of the narrowing has the commonly shared features of increased afterload on the left ventricle, exposure of the upper body to hypertension, flow disturbance in the thoracic aorta, and decreased perfusion to the lower body. Untreated coarctation carries a poor prognosis with average survival of 35 years of age; with 75% mortality by 46 years of age.[24] Long-term complications are the consequence of long-term hypertension, including premature coronary artery disease, stroke, endocarditis, aortic dissection, and heart failure.[29] Furthermore, recurrent coarctation and future aneurysm formation can occur following successful surgical and endovascular repair, which mandates long-term close surveillance.

Indications for relief of obstruction include peak-to-peak coarctation gradient of 20 mm Hg or more; which is the difference in peak pressure proximal and beyond the narrowed segment. Furthermore, intervention is also recommended if the gradient is less than 20 mm Hg in the presence of radiologic evidence of significant collateral flow, particularly in those with evidence of left ventricular dysfunction. In most centers, the overwhelming majority of adult patients with CoA undergo transcatheter repair, either using balloon angioplasty or stent implantation, with excellent results. Surgical repair is usually reserved for patients with complex arch lesions, such as arch hypoplasia, long-segment coarctation, aortic aneurysms/dissection, aortic root dilatation, and aortic valve stenosis/regurgitation. Surgical complications are generally more common in adults than children, and can be detrimental as surgical repair is associated with extended recovery time, potential phrenic nerve and recurrent laryngeal nerve injury, and the serious, although uncommon, lower body paralysis secondary to ischemic spinal cord injury.

Balloon angioplasty has been an acceptable technique for 3 decades for the relief of coarctation.[30] It produces controlled tear of the intima and part of the media, which results in an improvement of the vessel diameter. The size of the balloon selected should be no more than 1 to 2 mm larger in diameter than the smallest normal aortic diameter proximal to the coarctation. In cases of recurrent coarctation, the size of the balloon should not be larger than the size of the aorta at the level of the diaphragm. The procedure is successful in reducing the gradient to less than 20 mm Hg in 85% of patients, with a restenosis rate of 8%. Due to the high incidence of future aneurysm formation (up to 9%) and recoarctation,[31] as well as the availability of stents in most centers, balloon angioplasty fell out of favor as first-line therapy in endovascular repair.

Primary stent implantation may theoretically overcome some of the shortcomings of balloon angioplasty and is the procedure of choice for treatment of CoA (**Fig. 9**). It reduces the complications, improves luminal diameter, results in minimal residual gradient, and sustains hemodynamic benefit as compared with balloon angioplasty.[23,32,33] Additionally, stents may reduce the incidence of subsequent aneurysm formation by allowing both the use of smaller-dilatation balloons as well as graded inflations in staged procedures. Data from a multicenter case series of more than 500 patients demonstrated the efficacy and relative safety of stent placement for both native and recurrent coarctation with success rate exceeding 98%.[33,34] Several different endovascular stents are commercially available; however, very few are expandable to the average diameter of a large adult aorta (21.1 ± 3.2 mm for women, 26.1 ± 4.3 mm for men). The choice of stent depends on the coarctation anatomy, size of the patient, the preference of the operator, and availability. Balloon-expandable bare-metal stents are the most commonly used and are made from stainless steel (Palmaz Genesis, Johnson and Johnson, Miami, FL; Mega LD and Maxi LD series, ev3, Plymouth, MN), platinum-iridium alloy (Cheatham-Platinum stent; NuMED, Hopkinton, NY), or chromium-cobalt alloy (AndraStent XL and XXL; Andramed, Reutlingen, Germany). The use of covered stents has added further safety to the short-term and long-term outcomes in these patients. It has been proposed that the use of covered stents reduces the risk of aneurysms; however, in a randomized trial of 120 patients with severe native coarctation, there was no difference in the rate of recoarctation and pseudoaneurysm formation after 31 months of follow-up between patients who underwent implantation using a bare-metal stent and those with a covered stent.[35] Nevertheless, covered stents offer the advantage of excluding any stretch-induced wall trauma from the endoluminal aspect of the aorta, particularly in the catastrophic event of aortic rupture.

### Branch pulmonary artery stenosis

Pulmonary artery stenosis (PAS) may occur anywhere in the pulmonary vascular tree from the

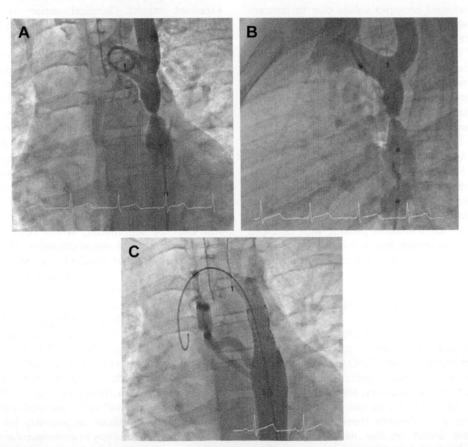

**Fig. 9.** Stenting of native aortic coarctation. Angiogram in the descending aorta in 40° LAO (*A*) and 90° LAO (*B*) demonstrating tight coarctation and presence of many collaterals. Repeat final angiogram after implantation of an ev3 MAX-LD stent (*C*) demonstrating good stent position and no residual narrowing.

main pulmonary artery to the distal-most branches. It is typically associated with other congenital defects or may occur in isolation. Additionally, PAS may result as a sequela of surgical intervention, such as tetralogy of Fallot repair, Blalock-Taussig shunt placement, arterial switch, or right ventricle to pulmonary artery conduit placement for truncus arteriosus repair or pulmonary atresia, which may all lead to branch PAS at suture lines. Many of these sites become technically very difficult to repair surgically and can be effectively treated in the catheterization laboratory with balloon angioplasty or stent placement. All patients with a history of these types of palliative repairs should be fully evaluated for branch pulmonary stenosis, as this is a common reason for right ventricular deterioration in previously well-palliated patients. Patients with any evidence of stenosis or increased right ventricular pressure should receive a pulmonary perfusion scan to quantify the degree of branch PAS. Indications for intervention in PAS include presence of right ventricular pressure greater than 50% of systemic levels or lesser pressure in the setting of symptoms, shunt-mediated cyanosis, subpulmonary ventricular dysfunction, pulmonary flow imbalance with less than 20% to 25% total flow to a single lung, pulmonary hypertension in unaffected lung arterial segments, or severe pulmonary regurgitation.

Balloon angioplasty of branch PAS has a variable success rate. Approximately 60% of procedures are technically successful, but midterm follow-up suggests that up to two-thirds have significant residual stenosis.[36] The restenosis rate approaches 15% and there is a 3% to 4% incidence of aneurysm formation.[37,38] This has led interventionalists to treat branch PA stenosis with primary stent placement. Stents that can be expanded to accommodate branch pulmonary artery size should be used (see the section "Coarctation of aorta"). Patients who require a surgical procedure and have distal pulmonary stenosis also can be treated with pulmonary artery stenting in the operating room. The sites of the stenosis need to be well established before the surgical repair. The surgical field allows relatively easy access to the central pulmonary arteries. A stent can then be advanced into the more distal pulmonary artery and expanded under direct vision and palpation. This technique is useful for patients who have failed attempts at stent placement in the catheterization laboratory or for patients without suitable venous access.

The results of stent placement have been impressive, with up to a 97% success rate with a 2% complication rate.[39,40] New stent technology will undoubtedly improve the results and allow smaller catheters and sheaths to be used. Future directions include self-expanding nitinol stents that can enlarge with the patient's growth and bioabsorbable stent material.

### Complex Congenital Heart Disease
#### D-transposition of the great vessels
The success of the Senning and Mustard-type venous switches for the treatment of the transposition of the great arteries has led to the long-term survival of many of these patients. These intra-atrial surgical baffles allow the systemic venous return to flow through the atria and cross the mitral valve to fill the left ventricle. The left ventricle then pumps the blood to the pulmonary arteries. The fully oxygenated blood returns to the left atrium and flows over the other side of the baffle to the right ventricle and out the aorta. Baffle obstruction is observed in up to 15% of patients undergoing atrial switch procedures. The surgical results of repair of the baffles obstruction were not favorable; therefore, transcatheter therapy with balloon dilation and stenting emerged as the preferred therapy of choice with low complication rates and superior results.[41,42] Complete obstructions can be perforated and residual narrowings treated by using single or multiple stents (**Fig. 10**). Redilatation for neointimal hyperplasia–induced stenosis following stent placement is also successful.[43] Furthermore, up to 25% of patients undergoing Mustard or Senning operations will demonstrate late baffle leaks, likely as the result of suture dehiscence. Although many of these shunts are hemodynamically unapparent and do not require therapy, closure is indicated for large defects resulting in significant intracardiac shunting. Baffle leaks can be treated successfully using percutaneous techniques, including covered stents or occlusion devices.

#### Post-Fontan
The growing number of patients who have palliated single-ventricle physiology is a group with significant adult-onset complications. These patients typically have undergone a variation of the Fontan procedure to redirect all the systemic venous blood directly into the pulmonary arteries. Common indications for catheterization in the adults with Fontan palliation are for hemodynamic evaluation in case of clinical status change, like dysrhythmia, and for preoperative assessment before Fontan revision or cardiac transplantation. During catheterization, it is important to record pulmonary, Fontan,

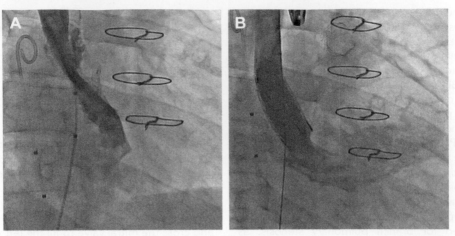

Fig. 10. Stenting of Mustard superior vena cava (SVC) baffle narrowing. (A) Angiogram in the SVC in 20° right axial oblique view demonstrating SVC baffle narrowing. (B) Repeat angiogram after stent implantation showing no residual narrowing.

and aortic pressures, as well as to evaluate for the presence of shunting (right-to-left or left-to-right) with oxygen saturation assessment at various levels. Angiograms should be performed to define the anatomic details of the great vessels, collateral vessels, and the systemic venous drainage, as well as the left ventricular volume and ejection fraction. The low, nonpulsatile flow in the systemic venous circulation and multiple suture lines can lead to significant stenosis within the Fontan circulation (Fig. 11). The same techniques of balloon angioplasty and stent placement are applied to relieve any anatomic obstruction in this complicated patient population. Similarly, transcatheter closure using coils and occlusion devices

are applied for abnormal vascular connections closure that may cause right-to-left (causing cyanosis and paradoxic embolism) or left-to-right shunting (causing systemic ventricular volume overload).

### Miscellaneous conditions

Coronary artery disease becomes more prevalent as the ACHD population ages. Thus, coronary angiography should be performed when ventricular dysfunction is encountered to rule out ischemia as a cause. Coronary stenting should be performed if indicated by operators with expertise in percutaneous coronary interventions.

Balloon atrial septoplasty may be considered in patients with refractory severe pulmonary

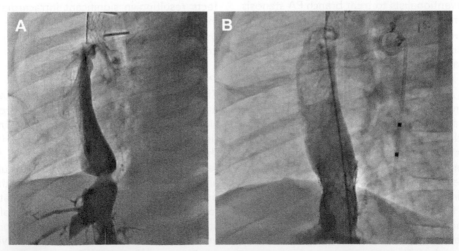

Fig. 11. Angiogram in straight lateral projection in the Fontan conduit demonstrating (A) narrowing in its proximal portion. (B) Repeat angiogram after stent implantation demonstrating no residual stenosis.

arterial hypertension and right ventricular failure, despite aggressive advanced therapy and maximal diuretic therapy. The resultant right-to-left shunting and consequent arterial desaturation that follow the procedure are offset by increased cardiac output and augmentation of systemic oxygen delivery. However, procedure-related mortality may be as high as 15% to 20%.[44] Restenosis of the interatrial septum is common, and fenestrated closure devices are becoming available with the hope of improving long-term patency.

## SUMMARY

Patients with ACHD form a large and complicated group, presenting unique challenges to caregivers. These patients require specialized care by physicians familiar with CHD, adult medicine, dysrhythmias, and interventional procedures. Management of patients with CHD requires a multidisciplinary approach with collaboration between adult congenital heart specialists, pediatric/adult congenital interventionalists, and congenital heart surgeons. Advances in catheterization-based interventions have changed the therapeutic strategy for many patients with CHD. The future holds many promises with advancements in catheter-based interventions as well as hybrid surgical techniques that will improve the survival and quality of life of this complicated patient population.

## REFERENCES

1. Warnes CA, Liberthson R, Danielson GK, et al. Task force 1: the changing profile of congenital heart disease in adult life. J Am Coll Cardiol 2001;37(5): 1170–5.
2. Brickner ME, Hillis LD, Lange RA. Congenital heart disease in adults. First of two parts. N Engl J Med 2000;342(4):256–63.
3. Landzberg MJ, Murphy DJ Jr, Davidson WR Jr, et al. Task force 4: organization of delivery systems for adults with congenital heart disease. J Am Coll Cardiol 2001;37(5):1187–93.
4. Engelfriet P, Boersma E, Oechslin E, et al. The spectrum of adult congenital heart disease in Europe: morbidity and mortality in a 5 year follow-up period. The Euro Heart Survey on adult congenital heart disease. Eur Heart J 2005;26(21):2325–33.
5. Webb G, Gatzoulis MA. Atrial septal defects in the adult: recent progress and overview. Circulation 2006;114(15):1645–53.
6. Campbell M. Natural history of atrial septal defect. Br Heart J 1970;32(6):820–6.
7. Hijazi ZM, Hakim F, Haweleh AA, et al. Catheter closure of perimembranous ventricular septal defects using the new Amplatzer membranous VSD occluder: initial clinical experience. Catheter Cardiovasc Interv 2002;56(4):508–15.
8. Carminati M, Butera G, Chessa M, et al. Transcatheter closure of congenital ventricular septal defects: results of the European Registry. Eur Heart J 2007;28(19):2361–8.
9. Predescu D, Chaturvedi RR, Friedberg MK, et al. Complete heart block associated with device closure of perimembranous ventricular septal defects. J Thorac Cardiovasc Surg 2008;136(5):1223–8.
10. Tzikas A, Ibrahim R, Velasco-Sanchez D, et al. Transcatheter closure of perimembranous ventricular septal defect with the Amplatzer((R)) membranous VSD occluder 2: initial world experience and one-year follow-up. Catheter Cardiovasc Interv 2014;83(4):571–80.
11. Kharouf R, Cao QL, Hijazi ZM. Transcatheter closure of coronary artery fistula complicated by myocardial infarction. J Invasive Cardiol 2007; 19(5):E146–9.
12. Warnes CA, Williams RG, Bashore TM, et al. ACC/AHA 2008 guidelines for the management of adults with congenital heart disease: a report of the American College of Cardiology/American Heart Association Task Force on Practice Guidelines (Writing Committee to Develop Guidelines on the Management of Adults With Congenital Heart Disease). Developed in Collaboration With the American Society of Echocardiography, Heart Rhythm Society, International Society for Adult Congenital Heart Disease, Society for Cardiovascular Angiography and Interventions, and Society of Thoracic Surgeons. J Am Coll Cardiol 2008;52(23):e143–263.
13. Mullins CE, Nihill MR, Vick GW 3rd, et al. Double balloon technique for dilation of valvular or vessel stenosis in congenital and acquired heart disease. J Am Coll Cardiol 1987;10(1):107–14.
14. Malekzadeh-Milani S, Ladouceur M, Cohen S, et al. Results of transcatheter pulmonary valvulation in native or patched right ventricular outflow tracts. Arch Cardiovasc Dis 2014;107(11):592–8.
15. O'Byrne ML, Glatz AC, Mercer-Rosa L, et al. Trends in pulmonary valve replacement in children and adults with tetralogy of Fallot. Am J Cardiol 2015; 115(1):118–24.
16. Quail MA, Frigiola A, Giardini A, et al. Impact of pulmonary valve replacement in tetralogy of Fallot with pulmonary regurgitation: a comparison of intervention and nonintervention. Ann Thorac Surg 2012;94(5):1619–26.
17. Baumgartner H, Bonhoeffer P, De Groot NM, et al. ESC Guidelines for the management of grown-up congenital heart disease (new version 2010). Eur Heart J 2010;31(23):2915–57.

18. Silversides CK, Kiess M, Beauchesne L, et al. Canadian Cardiovascular Society 2009 Consensus Conference on the management of adults with congenital heart disease: outflow tract obstruction, coarctation of the aorta, tetralogy of Fallot, Ebstein anomaly and Marfan's syndrome. Can J Cardiol 2010;26(3):e80–97.

19. Warnes CA, Williams RG, Bashore TM, et al. ACC/AHA 2008 guidelines for the management of adults with congenital heart disease: a report of the American College of Cardiology/American Heart Association Task Force on Practice Guidelines (writing committee to develop guidelines on the management of adults with congenital heart disease). Circulation 2008;118(23):e714–833.

20. Lee C, Kim YM, Lee CH, et al. Outcomes of pulmonary valve replacement in 170 patients with chronic pulmonary regurgitation after relief of right ventricular outflow tract obstruction: implications for optimal timing of pulmonary valve replacement. J Am Coll Cardiol 2012;60(11):1005–14.

21. Brown DW, McElhinney DB, Araoz PA, et al. Reliability and accuracy of echocardiographic right heart evaluation in the U.S. Melody Valve Investigational Trial. J Am Soc Echocardiogr 2012;25(4):383–92.e4.

22. Cheatham SL, Holzer RJ, Chisolm JL, et al. The Medtronic Melody(R) transcatheter pulmonary valve implanted at 24-mm diameter–it works. Catheter Cardiovasc Interv 2013;82(5):816–23.

23. Chessa M, Carrozza M, Butera G, et al. Results and mid-long-term follow-up of stent implantation for native and recurrent coarctation of the aorta. Eur Heart J 2005;26(24):2728–32.

24. Warnes CA, Williams RG, Bashore TM, et al. ACC/AHA 2008 guidelines for the management of adults with congenital heart disease: executive summary: a report of the American College of Cardiology/American Heart Association Task Force on Practice Guidelines (writing committee to develop guidelines for the management of adults with congenital heart disease). Circulation 2008;118(23):2395–451.

25. Phan K, Wong S, Phan S, et al. Transcatheter aortic valve implantation (TAVI) in patients with bicuspid aortic valve stenosis–systematic review and meta-analysis. Heart Lung Circ 2015;24(7):649–59.

26. Perlman GY, Blanke P, Dvir D, et al. Bicuspid aortic valve stenosis: favorable early outcomes with a next-generation transcatheter heart valve in a multicenter study. JACC Cardiovasc Interv 2016;9(8):817–24.

27. Reller MD, Strickland MJ, Riehle-Colarusso T, et al. Prevalence of congenital heart defects in metropolitan Atlanta, 1998-2005. J Pediatr 2008;153(6):807–13.

28. Hoffman JI, Kaplan S. The incidence of congenital heart disease. J Am Coll Cardiol 2002;39(12):1890–900.

29. Jenkins NP, Ward C. Coarctation of the aorta: natural history and outcome after surgical treatment. QJM 1999;92(7):365–71.

30. Singer MI, Rowen M, Dorsey TJ. Transluminal aortic balloon angioplasty for coarctation of the aorta in the newborn. Am Heart J 1982;103(1):131–2.

31. Shaddy RE, Boucek MM, Sturtevant JE, et al. Comparison of angioplasty and surgery for unoperated coarctation of the aorta. Circulation 1993;87(3):793–9.

32. Hamdan MA, Maheshwari S, Fahey JT, et al. Endovascular stents for coarctation of the aorta: initial results and intermediate-term follow-up. J Am Coll Cardiol 2001;38(5):1518–23.

33. Forbes TJ, Moore P, Pedra CA, et al. Intermediate follow-up following intravascular stenting for treatment of coarctation of the aorta. Catheter Cardiovasc Interv 2007;70(4):569–77.

34. Forbes TJ, Garekar S, Amin Z, et al. Procedural results and acute complications in stenting native and recurrent coarctation of the aorta in patients over 4 years of age: a multi-institutional study. Catheter Cardiovasc Interv 2007;70(2):276–85.

35. Sohrabi B, Jamshidi P, Yaghoubi A, et al. Comparison between covered and bare Cheatham-Platinum stents for endovascular treatment of patients with native post-ductal aortic coarctation: immediate and intermediate-term results. JACC Cardiovasc Interv 2014;7(4):416–23.

36. Kan JS, Marvin WJ Jr, Bass JL, et al. Balloon angioplasty–branch pulmonary artery stenosis: results from the Valvuloplasty and Angioplasty of Congenital Anomalies Registry. Am J Cardiol 1990;65(11):798–801.

37. Bush DM, Hoffman TM, Del Rosario J, et al. Frequency of restenosis after balloon pulmonary arterioplasty and its causes. Am J Cardiol 2000;86(11):1205–9.

38. Baker CM, McGowan FX Jr, Keane JF, et al. Pulmonary artery trauma due to balloon dilation: recognition, avoidance and management. J Am Coll Cardiol 2000;36(5):1684–90.

39. O'Laughlin MP, Slack MC, Grifka RG, et al. Implantation and intermediate-term follow-up of stents in congenital heart disease. Circulation 1993;88(2):605–14.

40. Hijazi ZM, al-Fadley F, Geggel RL, et al. Stent implantation for relief of pulmonary artery stenosis: immediate and short-term results. Cathet Cardiovasc Diagn 1996;38(1):16–23.

41. Chatelain P, Meier B, Friedli B. Stenting of superior vena cava and inferior vena cava for symptomatic narrowing after repeated atrial surgery for D-transposition of the great vessels. Br Heart J 1991;66(6):466–8.

42. Ward CJ, Mullins CE, Nihill MR, et al. Use of intravascular stents in systemic venous and systemic venous baffle obstructions. Short-term follow-up results. Circulation 1995;91(12):2948–54.

43. Trerotola SO, Lund GB, Samphilipo MA, et al. Palmaz stent in the treatment of central venous stenosis: safety and efficacy of redilation. Radiology 1994;190(2):379–85.

44. Reichenberger F, Pepke-Zaba J, McNeil K, et al. Atrial septostomy in the treatment of severe pulmonary arterial hypertension. Thorax 2003;58(9): 797–800.

# Alcohol Septal Ablation to Reduce Heart Failure

Joshua McKay, MD, Sherif F. Nagueh, MD*

---

## KEYWORDS

- Hypertrophic cardiomyopathy • Alcohol septal ablation • Heart failure

---

## KEY POINTS

- Hypertrophic cardiomyopathy (HCM) is the most common inheritable cardiac disorder with variable phenotypic expression.
- HCM can induce heart failure via left ventricular outflow tract obstruction, mitral regurgitation, diastolic dysfunction, and systolic dysfunction, as well as secondary pulmonary hypertension and atrial fibrillation.
- Severely symptomatic patients, despite optimal medical therapy, should be considered for invasive septal reduction techniques.
- Alcohol septal ablation can reverse the various mechanisms of heart failure in HCM and lead to clinical improvement with excellent short and intermediate results. Long-term results are promising but lacking in number, so more work is needed to describe the sustainability of the results in various patient populations.

---

## INTRODUCTION

Hypertrophic cardiomyopathy (HCM) is the most common inheritable cardiac disorder, with an estimated prevalence of 0.2%, or 1 case in 500 individuals[1,2]. Most of these patients have no or mild symptoms, but around 10% will develop heart failure symptoms refractory to medical therapy.[3] These patients are frequently considered for invasive septal reduction techniques: either surgical septal myectomy or alcohol septal ablation (ASA).[4] This article discusses the various mechanisms through which HCM induces heart failure, how ASA can reverse each of these mechanisms, and the evidence for clinical improvement and sustainability after the procedure.

## MECHANISMS OF HEART FAILURE IN HYPERTROPHIC CARDIOMYOPATHY

### Left Ventricular Outflow Tract Obstruction

The hallmark finding of symptomatic obstructive HCM is the presence of left ventricular outflow tract (LVOT) dynamic obstruction. About one-third of patients will have a significant LVOT gradient (defined as a gradient ≥30 mm Hg) at rest; one-third will have a significant gradient only with provocation, and the final one-third will not have a significant gradient at rest or with provocation.[5] Systolic contraction of the hypertrophied basal septal segment was initially thought to be the cause of this dynamic obstruction, but further studies have shown that drag forces imposed on an abnormal mitral apparatus leading to systolic anterior motion (SAM) of the anterior mitral leaflet are the cause of LVOT obstruction.[6–9] Mitral apparatus abnormalities that have been correlated with LVOT obstruction include mitral valve leaflet elongation, abnormal chordal attachment, anterior displacement of the papillary muscles, and bifid papillary muscle.[9,10] This helps explain the presence of severe LVOT obstruction in some patients in the absence of severe septal hypertrophy.

---

Department of Cardiology, Methodist DeBakey Heart and Vascular Center, Houston Methodist Hospital, 6550 Fannin, Smith Tower 677, Houston, TX 77030, USA

* Corresponding author. Methodist Debakey Heart and Vascular Center, 6550 Fannin, SM-677, Houston, TX 77030.

E-mail address: snagueh@houstonmethodist.org

Intervent Cardiol Clin 6 (2017) 445–452
http://dx.doi.org/10.1016/j.iccl.2017.03.012
2211-7458/17/© 2017 Elsevier Inc. All rights reserved.

## Mitral Regurgitation

Mitral regurgitation has long been correlated with obstructive HCM. In the majority of cases, the regurgitation is a secondary process directly related to the SAM of the mitral leaflet. This has been described in angiographic studies with an eject-obstruct-leak timing of events.[9,11] Thus, the onset of mitral leaflet–septal contact is one of the determinants of the severity of obstruction as well as the prolongation of ejection time and the extent of mitral regurgitation.[9,11–13] Hemodynamic conditions that affect LVOT obstruction often have a similar effect on mitral regurgitation severity. Given the link between obstruction and mitral regurgitation, afterload reduction and diuretics can lead to worsening of mitral regurgitation in this setting. The mitral regurgitation jet is directed posteriorly and laterally and occurs in mid to late systole. Centrally or anteriorly located regurgitant jets, or holosystolic regurgitation, should be further investigated for primary mitral valve disease.

## Diastolic Dysfunction

Diastolic dysfunction represents a significant and largely misunderstood cause of heart failure in HCM. Observational studies have shown that diastolic dysfunction starts early and will progress in HCM patients over time, and that advanced diastolic dysfunction (defined as a restrictive filling pattern on echo-Doppler interrogation) is an independent predictor of death and need of heart transplantation.[14] HCM can affect diastolic filling via increased left ventricular (LV) chamber stiffness, impaired relaxation and/or diminished residual chamber dimensions from massive hypertrophy (the latter works through increased LV chamber stiffness). It was initially believed that increased chamber stiffness due to hypertrophy and myocardial fibrosis was the cause of diastolic dysfunction in HCM patients. Although this does play a role, it has become increasingly evident that impaired relaxation also plays a large and more complex role. The systolic load from outflow tract obstruction, delayed inactivation from increased sarcoplasmic calcium, and nonuniformity of systolic and diastolic ventricular loads cause the impairment in ventricular relaxation.[4,9,12,15–18] Already a difficult to treat condition, diastolic dysfunction in HCM can be exceedingly challenging, as diuretics are the baseline for therapy but can actually worsen symptoms via increased outflow tract obstruction.

## Systolic Dysfunction

LV ejection fraction (EF) is usually normal to hyperdynamic in patients with HCM, but in end-stage or "burnt-out" HCM, depressed EF occurs.[19,20] Replacement fibrosis is usually present in these patients and may be related to the underlying myocardial fiber disarray, myocardial ischemia and/or infarction due to micro or macrovascular disease, or some combination of these components. At this stage of the disease, LVOT obstruction is usually absent despite a progression in clinical symptoms and worsened prognosis. LV systolic dysfunction represents a minority of cases, but with a grave prognosis, with a hazard ratio for death or cardiac transplantation reported as high as 25.[14,21] At this end stage, limited therapeutic options are available, so patients should be considered for $Vo_2$ testing in preparation for heart transplantation.

### Pulmonary hypertension

It is not uncommon for HCM patients to have pulmonary hypertension. This is due to the elevated LA pressure because of LV diastolic dysfunction, and in the setting of dynamic obstruction, mitral regurgitation. Mean PA pressure usually decreases as LA pressure decreases after successful septal reduction therapy, and there are several examples of patients having a dramatic decline in PA pressure after alcohol septal ablation.

Notwithstanding, it is important to carefully consider the etiology of pulmonary hypertension in HCM patients and determine the actual contribution of elevated LA pressure. This is possible with right heart catheterization where the transpulmonary gradient is measured along with pulmonary vascular resistance. Pulmonary hypertension (not type II), in and of itself, is not a reason to withhold septal reduction therapy, even if it were due to pulmonary parenchymal or vascular disease. This is due to the contribution of increased LA pressure to the elevated PA pressures. Thus, some decline in mean PA pressure occurs, albeit the elevated PA pressures are not normalized in these patients. Conversely, if HCM patients have pulmonary hypertension largely due to elevated LA pressure, it is not advisable to use pulmonary vasodilators, as they can lead to pulmonary edema in this setting.

### Atrial fibrillation

HCM patients with LA enlargement (due to diastolic dysfunction and mitral regurgitation) have a higher risk of atrial fibrillation. The arrhythmia in turn increases the risk for systemic embolic events and for the development of acute heart failure. Given the presence of LV diastolic dysfunction and reduced early diastolic LV filling, LA contraction plays an important role in maintaining lower LA pressure and higher LV stroke volume. Therefore, atrial fibrillation, particularly with a fast ventricular response, results in increased LA pressure and in reduced LV stroke volume. Maintenance of sinus rhythm is of paramount importance in patients who develop atrial fibrillation with pulmonary congestion signs and symptoms and with reduced peripheral perfusion.

There are few studies that have examined the effects of alcohol septal ablation on LA size and LV filling.[22] These have shown a significant decrease in LA volumes, LA ejection force, and LA kinetic energy. Importantly, LV passive filling volume (LV filling in early diastole before LA contraction) increased after ablation and was directly related to the improvement in exercise tolerance. Given the beneficial effects of alcohol septal ablation on decreasing LA volumes, one can speculate that the incidence of atrial fibrillation could decrease as well, although additional data are needed to support this hypothesis.

## ALCOHOL SEPTAL ABLATION
### History
Sigwart first described alcohol septal ablation (ASA) in 1995,[23] after performing the first procedure in 1994 (**Figs. 1–4**). He showed temporary improvement in LVOT obstruction with balloon occlusion of the first septal perforator in 3 patients with HCM refractory to conventional medical therapy. He then went on to show those effects to be sustained when absolute alcohol was injected into the septal perforator arteries. The alcohol injected induces a localized myocardial infarction. Subsequent scarring and thinning of the infarcted area results in an effective widening of the LVOT. The procedural steps are listed in brief:

1. A guiding catheter is used to engage the left main coronary artery, and a coronary wire is preferentially placed into the first septal perforator.
2. An angioplasty balloon is advanced into the septal perforator and then inflated.
3. The wire is removed, and contrast is injected through the balloon as transthoracic echocardiography is used to verify the territory at risk.
4. Absolute alcohol is lastly injected slowly through the inflated balloon lumen to induce localized myocardial infarction.

Currently, invasive septal reduction is recommended for severely symptomatic patients with LVOT obstruction refractory to optimal medical therapy.[4] Surgical myectomy is listed as the preferred choice in US guidelines, but not in European guidelines, due to the duration of experience and documented long-term results;

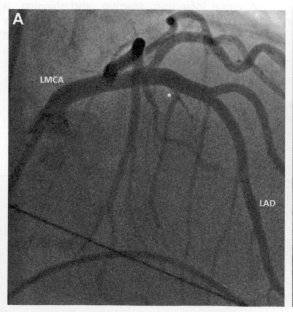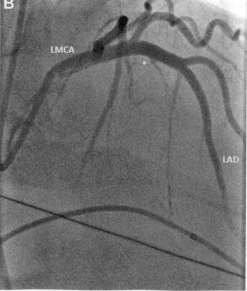

Fig. 1. Coronary angiogram before and after alcohol septal ablation from a 65-year-old woman who presented with pulmonary congestion symptoms, NYHA Class III. (A) Coronary angiography prior to alcohol septal ablation. (B) Coronary angiography after alcohol septal ablation showing occlusion of the first septal perforator. Asterisk, first septal perforator; LAD, left anterior descending artery; LMCA, left main coronary artery.

**Before Alcohol Septal Ablation**          **After Alcohol Septal Ablation**

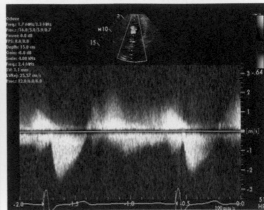

Fig. 2. LV outflow gradient (by continuous wave Doppler) caused by systolic anterior motion of the mitral valve from the same patient in Fig. 1. Before ablation, gradient was 115 mm Hg. After ablation, there is no outflow obstruction, with velocity peaking early at 2 m/s.

however, the desire for a less-invasive procedure has resulted in ASA being performed more often in the last several years globally.[24]

## EVIDENCE OF BENEFIT
### Decrease of Left Ventricular Outflow Tract Obstruction

The primary goal of ASA (similar to surgical myectomy) is to reduce the gradient across the LVOT, which should also reduce medication refractory symptoms in the appropriate patient population. In the initial description of the procedure, Sigwart described 3 cases of almost immediate abolishment of LVOT obstruction.[23]

Larger early case series showed more modest immediate reductions in LVOT gradient, with average residual mean gradient of 16 to 26 mm Hg at 3-month follow-up.[25–27] Although 1 study showed that the gradient continued to decrease up to 2 years after the procedure with ultimate gradient less than 10 mm Hg,[26,27] the delay to optimal reduction may result in delay to symptom relief. The efficacy of ASA was affected by patient anatomic factors. The amount of alcohol injected, and thus the amount of septal infarction, scarring, and thinning, is directly related to the size, location, and territory of perfusion of the first septal perforator. In

**Before Alcohol Septal Ablation**          **After Alcohol Septal Ablation**

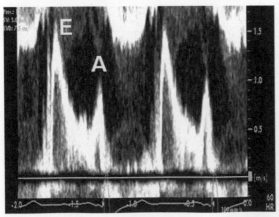
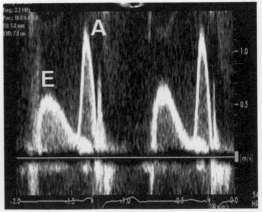

Fig. 3. Mitral inflow before and after alcohol septal ablation from the same patient in Fig. 1. Before ablation, E/A ratio is >1 with peak E velocity at 1.5 m/s. After ablation, E/A ratio is <1 with peak E velocity at 60 to 65 cm/s. This finding is consistent with reduced left atrial pressure. After the ablation the patient was asymptomatic. A, mitral atrial or late diastolic velocity; E, mitral early diastolic velocity.

## Before Alcohol Septal Ablation        After Alcohol Septal Ablation

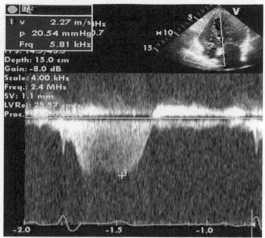

**Fig. 4.** Peak tricuspid regurgitation velocity (TR) by continuous wave Doppler before and after alcohol septal ablation from the same patient in **Fig. 1**. The peak velocity before ablation corresponds to pulmonary artery systolic pressure of 48 mm Hg (assuming right atrial pressure of 0 mm Hg). After ablation, peak TR velocity corresponds to pulmonary artery systolic pressure of 21 mm Hg, assuming right atrial pressure of 0 mm Hg. This is consistent with the change seen in the mitral inflow pattern and NYHA Class I the patient was in after alcohol septal ablation.

patients with small or multiple proximal septal perforators, ablation through the first perforator only often does not result in optimal relief of LVOT obstruction. Similarly, in patients with bifurcating septal perforators, ablation through a single branch may be limited. However, the counterargument that more extensive ablations were more likely to develop complications was recognized early as well. The addition of contrast echocardiography to the procedure was a major advancement in ASA efficacy and safety. The injection of contrast through the ablation balloon allows for direct visualization by echocardiography of the territory perfused. This technique allows for the more precise selection of perforator(s) or branches and/or a more effective ablation of hypertrophied septal segments and in an early case series showed immediate reductions in LVOT gradient to less than 10 mm Hg.[28] Other technological advances such as softer and more steerable coronary wires and more deliverable coronary balloons allowed for higher procedural success and lower complication rates, which furthered the widespread use of ASA.

### Regression of Septal Hypertrophy

A reduction in septal hypertrophy is expected with ASA due to the thinning of infarcted myocardium. In addition, LV remodeling occurs and results in wall thickness reduction in remote segments. Reduction of septal hypertrophy is an important predictor of procedural success. The early case series showed 30% to 40% reductions

in septal thickness, with results approaching normal septal thickness in many patients.[25–29] Similar to LVOT obstruction, the septal thickness continued to regress over time up to 5 years after procedure.[26]

### Improvement of Mitral Regurgitation

As previously discussed, mitral regurgitation in HCM is related to SAM of the anterior mitral leaflet. The SAM of the leaflet is the major causative factor for LVOT obstruction. These underlying mechanisms form the basis for the improvement in mitral regurgitation with ASA. Echocardiographic analysis has shown that the septal thinning after ASA results in a widening of the LVOT and an increased distance between the basal septum and anterior leaflet of the mitral valve.[29] The systolic distance between the septum and anterior leaflet was greater than 1 cm in 80% of patients, with no patients having septal leaflet contact. This has been demonstrated to reduce mitral regurgitation qualitatively to trace in two-thirds of patients and trace to mild in all patients without primary mitral valve disease.[22,26] Using quantitative methods, a 50% reduction in mitral regurgitation volume has been demonstrated.[22] The reduction in MR severity is important in reducing left atrial pressure and pulmonary congestion symptoms.

### Improvement of Diastolic Dysfunction

Diastolic dysfunction occurs primarily because of increased chamber stiffness and impaired relaxation, as previously discussed. An improvement in these parameters would improve the overall diastolic function of the left ventricle. ASA has been shown to improve diastolic dysfunction via changes in both parameters. The systolic load that is present with underlying LVOT obstruction by itself causes abnormal relaxation. The immediate reduction of LVOT gradient seen with ASA also leads to an acute improvement in LV relaxation as evidenced by shorter isovolumic relaxation times (IVRT) and shorter left ventricular relaxation time constant ($\tau$).[17] At short-term follow-up within 6 months of the procedure, further reductions in both the IVRT and $\tau$ were noted in addition to shorter acceleration time of early diastolic filling.[30] Indices of improved diastolic function have also been demonstrated by cardiac MRI.[31] Nonuniformity in regional ventricular loads is another contributor to impaired relaxation. ASA abolishes some of the regional load differences by relieving the LVOT gradient. The systolic contraction load of the LVOT is reduced after relief of obstruction, which eliminates some of the asynchrony between the LV outflow and inflow tracts and leads to an improvement in global LV diastolic dysfunction.

Chamber stiffness in HCM is increased secondary to hypertrophy and myocardial fibrosis. ASA reduces septal hypertrophy and increases LV end-diastolic volume,[28,30] which indicates the occurrence of a remodeling process after ASA. In further support of a remodeling process, reductions in nonseptal hypertrophy and nonseptal LV mass are present as early as 1 month after the procedure, with a 20% reduction at 6 months.[32] The reduced LV mass/volume ratio results in increased wall tension, which promotes passive diastolic filling.[22] Importantly, the early diastolic intraventricular pressure gradient (IVPG), which is directly related to the diastolic suction force, increased by 70% after ASA.[33] LV hypertrophy in HCM may be induced by cardiac TNF-$\alpha$, a cytokine expressed in response to pressure and/or volume overload and capable of inducing hypertrophy and cardiomyopathy. Myocardial levels of TNF-$\alpha$ are elevated in HCM patients and have been shown to be significantly reduced after ASA. Likewise, myocytes' diameter and interstitial collagen content are also reduced after ASA and contribute to the improved diastolic function.[34]

## Functional Status and Mortality

The most clinically relevant outcome measure after ASA is the improvement in functional status. Improvement in symptoms or functional class

can be described in terms of New York Heart Association (NYHA) class, Canadian Cardiovascular Society (CCS) grading of angina, exercise time, and maximal oxygen consumption (MVO2). These outcome measures can be further divided into early (defined as <1 year after the procedure) and intermediate (1–3 years after the procedure) results. The earlier case series showed significant early improvement in NYHA functional class, with 85% to 95% of patients having NYHA III-IV symptoms at baseline but 85% of patients reduced to asymptomatic or NYHA I symptoms after ASA.[25,28] These results were supported by larger case series, with results persisting out to at least 3 years.[26,27] In likely a closer representation of real-world results, a larger and more recent north American, multicenter registry reported the vast majority of patients in NYHA class I or II and 95% of patients with NYHA II or less symptoms at intermediate follow-up.[35] Similar to NYHA functional class, CCS improved after ASA, with greater than 90% of patients being angina free.[26,27,35] Exercise duration increased by 35% to 50% within the first 6 weeks after ASA, and MVO2 improved by 25%, with sustained improvement in these measures at intermediate follow-up.[25–28] In another marker of functional status, and certainly from the perspective of patient satisfaction with quality of life, 80% of patients stopped taking all HCM-specific medications after ASA.[28] Across multiple series, mortality after ASA (in addition to standard medical therapy and implantable cardiac defibrillators) has been shown to be similar to the general population, with survival rates of 97% at 1 year, 86% to 94% at 5 years, and 74% to 82% at 10 years.[3,26,27,35–39] Although not generally thought to have a mortality benefit, when compared with obstructive HCM patients who did not undergo septal reduction therapy, ASA patients have better survival at 1 (97% vs 90%), 5 (86% vs 79%), and 10 years (74% vs 61%).[35] It should be noted that no randomized controlled trials comparing ASA with surgical myectomy have been performed and likely will never be performed. Well-done comparative studies and meta-analyses have shown similar results between the 2 therapies in terms of mortality, functional class, and LVOT gradients, indicating that relief of obstruction, rather than the mechanism of that relief, is the determining factor.

## Longevity

As previously mentioned, the current American guidelines prefer surgical myectomy over ASA in most HCM patients because of documented long-term results. To date, long-term studies of ASA have shown persistent benefit in echocardiographic, symptomatic, and mortality outcomes with 10- to 12-year follow-up,[27,37] prompting a more aggressive European guideline stance. Large international registries have also been established to address this deficiency and other areas of investigation.

## SUMMARY

HCM is a complex disease with multiple pathologic processes needing to be addressed in the symptomatic patient. Asymmetric septal hypertrophy and LVOT obstruction are the pathognomonic signs of obstructive HCM, but mitral valve abnormalities and diastolic dysfunction are significant contributors to morbidity. For the symptomatic patient refractory to medical management, ASA use has grown since it was first reported in 1995. Extensive work has been done to describe the benefit of ASA across the spectrum of heart failure causes in HCM. Excellent short and intermediate follow-up results have been reported, but more work is needed to describe the long-term sustainability of these results in various patient populations. Because of the advancements that have already been made in ASA, when combined with medical therapy and implantable cardiac defibrillators, HCM survival is now similar to that of the general population.

## REFERENCES

1. Maron BJ, Gardin JM, Flack JM, et al. Prevalence of hypertrophic cardiomyopathy in a general population of young adults. echocardiographic analysis of 4111 subjects in the CARDIA study. Coronary artery risk development in (young) adults. Circulation 1995;92(4):785–9.
2. Zou Y, Song L, Wang Z, et al. Prevalence of idiopathic hypertrophic cardiomyopathy in china: a population-based echocardiographic analysis of 8080 adults. Am J Med 2004;116(1):14–8.
3. Maron BJ, Rowin EJ, Casey SA, et al. Hypertrophic cardiomyopathy in adulthood associated with low cardiovascular mortality with contemporary management strategies. J Am Coll Cardiol 2015; 65(18):1915–28.
4. Gersh BJ, Maron BJ, Bonow RO, et al. 2011 ACCF/AHA guideline for the diagnosis and treatment of hypertrophic cardiomyopathy: a report of the American College of Cardiology Foundation/American Heart Association task force on practice guidelines. Developed in collaboration with the American Association for Thoracic Surgery,

American Society of Echocardiography, American Society of Nuclear Cardiology, Heart Failure Society of America, Heart Rhythm Society, Society for Cardiovascular Angiography and Interventions, and Society of Thoracic Surgeons. J Am Coll Cardiol 2011;58(25):e212–60.
5. Maron MS, Olivotto I, Zenovich AG, et al. Hypertrophic cardiomyopathy is predominantly a disease of left ventricular outflow tract obstruction. Circulation 2006;114(21):2232–9.
6. Sherrid MV, Gunsburg DZ, Moldenhauer S, et al. Systolic anterior motion begins at low left ventricular outflow tract velocity in obstructive hypertrophic cardiomyopathy. J Am Coll Cardiol 2000;36(4):1344–54.
7. Sherrid MV, Chu CK, Delia E, et al. An echocardiographic study of the fluid mechanics of obstruction in hypertrophic cardiomyopathy. J Am Coll Cardiol 1993;22(3):816–25.
8. Shah PM, Taylor RD, Wong M. Abnormal mitral valve coaptation in hypertrophic obstructive cardiomyopathy: proposed role in systolic anterior motion of mitral valve. Am J Cardiol 1981;48(2):258–62.
9. Wigle ED, Rakowski H, Kimball BP, et al. Hypertrophic cardiomyopathy. clinical spectrum and treatment. Circulation 1995;92(7):1680–92.
10. Patel P, Dhillon A, Popovic ZB, et al. Left ventricular outflow tract obstruction in hypertrophic cardiomyopathy patients without severe septal hypertrophy: implications of mitral valve and papillary muscle abnormalities assessed using cardiac magnetic resonance and echocardiography. Circ Cardiovasc Imaging 2015;8(7):e003132.
11. Adelman AG, McLoughlin MJ, Marquis Y, et al. Left ventricular cineangiographic observations in muscular subaortic stenosis. Am J Cardiol 1969;24(5):689–97.
12. Wigle ED, Sasson Z, Henderson MA, et al. Hypertrophic cardiomyopathy. the importance of the site and the extent of hypertrophy. A review. Prog Cardiovasc Dis 1985;28(1):1–83.
13. Wigle ED, Adelman AG, Auger P, et al. Mitral regurgitation in muscular subaortic stenosis. Am J Cardiol 1969;24(5):698–706.
14. Pinamonti B, Merlo M, Nangah R, et al. The progression of left ventricular systolic and diastolic dysfunctions in hypertrophic cardiomyopathy: clinical and prognostic significance. J Cardiovasc Med (Hagerstown) 2010;11(9):669–77.
15. Bonow RO, Vitale DF, Maron BJ, et al. Regional left ventricular asynchrony and impaired global left ventricular filling in hypertrophic cardiomyopathy: effect of verapamil. J Am Coll Cardiol 1987;9(5):1108–16.
16. Inoue T, Morooka S, Hayashi T, et al. Global and regional abnormalities of left ventricular diastolic

filling in hypertrophic cardiomyopathy. Clin Cardiol 1991;14(7):573–7.

17. Park TH, Lakkis NM, Middleton KJ, et al. Acute effect of nonsurgical septal reduction therapy on regional left ventricular asynchrony in patients with hypertrophic obstructive cardiomyopathy. Circulation 2002;106(4):412–5.

18. Wang J, Buergler JM, Veerasamy K, et al. Delayed untwisting: the mechanistic link between dynamic obstruction and exercise tolerance in patients with hypertrophic obstructive cardiomyopathy. J Am Coll Cardiol 2009;54(14):1326–34.

19. ten Cate FJ, Roelandt J. Progression to left ventricular dilatation in patients with hypertrophic obstructive cardiomyopathy. Am Heart J 1979;97(6):762–5.

20. Ciro E, Maron BJ, Bonow RO, et al. Relation between marked changes in left ventricular outflow tract gradient and disease progression in hypertrophic cardiomyopathy. Am J Cardiol 1984;53(8):1103–9.

21. Sen-Chowdhry S, Jacoby D, Moon JC, et al. Update on hypertrophic cardiomyopathy and a guide to the guidelines. Nat Rev Cardiol 2016;13(11):651–75.

22. Nagueh SF, Lakkis NM, Middleton KJ, et al. Changes in left ventricular filling and left atrial function six months after nonsurgical septal reduction therapy for hypertrophic obstructive cardiomyopathy. J Am Coll Cardiol 1999;34(4):1123–8.

23. Sigwart U. Non-surgical myocardial reduction for hypertrophic obstructive cardiomyopathy. Lancet 1995;346(8969):211–4.

24. Yacoub MH. Surgical versus alcohol septal ablation for hypertrophic obstructive cardiomyopathy: the pendulum swings. Circulation 2005;112(4):450–2.

25. Bhagwandeen R, Woo A, Ross J, et al. Septal ethanol ablation for hypertrophic obstructive cardiomyopathy: early and intermediate results of a Canadian referral centre. Can J Cardiol 2003;19(8):912–7.

26. Fernandes VL, Nagueh SF, Wang W, et al. A prospective follow-up of alcohol septal ablation for symptomatic hypertrophic obstructive cardiomyopathy—the Baylor experience (1996-2002). Clin Cardiol 2005;28(3):124–30.

27. Fernandes VL, Nielsen C, Nagueh SF, et al. Follow-up of alcohol septal ablation for symptomatic hypertrophic obstructive cardiomyopathy the Baylor and Medical University of South Carolina experience 1996 to 2007. JACC Cardiovasc Interv 2008;1(5):561–70.

28. Lakkis NM, Nagueh SF, Kleiman NS, et al. Echocardiography-guided ethanol septal reduction for hypertrophic obstructive cardiomyopathy. Circulation 1998;98(17):1750–5.

29. Flores-Ramirez R, Lakkis NM, Middleton KJ, et al. Echocardiographic insights into the mechanisms of relief of left ventricular outflow tract obstruction after nonsurgical septal reduction therapy in patients with hypertrophic obstructive cardiomyopathy. J Am Coll Cardiol 2001;37(1):208–14.

30. Nagueh SF, Lakkis NM, Middleton KJ, et al. Changes in left ventricular diastolic function 6 months after nonsurgical septal reduction therapy for hypertrophic obstructive cardiomyopathy. Circulation 1999;99(3):344–7.

31. Chen YZ, Duan FJ, Yuan JS, et al. Effects of alcohol septal ablation on left ventricular diastolic filling patterns in obstructive hypertrophic cardiomyopathy. Heart Vessels 2016;31(5):744–51.

32. van Dockum WG, Beek AM, ten Cate FJ, et al. Early onset and progression of left ventricular remodeling after alcohol septal ablation in hypertrophic obstructive cardiomyopathy. Circulation 2005;111(19):2503–8.

33. Rovner A, Smith R, Greenberg NL, et al. Improvement in diastolic intraventricular pressure gradients in patients with HOCM after ethanol septal reduction. Am J Physiol Heart Circ Physiol 2003;285(6):H2492–9.

34. Nagueh SF, Stetson SJ, Lakkis NM, et al. Decreased expression of tumor necrosis factor-alpha and regression of hypertrophy after nonsurgical septal reduction therapy for patients with hypertrophic obstructive cardiomyopathy. Circulation 2001;103(14):1844–50.

35. Nagueh SF, Groves BM, Schwartz L, et al. Alcohol septal ablation for the treatment of hypertrophic obstructive cardiomyopathy. A multicenter North American registry. J Am Coll Cardiol 2011;58(22):2322–8.

36. Sorajja P, Ommen SR, Holmes DR Jr, et al. Survival after alcohol septal ablation for obstructive hypertrophic cardiomyopathy. Circulation 2012;126(20):2374–80.

37. Veselka J, Jensen MK, Liebregts M, et al. Long-term clinical outcome after alcohol septal ablation for obstructive hypertrophic cardiomyopathy: results from the euro-ASA registry. Eur Heart J 2016;37(19):1517–23.

38. Fortunato de Cano S, Nicolas Cano M, de Ribamar Costa J Jr, et al. Long-term clinical follow-up of patients undergoing percutaneous alcohol septal reduction for symptomatic obstructive hypertrophic cardiomyopathy. Catheter Cardiovasc Interv 2016;88(6):953–60.

39. Liebregts M, Steggerda RC, Vriesendorp PA, et al. Long-term outcome of alcohol septal ablation for obstructive hypertrophic cardiomyopathy in the young and the elderly. JACC Cardiovasc Interv 2016;9(5):463–9.

# Renal Denervation to Modify Hypertension and the Heart Failure State

Ming Zhong, MD[a], Luke K. Kim, MD[a],
Rajesh V. Swaminathan, MD[b],
Dmitriy N. Feldman, MD[a,*]

## KEYWORDS

- Renal denervation • Resistant hypertension • Renal sympathetic activation
- Renal artery ablation

## KEY POINTS

- Overactivation of renal afferent and efferent nerve fibers have been implicated in the pathophysiology of resistant hypertension, systolic heart failure, and diastolic heart failure.
- Percutaneous renal denervation may be used as adjunctive treatment in resistant hypertension and systolic and diastolic heart failure.
- Future randomized controlled trials are needed to further evaluate the role of percutaneous renal denervation in the treatment of resistant hypertension and systolic and diastolic heart failure.

## INTRODUCTION

Sympathetic activation of renal afferent and efferent nerve fibers has long been implicated in the development and maintenance of several cardiovascular disease states. In recent years, the advancement of catheter-based interventional techniques has led to the development of minimally invasive procedures intended to directly and selectively target renal sympathetic nerve overactivation. The technique has been extensively examined in both preclinical and clinical studies, with potential applications in both hypertension and heart failure. By affecting one of the underlying mechanisms of cardiovascular disease states, renal denervation (RDN) has the potential to shift our treatment paradigm for hypertension and heart failure. This review examines the current literature behind RDN and its ability to modify hypertension and the heart failure state.

## RENAL DENERVATION AND RESISTANT HYPERTENSION

An area of primary attention with regard to RDN has been its potential role in the treatment of resistant hypertension. Resistant hypertension is frequently defined as blood pressure above goal, often defined as blood pressure higher than 140/90 mm Hg, despite treatment with full doses (or highest tolerated doses) of 3 or more antihypertensive medications from different drug classes, including at least 1 diuretic.[1] Resistant hypertension includes those patients who achieve blood pressure control but require 4 or more antihypertensive agents to do so. Furthermore, causes of secondary

Disclosure Statement: No relevant conflicts.
[a] Division of Cardiology, Interventional Cardiology and Endovascular Laboratory, Weill Cornell Medical College, New York Presbyterian Hospital, 520 East 70th street, New York, NY 10021, USA; [b] Division of Cardiology, Duke University Medical Center, Duke Clinical Research Institute, 2400 Pratt Street, Durham, NC 27705, USA
* Corresponding author.
E-mail address: dnf9001@med.cornell.edu

Intervent Cardiol Clin 6 (2017) 453–464
http://dx.doi.org/10.1016/j.iccl.2017.03.013
2211-7458/17/© 2017 Elsevier Inc. All rights reserved.

hypertension, including renovascular hypertension, chronic kidney disease, mineralocorticoid excess, and obstructive sleep apnea must be excluded. The prevalence of resistant hypertension is difficult to accurately measure and may be underappreciated. Recently, the National Health and Nutrition Examination Survey (NHANES) dataset estimated the prevalence to be 8.9% of all adults in the United States with hypertension.[2] Even more troubling, the estimated prevalence of resistant hypertension has been steadily increasing since the 1980s, and is likely to continue rising with rates of obesity and the aging population.[3] Importantly, studies have indicated that patients with resistant hypertension are at higher risk compared with those with nonresistant hypertension for diabetes, chronic kidney disease, and cardiovascular events, including death, myocardial infarction, heart failure, and stroke.[4] As patients with true treatment resistance are unable to control their blood pressure with medication use alone, RDN may represent an attractive therapeutic adjunct to medical therapy.

## Pathogenesis

Resistant hypertension revolves around the role of renal sympathetic tone in the development and maintenance of hypertension. The renal sympathetic nervous system is composed of a network of afferent and efferent fibers that primarily follow the course of the renal artery, located within the adventitia.[5] These afferent and efferent fibers communicate directly with the autonomic centers of the central nervous system, thereby allowing cross-talk between the brain and kidneys to regulate overall sympathetic tone. It is believed that these renal sympathetic nerves directly contribute to the hypertensive state by decreasing renal blood flow via vasoconstriction, thereby increasing renal tubular sodium and water absorption, as well as increasing rates of renin secretion.[6] The extent to which these effects occur is thought to depend heavily on the degree of renal sympathetic activation. Furthermore, afferent signals from the kidney have a direct influence on central nervous system sympathetic outflow, thereby contributing to neurogenic hypertension.[7] In examining the role of sympathetic tone in the development and maintenance of hypertension, several studies have used norepinephrine spillover as a surrogate for sympathetic activation. Compared with controls, total norepinephrine spillover was found to be increased in patients with essential hypertension.[8] Furthermore, approximately 50% of the increase

in norepinephrine spillover was attributable to increased norepinephrine overflow from the kidneys and heart, whereas there was no substantial increase in norepinephrine release from the hepatomesenteric or pulmonary circulation, suggesting that increased renal sympathetic nervous activity plays a central role in the pathogenesis of hypertension.

### Renal Denervation in Experimental Animal Models of Resistant Hypertension

Several animal studies have demonstrated that disruption of this sympathetic network can provide effective means of modulating blood pressure.

In the rat model, upregulation of renal sympathetic activity was found to be associated with increased blood pressure.[9] In this model, renal injury was induced via intrarenal injection of phenol and increased levels of renal sympathetic activity was documented with direct renal nerve recordings and plasma norepinephrine levels. Up to 3 weeks after injury, there was a substantial increase in blood pressure, which was attenuated by surgical RDN and treatment with clonidine.

Beyond inducing hypertension via the upregulation of sympathetic activity, several animal studies have demonstrated a reduction in blood pressure with denervation. In the swine model, pigs undergoing surgical RDN had mean arterial blood pressure measured and compared before and after surgery.[10] Following denervation, mean arterial blood pressure was found to be substantially decreased from 141 ± 6 to 121 ± 3 mm Hg, a reduction that persisted by 3 weeks after the procedure, demonstrating a clinically meaningful reduction in blood pressure with disruption of renal adventitial nerves.

These results were further corroborated in the canine model, in which dogs undergoing bilateral RDN were compared with a control group, after being fed a high-fat diet for 5 weeks.[11] In response to the high-fat diet, both groups demonstrated increased body weight and heart rate compared with baseline. However, the control group had a significant increase in arterial blood pressure, which was mitigated in the group undergoing RDN.

### Surgical Renal Denervation

Before the advent of multiple classes of antihypertensives, surgical RDN was used as a final treatment option for refractory hypertension. Surgical denervation for resistant hypertension was described as early as 1935, where patients underwent bilateral denervation via splanchnicectomy, radical surgical sympathectomy, or even nephrectomy in patients with end-stage renal disease and difficult-to-manage hypertension.[12] Despite the invasiveness of the procedure, surgical denervation proved to be an effective means of controlling hypertension. A large observational study of 1266 patients undergoing surgical sympathectomy revealed a significant improvement in blood pressure control when compared with patients treated with conventional medical therapy alone. Furthermore, surgical sympathectomy was associated with decreased 5-year mortality in patients with resistant, malignant hypertension.[13] However, despite the effectiveness of the procedure, overall operative mortality was found to be as high as 3%.[14] In addition, patients frequently developed significant side effects, including orthostasis, anhidrosis, gastrointestinal dysfunction, incontinence, neuralgic back pain, and sexual dysfunction. Furthermore, although some patients showed significant improvement in blood pressure with sympathectomy, the results were not uniform across all patients.[14] As a result of the difficulty in identifying the patients who would benefit most significantly, along with the high associated morbidity and mortality, surgical sympathectomy increasingly fell out of favor with the development of safe and effective pharmacotherapies in the 1960s. Although no longer widely used, surgical denervation proved that renal sympathectomy can be an effective means of blood pressure control; a concept that ultimately led to the rise of a catheter-based approach.

## Catheter-Based Renal Denervation

With the recent rise in prevalence of resistant hypertension and multiple animal and human studies indicating improved blood pressure control with renal sympathetic denervation, there has been renewed interest in developing minimally invasive methods of sympathectomy. With the challenge of downregulating renal sympathetic activity, without causing unwanted side effects by disrupting sympathetic innervation to other organs, percutaneous catheter-based approaches to RDN have emerged as a minimally invasive and safe technique.

With catheter-based RDN, successive ablations are made from the distal to proximal end of the renal artery to make circumferential lesions. In radiofrequency ablations, heat is used to disrupt the sympathetic fibers coursing through the adventitia of the renal artery,[5] thereby reducing sympathetic afferent and efferent activity to the kidney. Although radiofrequency ablation is the most common technique for percutaneous RDN,

ablation of the renal sympathetic network also may be achieved by using ultrasound energy and tissue-directed pharmacologic injections.[15]

In one of the earliest, large clinical trials investigating catheter-based RDN, the SYMPLICITY HTN-1 trial was a proof-of-concept and safety trial, enrolling a cohort of 45 patients with resistant hypertension (defined as systolic blood pressure >160 mm Hg while being treated with 3 or more antihypertensives, including a diuretic).[16] Patients in this study underwent bilateral radiofrequency ablation of the renal arteries and were found to have a substantial decrease in office blood pressures, as early as 1 month postprocedure, with effects durable up to 24 months postprocedure, with office blood pressures reduced by an average of 14/10 mm Hg at 1 month and 27/17 mm Hg at 12 months. Total body and renal norepinephrine production were measured and found to be significantly reduced after ablation, indicating successful downregulation of renal sympathetic activity. Importantly, 97% of patients did not experience significant complications, although 3 cases of pseudoaneurysms and 1 case of renal artery dissection were reported.

With encouraging results from SYMPLICITY HTN-1, the SYMPLICITY HTN-2 trial was a multicenter, prospective randomized study in which patients with resistant hypertension were randomly assigned to catheter-based RDN plus conventional medical therapy versus medical therapy alone, with a primary endpoint of office systolic blood pressure at 6 months.[17] Similar to HTN-1, the study found that RDN was associated with improved blood pressure control, with an average in office reduction in blood pressure of 32/12 mm Hg in the denervation cohort at 6 months, compared with no significant blood pressure reduction in the medical therapy group. This reduction was found to be durable up to 12 months postprocedure. Similar to the HTN-1 study, major adverse events were rare, comprising pseudoaneurysm and transient hypotension and bradycardia. Although results were once again encouraging, the study received criticism for lacking a sham control and not blinding the physicians performing blood pressure measurements. Furthermore, the magnitude of reduction in ambulatory blood pressure following denervation was significantly smaller than that of office blood pressure.

In an effort to address these concerns, the SYMPLICITY HTN-3 trial was a randomized, blinded and sham-controlled trial, in which patients with resistant hypertension received catheter-based RDN or sham procedure.[18] The study found no significant difference in mean change in systolic blood pressure between the 2 groups at 6 months. There was also no significant difference in mean change in 24-hour ambulatory systolic blood pressures between groups. As a result, although the trial met its primary safety end point in terms of mortality, end-stage renal disease, embolic events, vascular complications, and renal artery stenosis, it failed to meet its primary and major secondary efficacy end points. In many ways, these results were surprising, especially in light of previous study findings.

More recently, the Renal Denervation for Hypertension (DEHERHTN) trial enrolled 106 patients who were randomized to either radiofrequency-based denervation plus a standardized stepped-care antihypertensive treatment (SSAHT) regimen versus SSAHT alone.[19] In this study, patients were confirmed to have resistant hypertension based on ambulatory blood pressure monitoring for 4 weeks before randomization, while taking a standardized antihypertensive regimen. At 6 months, the mean change in daytime ambulatory systolic blood pressure was greater in the denervation group (−15.8 mm Hg, 95% confidence interval [CI] −19.7 to −11.9 mm Hg), compared with the control group (−9.9 mm Hg, 95% CI −13.6 to −0.5 mm Hg) for a baseline adjusted difference of −5.9 mm Hg ($P = .0329$).

Given that the negative findings from the SYM-PLICITY HTN-3 trial regarding the efficacy of catheter-based RDN in the treatment of resistant hypertension were in many ways surprising and disappointing, several explanations have been proposed to explain the findings. Specifically, investigators have questioned whether suboptimal denervation was achieved in some study participants due to the design of the single-tip catheter, potentially limited operator experience, and the inherent steep learning curve of producing patterned lesions in a 3-dimensional artery.[20] Furthermore, it is unclear whether study participants truly had resistant hypertension and whether increasing oral antihypertensive regimens during the trial masked the effect of denervation.[21] Last, as the trial was primarily designed to assess for blood pressure reduction, it did not provide any additional information regarding the potentially clinically important, pleiotropic effects of RDN on cardiac mass, end-diastolic ventricular and atrial pressures, natriuresis, glucose tolerance, and arrhythmias.[20] Although current societal guidelines do not recommend RDN as a treatment for resistant hypertension,[22] many people believe the results of HTN-3 neither proved nor disproved the efficacy of RDN, but rather highlighted the need for further ongoing research. One such study currently enrolling is SPYRAL HTN, which seeks to address the concerns regarding the previous RDN studies.[23] SPYRAL HTN aims to investigate the efficacy and safety of denervation compared with a sham procedure in both the absence of antihypertensives and in the presence of a standardized triple antihypertensive therapy (Table 1). However, until future studies are able to definitively demonstrate the efficacy of RDN in resistant hypertension, it remains a promising but unproven therapy.

## RENAL DENERVATION AND HEART FAILURE

Beyond the potential therapeutic benefits in resistant hypertension, recently there has been research interest in the application of RDN to other disease states, notably heart failure and its various comorbidities. By affecting the autonomic neural regulation of renal function, water and sodium retention, and peripheral vascular tone, catheter-directed ablation of renal afferent and efferent fibers may disrupt the progression and maintenance of the heart failure state. Similar to the physiology of resistant hypertension, it is believed that sympathetic overactivation plays a major role in the development of heart failure, whereby modulation of this sympathetic activity could yield clinical benefit and become a viable treatment modality.

### Pathogenesis

Congestive heart failure is often thought to be a state of generalized sympathetic activation as a response to changes in cardiac and peripheral hemodynamics.[24] In the normal state, the heart and kidneys interact with regard to hemodynamics and neurohormonal regulatory mechanisms to maintain homeostasis. However, perturbations of these regulatory mechanisms can lead to the development of congestive heart failure. One such way in which this may occur is by overstimulation of the renal sympathetic nervous system. Activation of renal sympathetic nerves can cause reduced renal blood flow, leading to increased renin release, elevated levels of angiotensin II, and sodium and water retention.[25] Similarly, activation of renal sensory nerves may cause a reflex increase in sympathetic tone, thereby resulting in peripheral vasoconstriction and elevation of peripheral vascular resistance, hallmark changes in the development of heart failure.[26]

**Table 1**
**Ongoing trials of renal denervation in resistant hypertension**

| Title | Study Design | Primary Outcome | Secondary Outcome |
|---|---|---|---|
| SPYRAL HTN-ON MED Study | Patients with office SBP <150 mm Hg and <180 mm Hg and DBP >90 mm Hg off medications with 24-h ambulatory SBP averages >140 mm Hg and <170 mm Hg randomized to renal denervation or sham procedure | Short-term and long-term safety as evaluated by incidence of major adverse events; change in 24-h ambulatory measure of SBP | Change in office SBP; incidence of achieving target SBP <140 mm Hg or <130 mm Hg in patients with diabetes; change in office DBP; change in 24-h ambulatory measure of DBP |
| SPYRAL HTN-OFF MED Study | Patients with office SBP >150 mm Hg and <180 mm Hg and DBP >90 mm Hg off medications with 24-h ambulatory SBP averages >140 mm Hg and <170 mm Hg, who are willing to discontinue antihypertensives, are randomized to renal denervation or sham procedure with discontinuation of antihypertensives before angiography | Short-term and long-term safety as evaluated by incidence of major adverse events; change in 24-h ambulatory measure of SBP | Change in office SBP; incidence of achieving target SBP <140 mm Hg or <130 mm Hg in patients with diabetes; change in office DBP; change in 24-h ambulatory measure of DBP |
| Renal Denervation on Quality of 24-h BP Control by Ultrasound in Resistant HTN (REQUIRE) | Patients with office SBP >150 mm Hg and DBP >90 mm Hg with 24-h ambulatory SBP >140 mm Hg are randomized to ultrasound ablation of bilateral renal arteries or sham procedure | Decrease in 24-h ambulatory DBP from baseline | Decrease in average ambulatory daytime and nighttime SBP; decrease in average ambulatory daytime and nighttime DBP; decrease in average office SBP and DBP |
| Renal Denervation Therapy for Resistant Hypertension in Type 2 Diabetes Mellitus (HTN2DM) | Patients with resistant hypertension and office BP >150/90 with type 2 diabetes mellitus on an oral hypoglycemic are assigned to renal denervation | Change in office SBP and DBP from baseline at 6 mo | Change in office SBP and DBP up to 3 y; change in insulin sensitivity; change in glucose metabolism |

*Abbreviations:* BP, blood pressure; DBP, diastolic BP; SBP, systolic BP.

Using plasma norepinephrine levels as a surrogate measure for sympathetic nervous activity of the body and individual organs, patients with reduced ejection fraction were found to have elevated levels of circulating norepinephrine.[27] Although increased neurohormonal levels were found in all patients with left ventricular dysfunction, those with symptoms were found to have the highest levels, suggesting that sympathetic stimulation contributes to symptomatology of the heart failure syndrome. These higher levels of neurohormones were later discovered to be due to both increased spillover and reduced clearance. When assessing rates of norepinephrine spillover from individual organs, cardiac and renal spillover in the setting of systolic dysfunction was found to be increased by 540% and 206%, respectively, accounting for more than 62% of the increased total body norepinephrine levels.

Furthermore, several studies have suggested that the degree of sympathetic activation may predict clinical outcomes. In patients with symptomatic moderate to severe congestive heart failure, plasma norepinephrine levels were found to be independently related to risk of mortality, whereby most patients died from progressive heart failure, rather than sudden cardiac death.[28] Similarly, even in patients with asymptomatic reduced ejection fraction, plasma norepinephrine level was found to be the strongest predictor of clinical events, with elevated risk of all-cause mortality, cardiovascular mortality, hospitalization for heart failure, and myocardial ischemia.[29] When applied to all patients with reduced ejection fraction, New York Heart Association (NYHA) Class I through IV, among several factors including renal function, cardiac index, heart failure etiology, and age, increased renal norepinephrine spillover was independently associated with an increased relative risk of both death and heart transplantation.[30]

To a large extent, attenuation of renal sympathetic activation has already become a therapeutic target in heart failure. Angiotensin-converting enzyme (ACE) inhibitors and beta blockers have long been a mainstay of medical therapy in systolic heart failure, with much of the benefit thought to be derived from reducing the harmful effects of sympathetic activation.[31,32] Furthermore, the greatest survival benefit in treatment with ACE inhibitors, when compared with combination of hydralazine and isosorbide dinitrate, was found to be in the cohort of patients with the highest plasma norepinephrine levels.[33] Such observations have fueled the hypothesis that denervation of the renal sympathetic nerves via a catheter-based approach may be able to offer additive benefits.

## Renal Denervation in Experimental Animal Models of Heart Failure

With the observation that sympathetic denervation results in a marked reduction in renal norepinephrine spillover, affects sodium and water balance regulation, and decreases plasma renin activity,[34] several animal models have attempted to investigate the effects of denervation on the heart failure state.

Most studies have used various models of ischemic cardiomyopathy, in which RDN has been found to improve several markers of clinical status. In the rat model, heart failure was induced by myocardial infarction from ligation of the left anterior descending artery. In these animals, renal sympathetic nerve activity was markedly elevated compared with controls, but RDN was found to significantly improve volume status by decreasing cumulative sodium balance[35] and plasma B-type natriuretic peptide levels,[36] and increasing urine output and urinary sodium excretion rate.[37] By improving natriuretic response and surrogate markers of volume status, it is believed that renal sympathetic activity is heavily involved in sodium and fluid balance in chronic, ischemic heart failure. Furthermore, these observations were not limited to only ischemic cardiomyopathy. In the canine model of high-output heart failure from arteriovenous fistula formation, RDN resulted in a similar increase in urinary sodium excretion following an oral salt load.[38]

In addition, RDN has not only been shown to simply affect fluid retention, it has also been associated with improved left ventricular performance. In post–myocardial infarction rat models, RDN was associated with a significant improvement in left ventricular ejection fraction to normal levels, compared with controls that did not undergo denervation.[32] These findings were consistent regardless of the temporal relationship between denervation and myocardial infarction.

Similar to ischemic cardiomyopathy, denervation also was found to be beneficial in models for chronic, nonischemic cardiomyopathy. Specifically, in pacing-induced heart failure, sympathetic denervation was found to not only affect renal hemodynamics, but it also was shown to alter the expression of several renal angiotensin receptors, providing a possible mechanism to modulate the pathophysiology of cardiorenal syndrome.[39]

## Renal Denervation in Heart Failure with Reduced Ejection Fraction

Beyond benefits seen in experimental models, there is evidence to suggest that attenuation of renal sympathetic activity may produce similar benefits in patients with systolic heart failure. In a series of patients with reduced ejection fraction treated with intravenous diuretics, decreased levels of plasma norepinephrine and renin, surrogate markers for sympathetic activity, were associated with augmentation of diuresis.[40] In light of these observations, it is hypothesized that tempering with renal sympathetic activity via a catheter-directed approach might alter the hemodynamic and neurohormonal dysfunction associated with heart failure.

As such, there are currently several randomized controlled trials under way to investigate the efficacy and safety of catheter-directed RDN in chronic systolic heart failure. In an initial pilot study of 7 patients with chronic systolic heart failure, on maximal tolerated medical therapy, bilateral RDN was performed and patients were observed for 6 months for any adverse effects.[41] Over a period of 6 months, there was no significant reduction in blood pressure or hypotensive or syncopal episodes reported. Furthermore, renal function remained preserved and patients even reported an improvement in symptoms, as supported by an increased 6-minute walk

| Table 2 | | | |
|---|---|---|---|
| Ongoing trials of renal denervation in heart failure with reduced ejection fraction | | | |
| Title | Study Design | Primary Outcome | Secondary Outcome |
| Renal Denervation in Patients with Chronic Heart Failure | Patients with LVEF 10%–40% with NYHA Class II-III symptoms randomized to renal denervation and maintenance of heart failure medications or maintenance of heart failure medications alone | Safety of renal denervation as measured by the number of periprocedural adverse events using the Symplicity catheter | Change in ventricular function as measured by echocardiography; change in renal function as measured by GFR; response in quality of life and symptoms |
| Renal Artery Denervation in Chronic Heart Failure Study (REACH) | Patients with LVEF <40% with NYHA Class II or higher symptoms randomized to renal denervation or sham procedure | Improvement in symptoms as measured by Kansas City Cardiomyopathy Questionnaire | Improvement in peak $Vo_2$ on exercise testing; improvement in 6-min walk distance; change in NYHA functional classification; incidence of major adverse events |
| Effect at 6 mo of Renal Denervation in Chronic Heart Failure (DENRENIC) | Patients with LVEF <35% with NYHA Class III-IV symptoms undergoing renal denervation using the EnligHTN Renal Denervation System | Significant improvement in 6-min walk test | Incidence of adverse events as measured by renal artery stenosis, aneurysm and change in renal function; quality of life as evaluated by EQ-5D |
| Renal Sympathetic Denervation for Patients with Chronic Heart Failure (RSD4CHF) | Patients with LVEF <35% with NYHA Class II-IV symptoms and adequate renal artery anatomy randomized to renal denervation with conventional therapy or conventional therapy alone | All-cause mortality and cardiovascular events (cardiac death, myocardial infarction, arrhythmia, angina) | Blood pressure as measured by ambulatory and home monitoring; quality of life as measured by SF-36; rehospitalization rate; recurrence rate of malignant arrhythmia; cardiac function as measured by LVEF, 6-min walk test, BNP, and NYHA class |
| Renal Denervation in Patients with Chronic Heart Failure and Renal Impairment Clinical Trial (SymplicityHF) | Patients with LVEF <40% and NYHA Class II or III symptoms undergoing renal denervation using the Symplicity catheter | Safety of renal denervation as measured by adverse events | Ventricular function as measured by echocardiography; renal function as measured by GFR |

Abbreviations: BNP, brain natriuretic peptide; EQ-5D, EuroQol-5D; GFR, glomerular filtration rate; LVEF, left ventricular ejection fraction; NYHA, New York Heart Association.

distance at 6 months (difference of $27.1 \pm 9.7$ m, $P = .03$) and a trend toward deescalation of diuretic therapy. Although not randomized, the results of the study suggested that RDN is safe in chronic heart failure and even may be associated with improved exercise capacity.

Similarly, the SYMPLICITY HF study is a larger, ongoing proof-of-concept trial. It is a multi-center prospective study, enrolling patients with NYHA Class II-III symptoms and impaired renal function.[42] The study seeks to evaluate the safety of denervation in this patient population, as well as any changes in cardiac function, as assessed by echocardiography, and changes in renal function, as assessed by estimated glomerular filtration rate. Although the investigation is ongoing, no significant vascular complications were reported during denervation.

**Table 3**
Ongoing trials of renal denervation in heart failure with preserved ejection fraction

| Title | Study Design | Primary Outcome | Secondary Outcome |
|---|---|---|---|
| Renal Denervation in Heart failure Patients with Preserved Ejection Fraction (RESPECT-HF) | Patients with LVEF >50% and NYHA Class II or higher symptoms with echocardiographic evidence of diastolic dysfunction and an episode of acute decompensated heart failure randomized to renal denervation and conventional therapy or conventional therapy alone | Change in left atrial volume index or left ventricular mass index on cardiac MRI | Change in exercise capacity as assessed by Vo$_{2max}$ and 6-min walk test; change in diastolic function as assessed by echocardiography; change in biomarkers of cardiac load and interstitial fibrosis; quality of life as assessed by Minnesota Living with Heart Failure Questionnaire; composite endpoint death or hospitalization with heart failure |
| Denervation of the Renal Sympathetic Nerves in Heart Failure with Normal LV Ejection Fraction (DIASTOLE) | Patents with LVEF >50% with signs or symptoms of heart failure, evidence of diastolic dysfunction, and hypertension on at least 2 antihypertensives randomized to renal denervation and conventional therapy or conventional therapy alone | Change in diastolic function as measured by E/E′ ratio on echocardiography | Number of adverse events |
| Renal Denervation in Heart Failure with Preserved Ejection Fraction (RDT-PEF) | Patients with LVEF >40% and NYHA Class II-III symptoms with evidence of HFPEF (on echocardiography, elevated filling pressures on cardiac catheterization or elevated BNP) randomized to renal denervation or conventional therapy | Change in quality of life as measured by Minnesota Living with Heart Failure Questionnaire; change in peak Vo$_2$; change in BNP level; change in LV filling pressure as measured by E/E′ ratio; change in LV mass index; change in LA volume index | Change in heart rate variability; change in autonomic function as measured by mIBG radiotracer assessment; change in neurohormone level; change in ambulatory blood pressure; change in endothelial function |

*Abbreviations:* BNP, brain natriuretic peptide; HFPEF, heart failure with preserved ejection fraction; LA, left atrial; LV, left ventricular; LVEF, left ventricular ejection fraction; mIBG, metaiodobenzylguanidine; NYHA, New York Heart Association.

In addition, several ongoing trials are currently under way to assess the efficacy of RDN in systolic heart failure, by investigating its effect on all-cause and cardiovascular death, hospitalization for heart failure, urinary sodium and water excretion, and change in symptomatology as measured by peak $Vo_2$, cardiopulmonary exercise testing, and change in NYHA functional classification[43–45] (Table 2).

In addition to potentially influencing left ventricular function and exercise tolerance, RDN may also provide benefit in the management of heart failure comorbidities, notably arrhythmias. Studies have observed that denervation has been associated with a reduced resting heart rate, leading to both improved rate control of atrial arrhythmias[46] and suppression of ventricular ectopy.[47]

## Renal Denervation in Heart Failure with Preserved Ejection Fraction

Similar to the case of heart failure with reduced ejection fraction, it is hypothesized that the sympathetic nervous system plays a significant role in the development and maintenance of heart failure with preserved ejection fraction (HFPEF). Clinically, HFPEF is characterized predominantly by impaired diastolic function and abnormal relaxation and filling of the left ventricle. Frequently, hypertension is a major cause of diastolic dysfunction, whereby chronic pressure overload leads to left ventricular hypertrophy and remodeling.[48] Studies have suggested that sympathetic overdrive not only plays a major role in the pathophysiology of hypertension, but also may contribute to the development of diastolic dysfunction.[49] As such, renal sympathetic denervation may prove particularly valuable in the treatment of HFPEF.

Studies of patients with resistant hypertension have long suggested that RDN not only improves blood pressure, but also is associated with positive left ventricular remodeling.[50] In addition, patients with HFPEF and concomitant hypertension have shown improvement in several echocardiographic parameters of diastolic function with denervation. In an investigation of patients with diastolic dysfunction and resistant hypertension, RDN was not only associated with a significant reduction in blood pressure, but also with a significant reduction in interventricular septal thickness, left ventricular mass index, and left ventricular filling pressures, as assessed by mitral valve lateral E/E' measurements.[51] Furthermore, these improvements in left ventricular filling and hypertrophy parameters were seen across all tertiles of systolic blood

pressure and heart rate, suggesting that the benefits seen may be independent of the effect on pulse and blood pressure.[52]

Most recently, a small randomized trial comparing RDN with medical therapy in an HFPEF cohort, observed denervation to be safe in this patient population, with no significant procedural complications or change in renal function between groups. However, there was no observed difference in left ventricular mass index, peak oxygen uptake during exercise, left atrial volume index, or diastolic relaxation, as assessed by E/E' measurements, between groups.[53] Although the study may have been underpowered to detect whether denervation affects left ventricular remodeling and exercise capacity in patients with HFPEF, it demonstrated the procedure to be safe in this population. As such, randomized controlled trials are currently under way to investigate the impact of RDN on exercise capacity, quality of life, and diastolic parameters, as measured by Doppler echocardiography and MRI, in the HFPEF population[54] (Table 3).

## SUMMARY

Sympathetic overdrive has been implicated in the pathogenesis of several cardiovascular disease states, from hypertension[7] to heart failure[35] to arrhythmias[44] and ischemia.[55] Targeted ablation of renal sympathetic fibers via catheter-based RDN has been proposed as a minimally invasive, adjunctive therapy for the treatment of both resistant hypertension and heart failure. Although early studies have shown promise, the only large sham-controlled study to date observed no difference in blood pressure compared with medical therapy.[16] Ongoing studies to better identify patient populations that may benefit from RDN along with improvements in device technology will shed light on the future promise of this field. If successful, RDN may shift the treatment paradigm for hypertension and heart failure, and potentially extend to a broad range of noncardiovascular diseases associated with sympathetic overactivity, such as chronic kidney disease,[56] arrhythmias,[57] diabetes,[58] and sleep apnea.[59]

## REFERENCES

1. Calhoun DA, Jones D, Textor S, et al, American Heart Association Professional Education Committee. Resistant hypertension: diagnosis, evaluation, and treatment: a scientific statement from the American Heart Association Professional Education

Committee of the Council for High Blood Pressure Research. Circulation 2008;117:e510–26.

2. Pimenta E, Calhoun DA. Resistant hypertension: incidence, prevalence and prognosis. Circulation 2012;125:1594–6.

3. Sarafidis PA, Georgianos P, Bakris GL. Resistant hypertension–its identification and epidemiology. Nat Rev Nephrol 2013;9:51–8.

4. Daugherty SL, Powers JD, Magid DJ, et al. Incidence and prognosis of resistant hypertension in hypertensive patients. Circulation 2012;125:1635–42.

5. Myat A, Redwood SR, Qureshi AC, et al. Renal sympathetic denervation therapy for resistant hypertension: a contemporary synopsis and future implications. Circ Cardiovasc Interv 2013;6:184–97.

6. Santos M, Carvalho H. Renal sympathetic denervation in resistant hypertension. World J Cardiol 2013;5(4):94 101.

7. Esler M. The sympathetic nervous system through the ages: from Thomas Willis to resistant hypertension. Exp Physiol 2011;96:611–22.

8. Esler M, Jennings G, Korner P, et al. Assessment of the human sympathetic nervous system activity from measurements of norepinephrine turnover. Hypertension 1988;11(1):3–20.

9. Ye S, Zhong H, Yanamadala V, et al. Renal injury caused by intrarenal injection of phenol increases afferent and efferent renal sympathetic nerve activity. Am J Hypertens 2002;15(8):717–24.

10. O'Hagan KP, Thomas GD, Zambraski EJ. Renal denervation decreases blood pressure in DOCA-treated miniature swine with established hypertension. Am J Hypertens 1990;3(1):62–4.

11. Kassab S, Kato T, Wilkins FC, et al. Renal denervation attenuates the sodium retention and hypertension associated with obesity. Hypertension 1995;25:893–7.

12. Page IH, Heuer GJ. The effect of renal denervation on the level of arterial blood pressure and renal function in essential hypertension. J Clin Invest 1935;14(1):27–30.

13. Smithwick RH, Thompson JE. Splanchnicectomy for essential hypertension; results in 1,266 cases. J Am Med Assoc 1953;152:1501–4.

14. Hoobler SW, Manning JT, Paine WG, et al. The effects of splanchnicectomy on the blood pressure in hypertension: a controlled study. Circulation 1951;4:173–83.

15. Gulati V, White WB. Novel approaches for the treatment of the patient with resistant hypertension: renal nerve ablation. Curr Cardiovasc Risk Rep 2013;7(5):401–8.

16. Symplicity HTN-1 Investigators. Catheter-based renal sympathetic denervation for resistant hypertension: durability of blood pressure reduction out to 24 months. Hypertension 2011;57(5):911–7.

17. Esler M, Krum H, Schneider R, et al. Renal sympathetic denervation for treatment of resistant hypertension: two-year update from the SYMPLICITY HTN-2 randomized controlled trial. J Am Coll Cadiol 2013;61:E1386.

18. Bhatt D, Kandzari DE, O'Neill WW, et al. A controlled trial of renal denervation for resistant hypertension. N Engl J Med 2014;370:1393–401.

19. Azizi M, Sapoval M, Gosse P, et al. Optimum and stepped care standardized antihypertensive treatment with or without renal denervation for resistant hypertension (DENERHTN): a multicenter, open-label, randomised controlled trial. Lancet 2015;385(9981):1957–65.

20. Papademetriou V, Tsioufis C, Doumas M. Renal denervation and SYMPLICITY HTN-3: "Dubium sapientiae initium" (doubt is the beginning of wisdom). Circ Res 2014;115(2):211–4.

21. Schmider RE. Hypertension: how should data from SYMPLICITY HTN-3 be interpreted? Nat Rev Cardiol 2014;11(7):375–6.

22. Rosendorff C, Lackland DT, Allison M, et al. Treatment of hypertension in patients with coronary artery disease. A scientific statement from the American Heart Association, American College of Cardiology, and American Society of Hypertension. J Am Coll Cardiol 2015;65(18):1998–2038.

23. Kandzari DE, Kario K, Mahfoud F, et al. The SPYRAL HTN global clinical trial program: rationale and design for studies of renal denervation in the absence (SPYRAL HTN OFF-MED) and presence (SPYRAL HTN ON-MED) of antihypertensive medications. Am Heart J 2016;171(1):82–91.

24. Hasking GJ, Esler MD, Jennings GL, et al. Norepinephrine spillover to plasma in patients with congestive heart failure: evidence of increased overall and cardiorenal sympathetic nervous activity. Circulation 1986;73(4):615–21.

25. Sobotka PA, Krum H, Böhm M, et al. The role of renal denervation in the treatment of heart failure. Curr Cardiol Rep 2012;14(3):285–92.

26. Triposkiadis F, Karayannis G, Giamouzis G, et al. The sympathetic nervous system in heart failure: physiology, pathophysiology, and clinical implications. J Am Coll Cardiol 2009;54(19):1747–62.

27. Francis GS, Benedict C, Johnstone DE, et al. Comparison of neuroendocrine activation in patients with left ventricular dysfunction with and without congestive heart failure: a substudy of the studies of left ventricular dysfunction (SOLVD). Circulation 1990;82:1724–9.

28. Cohn JN, Levine TB, Olivari MT, et al. Plasma norepinephrine as a guide to prognosis in patients with chronic congestive heart failure. N Engl J Med 1984;311(13):819–23.

29. Benedict CR, Shelton B, Johnstone DE, et al. Prognostic significance of plasma norepinephrine

in patients with asymptomatic left ventricular dysfunction: SOLVD investigators. Circulation 1996;94(4):690–7.

30. Petersson M, Friberg P, Eisenhofer G, et al. Long-term outcome in relation to renal sympathetic activity in patients with chronic heart failure. Eur Heart J 2005;26:906–13.

31. Effect of enalapril on survival in patients with reduced left ventricular ejection fractions and congestive heart failure. The SOLVD investigators. N Engl J Med 1991;325(5):293–302.

32. Krum H. Sympathetic activation and the role of beta-blockers in chronic heart failure. Aust N Z J Med 1999;29:418–27.

33. Francis GS, Cohn JN, Johnson G, et al. Plasma norepinephrine, plasma renin activity, and congestive heart failure. Relations to survival and the effects of therapy in V-HeFT II. The V-HeFT VA cooperative studies group. Circulation 1993;87: VI40–8.

34. Schlaich MP, Sobotka PA, Krum H, et al. Renal sympathetic nerve ablation for uncontrolled hypertension. N Engl J Med 2009;361(9):932–4.

35. DiBona GF. Role of the renal nerves in sodium retention and edema formation. Trans AM Clin Climatol Assoc 1990;101:38–45.

36. Hu J, Ji M, Niu C, et al. Effects of renal sympathetic denervation on post-myocardial infarction cardiac remodeling in rats. PLoS One 2012;7(9):e45986.

37. Souza DR, Mill JG, Cabral AM, et al. Chronic experimental myocardial infarction produces antinatriuresis by a renal nerve-dependent mechanism. Braz J Med Biol Res 2004;37:285–93.

38. Villarreal D, Freeman RH, Johnson RA, et al. Effects of renal denervation on postprandial sodium excretion in experimental heart failure. Am J Physiol 1994;266(5 Pt 2):R1599–604.

39. Clayton SC, Haack KK, Zucker IH, et al. Renal denervation modulates angiotensin receptor expression in the renal cortex of rabbits with chronic heart failure. Am J Physiol Renal Physiol 2011;300(1):F31–9.

40. Galiwango PJ, McReynolds A, Ivanov J, et al. Activity with ambulation attenuates diuretic responsiveness in chronic heart failure. J Card Fail 2011;17: 797–803.

41. Davies JE, Manisty CH, Petraco R, et al. First-in-man safety evaluation of renal denervation for chronic systolic heart failure: primary outcome from REACH-Pilot study. Int J Cardiol 2013;162(3): 189–92.

42. Krum E, Cohen SA. The SYMPLICITY HF feasibility study: twelve month outcomes of renal denervation in patients with chronic heart failure and renal impairment. Circulation 2015;132:A10452.

43. Taborsky M. Renal denervation in patients with heart failure and severe left ventricular

dysfunction. In: ClinicalTrials.gov [Internet]. Bethesda (MD): National Library of Medicine (US); 2000. Available at: https://clinicaltrials.gov/ct2/show/NCT01870310. NLM Identifier: NCT01870310. Accessed October 25, 2016.

44. Hernandez A. Study of renal denervation in patients with heart failure (PRESERVE). In: ClinicalTrials.gov [Internet]. Bethesda (MD): National Library of Medicine (US); 2000. Available at: https://clinicaltrials.gov/ct2/show/NCT01954160. NLM Identifier: NCT01954160. Accessed October 25, 2016.

45. Davies J. Renal artery denervation in chronic heart failure study (REACH). In: ClinicalTrials.gov [Internet]. Bethesda (MD): National Library of Medicine (US). 2000. Available at: https://clinicaltrials.gov/ct2/show/NCT01639378. NLM Identifier: NCT01639378. Accessed October 25, 2016.

46. Linz D, Mahfoud F, Schotten U, et al. Renal sympathetic denervation provides ventricular rate control but does not prevent atrial electrical remodeling during atrial fibrillation. Hypertension 2013;61: 225–31.

47. Linz D, Wirth K, Ukena C, et al. Renal denervation suppresses ventricular arrhythmias during acute ventricular ischemia in pigs. Heart Rhythm 2013; 10(10):1525–30.

48. Schlaich MP, Sobotka PA, Krum H, et al. Renal denervation as a therapeutic approach for hypertension: novel implications for an old concept. Hypertension 2009;54:1195–201.

49. Grassi G, Seravalle G, Quarti-Trevano F, et al. Sympathetic and baroreflex cardiovascular control in hypertension-related left ventricular dysfunction. Hypertension 2009;53(2):205–9.

50. De Sousa Almeida M, de Araújo Gonçalves P, Branco P, et al. Impact of renal denervation on left ventricular structure and function at 1-year follow-up. PLoS One 2016;11(3):e0149855.

51. Brandt MC, Mahfoud F, Reda S, et al. Renal sympathetic denervation reduces left ventricular hypertrophy and improves cardiac function in patients with resistant hypertension. J Am Coll Cardiol 2012; 59(10):901–9.

52. Schirmer SH, Sayed MM, Reil JC, et al. Improvements in left ventricular hypertrophy and diastolic function following denervation: effects beyond blood pressure and heart rate reduction. J Am Coll Cardiol 2014;63(18):1916–23.

53. Patel HC, Rosen SD, Hayward C, et al. Renal denervation in heart failure with preserved ejection fraction (RDT-PEF): a randomized controlled trial. Eur J Heart Fail 2016;18(6):703–12.

54. Verloop WL, Beeftink MM, Nap A, et al. Renal denervation in heart failure with normal left ventricular ejection fraction. Rationale and design of the DIASTOLE (Denervation of the Renal Sympathetic

Nerves in Heart Failure with Normal LV Ejection Fraction) trial. Eur J Heart Fail 2013;15(12):1429–37.

55. Graham LN, Smith PA, Huggett RJ, et al. Sympathetic drive in anterior and inferior uncomplicated acute myocardial infarction. Circulation 2004;109: 2285–9.

56. Converse RL, Jacobsen TN, Toto RD, et al. Sympathetic overactivity in patients with chronic renal failure. N Engl J Med 1992;327:1912–8.

57. Kosiuk J, Hilbert S, Pokushalov E, et al. Renal denervation for treatment of cardiac arrhythmias:

state of the art and future directions. J Cardiovasc Electrophysiol 2015;26(2):233–8.

58. Mahfoud F, Schlaich M, Kindermann I, et al. Effect of renal sympathetic denervation on glucose metabolism in patients with resistant hypertension: a pilot study. Circulation 2011;123(18):1940–6.

59. Witkowski A, Prejbisz A, Florczak E, et al. Effects of renal sympathetic denervation on blood pressure, sleep apnea course, and glycemic control in patients with resistant hypertension and sleep apnea. Hypertension 2011;58:559–65.

# SECTION III - Interventional Heart Failure

# Prioritizing and Combining Therapies for Heart Failure in the Era of Mechanical Support Devices

George S. Hanzel, MD[a], Simon Dixon, MBchB[b], James A. Goldstein, MD[c],*

---

### KEYWORDS

- Interventional strategies and tactics • Myocardial ischemic burden • Hemodynamic compromise
- Percutaneous ventricular support devices

---

### KEY POINTS

- Prioritizing and combining therapies for heart failure (HF) are based on pathophysiologic, clinical, and procedural perspectives, encompassing analysis of hemodynamic status, anatomic considerations, and technical challenges.
- Complex decision making is based on an anatomic-pathophysiologic-clinical foundation, classifying problems according to (1) underlying pathogenesis: primary coronary, myocardial, and valvular (and their common coexistence in individual patients); (2) active pathophysiology: presence and severity of hemodynamic compromise and acute myocardial ischemia; and (3) comorbidities.
- These considerations facilitate goal setting for both medical and interventional therapies based on the likelihood of definitive resolution of the underlying disease as definitive/destination, preservation/salvage, step-wise, bridge, or palliation. Establishing these goals then serves to strategize the therapeutic options and deployment in temporal sequence.

---

## GOALS DETERMINE PRIORITIZATION AND INTERVENTIONAL STRATEGY

Clinical and procedural tactics must be based on specific goals, which are determined by

- Presence of acute myocardial ischemia
- Presence and severity of hemodynamic compromise
- Likelihood of definitive resolution of the underlying disease(s), which allows goal stratification as definitive/destination, preservation/salvage, step-wise, bridge, or palliation)

Establishing these goals then serves to strategize the therapeutic options and deployment in a temporal sequence (eg, definitive interventions, such as single-setting percutaneous coronary intervention [PCI] + transcatheter aortic valve replacement [TAVR], stepwise escalation

---

Disclosure: Dr J.A. Goldstein is a consultant for Abimed, Inc, manufacturer of left ventricular and right ventricular support devices.

[a] Cardiac Catheterization Laboratory, Department of Cardiovascular Medicine, William Beaumont Hospital, 3601 West 13 Mile Road, Royal Oak, MI 48073, USA; [b] Department of Cardiovascular Medicine, William Beaumont Hospital, 3601 West 13 Mile Road, Royal Oak, MI 48073, USA; [c] Cardiovascular Research and Education, Department of Cardiovascular Medicine, William Beaumont Hospital, 3601 West 13 Mile Road, Royal Oak, MI 48073, USA

* Corresponding author.

E-mail address: James.Goldstein@beaumont.edu

Intervent Cardiol Clin 6 (2017) 465–480
http://dx.doi.org/10.1016/j.iccl.2017.03.015

to achieve initial hemodynamic stabilization for a subsequent intervention, such as balloon vavulo-plasty, bridge to TAVR, etc).

## ASSESSMENT OF HEMODYNAMIC STATUS AND MYOCARDIAL ISCHEMIA

Therapeutic intervention strategy is in great part determined by the hemodynamic and ischemic status of a patient, categorized by (1) the presence of acute myocardial ischemia and (2) the presence and severity of manifest hemodynamic compromise. These parameters can be easily ascertained by bedside evaluation and noninvasive echocardiography, together with invasive assessments.

### Assessment of Myocardial Ischemia

Assessing ischemia and whether it is acute or chronic exerts profound influence on decisions, strategies, and tactics. The presence of acute coronary syndrome (ACS) dramatically alters the strategy and temporal urgency of interventions, particularly in patients suffering ST segment elevation myocardial infarction (STEMI), and is discussed later; determination of ACS is straightforward by symptoms, ECG, and cardiac biomarkers. Evaluation of chronic ischemia is also straightforward by stress imaging and angiography, although in the setting of HF, myocardial viability testing data are also key in decision making for PCI (and for coronary artery bypass grafting).

### Assessment of Hemodynamic Status

Stabilizing the circulation is of primary concern. It is essential to perform detailed assessment of hemodynamics status combining bedside evaluation, noninvasive assessment by echocardiography, and potentially invasive hemodynamic interrogation as well. A basic approach should address each issue, including

- Is there hypotension/hypoperfusion?
- Is preload adequate?
- Is there pulmonary congestion?
- Is there systemic venous congestion?
- Is rhythm optimal?
- Are there mechanical defects?
- Is there renal dysfunction (which may confound/complicate dye-requisite interventions)?
- Does the patient have hematologic issues (significant anemia and/or bleeding diatheses
- Are there other HF precipitants (infection, thyroid disorder, and so forth)?

## CARDIOGENIC SHOCK: A SPECIAL CIRCUMSTANCE

Hypotension resulting in organ hypoperfusion is devastating (particularly to any organ supplied by stenotic arteries, such as the atherosclerotic coronary bed); therefore, defining cardiogenic shock [CS] and rapidly rectifying it are essential. CS is clinically defined as systemic tissue hypoperfusion (decreased urine output and cool extremities) secondary to inadequate cardiac output (CO) despite adequate circulatory volume and left ventricular (LV) filling pressure. The hemodynamic definition includes marked and persistent (>30 min) hypotension (systolic blood pressure [BP] <90 mm Hg) or a fall in mean arterial BP greater than 30 mm Hg below baseline, with a cardiac index of less than 1.8 L/min/m$^2$ without hemodynamic support or less than 2.2 L/min/m$^2$ with support and a pulmonary capillary wedge pressure (PCWP) greater than 15 mm Hg.

### Importance of Recognizing Preshock

Defining CS by these end-stage criteria alone misses critical upstream opportunities in patients with severe hemodynamic compromise who are suffering organ hypoperfusion but who may not yet manifest frank hypotension. Such cases may be categorized as preshock, meeting all criteria for shock (cool clammy mottled extremities, low urine output, compensatory sinus tachycardia, and pulmonary congestion), except the BP parameter, with adequate systolic pressure greater than 90 mm Hg to 100 mm Hg only maintained by intense neurohormonal stimulation (leading to compensatory but deleterious tachycardia, vasoconstriction, and expanded blood volume). Clearly such patients suffering profound pump failure and hemodynamic compromise and organ hypoperfusion may greatly benefit form that timely interventions.

## OPTIONS FOR PERCUTANEOUS MECHANICAL SUPPORT

The design, mechanisms, deployment, benefit, and risks of the various mechanical circulatory support devices are discussed later and in several excellent reviews.[1,2] Regarding prioritizing and combining therapies, a few points of emphasis are relevant:

- First, the intra-aortic balloon pump (IABP) is easy to insert, is inexpensive, and primarily provides BP support together with some modest indirect LV unloading. It has aggregate hemodynamic benefits, including augmentation of systemic perfusion in general as well as some lowering of LV filling pressure due to reduced afterload and increased forward CO. Patients with coronary artery disease (CAD) benefit from enhanced coronary blood flow which, together with reduced oxygen demand, relives myocardial ischemia to some extent, especially if they are suffering hemodynamic compromise. As discussed later, the IABP is useful as an initial support device in decompensated HF and in certain conditions can sufficiently stabilize BP, improve myocardial ischemia, and support complex PCI.

- Percutaneous ventricular assist devices (PVADs), including the Impella (Abiomed, Danvers, Massachusetts) and Tandem-Heart (Cardiac Assist Inc, Pittsburgh, PA), generate direct cardiac power and CO and directly unload the ventricle. Their hemodynamic benefits are superior to the IABP, including not only augmented mean aortic BP and improved systemic perfusion but also ventricular unloading, which further relieves congestion, reduces myocardial oxygen demand, and may serve to minimize requirement for vasopressor/intrope support. These devices achieve not only superior hemodynamic benefit but also, by virtue of their net benefit on oxygen supply-demand balance, reduce myocardial ischemia. The Impella can be easily and quickly placed with techniques analogous to an LV pigtail catheter and in modestly experienced hands should take no longer than the IABP; however, it is more expensive. TandemHeart is more challenging and time consuming to deploy, and requires greater operator technical expertise and an experienced team to insert and manage. The PVADs are higher-profile vascular access devices compared with IABP (eg, Impella 14F vs IABP 8F). The potential superiority of these devices versus the IABP in high-risk PCI and CS is discussed.

## CLINICAL SCENARIOS ILLUSTRATING ISCHEMIC HEART FAILURE STRATEGIES
### High-risk Percutaneous Coronary Intervention
Whereas modern coronary interventional technique and technology have made the vast majority of PCIs straightforward, successful, and safe, there is still attendant risk for adverse events (in particular, periprocedural hemodynamic instability). It is essential to identify such high-risk cases,[3–5] which may be stratified and predicted from a tripartite set of factors: (1) patient-specific, related to comorbidities, including depressed LV systolic function (particularly if recently decompensated), impaired renal function, diabetes mellitus, and peripheral arterial disease; (2) lesion-specific high risk factors, defined according to anatomic characteristics of the target lesion(s), including left main stenosis and other targets that supply a large territory of the residual functioning myocardium, bifurcation disease, disease in older degenerated saphenous vein grafts, ostial stenoses, heavily calcified lesions, and chronic total occlusions; and (3) clinical setting, specifically PCI in the setting of ACS, particularly in those with manifest hemodynamic compromise and especially CS.

### Prioritization Based on Hemodynamics and Acute Myocardial Ischemia
Decisions for prophylactic insertion of mechanical support or at minimum preparation for urgent application are determined by

- Whether there is active myocardial ischemia and the extent of residual viable myocardium so endangered by PCI
- Magnitude of depression of LVEF and presence of complicating mechanical lesions, for example, functional mitral regurgitation (MR)
- The hemodynamic condition of a patient at the time of referral for PCI, the anticipated risk of hemodynamic compromise during the procedure, and the likelihood of requisite hemodynamic support after revascularization

### Elective percutaneous coronary intervention—hemodynamically stable
In patients undergoing PCI, the presence of hemodynamic compromise is critical to consider. In hemodynamically stable patients undergoing elective PCI, those in whom benefit from prophylactic mechanical circulatory support has been demonstrated include cases of severe LV dysfunction (ejection fraction [EF] <30%), unprotected left main, or sole remaining vessel. In general, support devices allow for more complete revascularization with lesser likelihood of periprocedural hemodynamic deterioration.

Although feasibility for supporting high-risk PCI has been demonstrated for the IABP and TandemHeart devices, the Impella device has the most robust database, both in observational and randomized controlled data. The PROTECT II trial, the largest randomized controlled trial of mechanical support for high-risk PCI using any device, randomized patients to either IABP or Impella 2.5 support.[3–5] Although there was no difference in 30-day outcome between groups, secondary outcomes, including 90-day major adverse cardiac and cerebrovascular events and repeat revascularization, occurred with lower frequency with use of the Impella device. In general, it is thought that the hemodynamic stability provided by mechanical support (in particular a direct cardiac power source, such as the Impella vs the less robust power of IABP), allows an interventionist the safety and comfort of accomplishing more complete revascularization. After successful PCI, presuming the patient is stable, the device can be removed immediately.

### Hemodynamically unstable but non–acute coronary syndrome: sequenced or deferred percutaneous coronary interventions

Patients with manifest hemodynamic compromise but without acute myocardial ischemia should not undergo angiographic procedures (and thereby minimize the attendant stresses of contrast dye, ischemia, and coronary complications) unless clinical circumstances, that is, acute ischemia and intractable ischemic HF, do not allow their delay. Rather, patients with ischemic heart disease and hemodynamic compromise, but without active ischemia, should be optimized medically (vasodilators, diuretics, and inotropic agents if necessary), in some cases with the guidance of invasive right heart hemodynamic monitoring.

If, despite appropriate medical therapies, there is ongoing pulmonary congestion, intractable right HF, cardiorenal syndrome, and so forth, then escalation of care must be rapidly used, including pharmacologic support (inotropes) and early consideration of percutaneous mechanical support, either with an IABP or via direct mechanical support (Impella or TandemHeart) to achieve hemodynamic stability before planned elective PCI. Once hemodynamically optimized (defined by resolution of pulmonary congestion, stabilized systemic perfusion in general, and renal function, in particular), high-risk PCI can be carried out: depending on the magnitude of risk (typically high in such patients who were just decompensated), PCI should be performed with prophylactic use of percutaneous assist devices.

### Case illustration: high-risk percutaneous coronary intervention in ischemic cardiomyopathy

An 88-year-old man presented with acute pulmonary edema with a history of chronic ischemic LV systolic dysfunction EF less than 30% with moderate functional MR. Comorbidities included bifascicular block, peripheral vascular disease, renal dysfunction, and chronic obstructive pulmonary disease (COPD).

**Initial stabilization.** Urgent catheterization showed aortic pressure = 87/51 mm Hg (mean = 65 mm Hg); PCWP was 37 mm Hg. Intravenous (IV) furosemide was given and

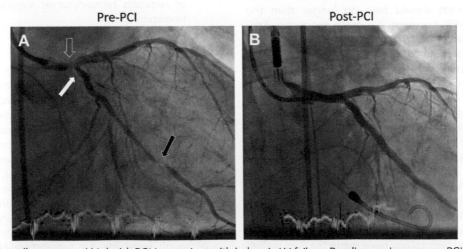

Pre-PCI          Post-PCI

**Fig. 1.** Impella-supported high-risk PCI in a patient with ischemic LV failure. Baseline angiogram pre-PCI (*A*) demonstrates hazy calcified severe distal left main stenosis (*open arrow*), significantly narrowed ostial circumflex lesion (*white arrow*), and diffuse disease in the distal circumflex culminating in a tight midstenosis (*black arrow*). Although the LAD appeared angiographically insignificant, intravascular ultrasound demonstrated a tight calcified lesion. Post-PCI angiogram (*B*) demonstrates successful Impella-supported revascularization of the left coronary artery, including circumflex and distal left main bifurcation.

Impella 2.5 was placed, after which BP improved (120/60 mm Hg, mean = 85 mm Hg) and PCWP was reduced to 24 mm Hg. Angiography documented severe (70%) eccentric heavily calcified left main stenosis (**Fig. 1A**). The ostium of the circumflex was significantly stenosed (70%); there was severe in-stent stenosis of the midobtuse marginal branch and moderate diffuse disease in the midvessel. Although the left anterior descending (LAD) ostium looked angiographically moderate, intravascular ultrasound revealed a tight (90%) heavily calcified lesion.

**Supported high-risk complex percutaneous coronary intervention.** On Impella support, successful complex high-risk PCI was performed, first stenting the circumflex lesions, after which stenting was performed to the distal left main and its bifurcation into the ostial circumflex and LAD using the culotte technique to the LAD (see **Fig. 1B**). The Impella device was then explanted in the catheterization laboratory.

**Hemodynamic instability during acute coronary syndrome.** Hemodynamic compromise in the setting of acute myocardial ischemia is a dangerous pathophysiologic scenario in which ischemia induces dysfunction (acute and chronic), with LV dysfunction exacerbating ischemia via the adverse effects of compensatory neurohormonal stimulation designed to maintain BP by sympathetic stimulation, catecholamines, and the renin-angiotensin-aldosterone system, which increases preload, afterload, heart rate, and contractility, thereby increasing myocardial oxygen demand in the setting of impaired supply attributable to coronary stenoses or occlusions. There are 3 exacerbating, calamitous, and disastrous hemodynamic parameters that contribute to the vicious cycle of perpetuating ischemic myocardial dysfunction: severe coronary stenosis, elevated LV filling pressure, and hypotension.

- The first consideration is the proximate cause of ischemia, diminished coronary blood flow due to severe coronary stenosis (or worse, total occlusion), which must be relieved rapidly in the setting of severe ischemia, in particular STEMI.
- Elevated LV filling pressure is deleterious as an ischemic driver, because the pressure drop across a severe stenosis results in lower distal driving force to perfuse through the myocardium to the subendocardial capillaries, which are compressed by elevated cavitary pressure (at the same time that increasing preload is itself a determinant of increased subendocardial oxygen demand); the contrast dye load requisite to guide PCI exacerbates this problem. Therefore, aggressive interventions (including IV diuretics, nitrates, and mechanical support) are critical to relieving ischemia, not only to reperfuse but also to directly reduce and optimize LV filling pressure.
- Hypotension is disastrous in the setting of any severe coronary stenosis, particularly in patients with manifest hemodynamic compromise. The flow dynamics across the coronary stenosis dictate that frictional and separation forces reduce downstream coronary perfusion pressure; under these conditions, systemic hypotension may drastically and disastrously further reduce perfusion and thereby exacerbate myocardial ischemic dysfunction, which is calamitous if the stenosis is in a precarious proximal location supplying a large territory of the functioning myocardium.
- Not only does hypotension result in hypoperfusion to all critical organs in the body but also, most important, inadequate aortic perfusion pressure exacerbates coronary ischemia across severe coronary stenoses that are critically dependent on optimal perfusion pressure to maintain whatever minimal flow may be possible through the narrowing per se. Furthermore, ischemic LV failure is typically associated with elevated LV diastolic pressure, which not only increases ischemia by virtue of increased demand but also compresses subendocardial capillary network supplied by stenotic epicardial vessels, thereby profoundly exacerbating ischemic LV dysfunction both with respect to adequate forward driving pressure across the coronary stenosis and a vascular waterfall effect, which compresses subendocardial perfusion.

In aggregate, these pathophysiologic considerations serve as the foundation for a tripartite therapeutic intervention in ischemic patients with hemodynamic compromise based on rapid restoration of optimal aortic perfusion pressure, reduction of LV filling pressure, and relief of coronary stenosis through PCI. Some of these goals may be accomplished by medical therapy alone (diuretics, vasodilators, inotropes, and vasopressors), but it is classically such patients who benefit from rapid institution of mechanical support.

**Intervention sequencing and escalation.** It is important to emphasize that PCI, even in the setting of STEMI, should be performed once hemodynamic stabilization has been at least initiated (but not necessarily fully accomplished). Prior to and during emergency percutaneous revascularization of STEMI, hemodynamic compromise due to ischemic LV pump failure must be rectified, not only to achieve hemodynamic stabilization but also to accommodate the contrast dye necessary to perform the intervention. Furthermore, in the setting of ACS in general, and STEMI in particular, coronary interventions hazard the risk of thrombotic embolization to the subtended myocardium further increase the risk of hemodynamic decompensation and cardiovascular collapse. In STEMI, reperfusion itself may cause myocardial damage, known as ischemia-reperfusion injury. Finally, these devices may have beneficial effects on reducing the LV work and, therefore, myocardial oxygen demand, which may reduce infarct size and/or reduce ischemic complications.

## Acute Coronary Syndrome Patients with Pulmonary Congestion but Intact Blood Pressure and Perfusion

- For patients with pulmonary congestion without manifest low output or hypotension, IV diuretics may suffice. Although primary reperfusion intervention should not be delayed, at an appropriate point insertion of right heart catheter to monitor optimization of filling pressure by diuresis is often clinically beneficial. In such patients with predominant pulmonary congestion and depressed LVEF, early administration of vasodilators is beneficial (including IV nitroglycerine and angiotensin-converting enzyme inhibitors).
- Furthermore, in patients not fully stabilized from a respiratory standpoint, consideration should be given to prophylactic intubation prior to PCI, because dye administration and ischemia may precipitate respiratory decompensation form worsening pulmonary congestion.

## Acute Coronary Syndrome Patients with Pulmonary Congestion and Intact Blood Pressure but Clinical Hypoperfusion: Preshock

- In patients with pulmonary congestion and clinical hypoperfusion (cool, mottled extermities, tachycardia, and low urine output), pharmacologic and mechanical support is paramount and should be instituted prior to PCI. IV diuretics are essential and inotropic agents may be initiated to achieve stabilization (preferably milrinone, which is an inodilator and has the least adverse effects on myocardial ischemia).

- In all such cases, a right heart catheter facilitates more precise hemodynamic optimization, but this may be reasonably delayed to follow emergency percutaneous revascularization in the setting of profound ischemia and STEMI, in particular.

- All such cases are by definition prime candidates for prophylactic mechanical support to facilitate PCI, which is by definition high risk based on patient factors (even if the target lesion is straightforward). Mechanical support should be considered, including in patients who achieve rapid hemodynamic stabilization with such initial medical therapies.

- It is critical that mechanical support be implemented prior to reperfusion, because coronary angiography and intervention require contrast dye, which exacerbates ischemic LV failure and hemodynamic instability, and intervention may disrupt plaque, causing downstream embolization, and in those with STEMI reperfusion injury may exacerbate hemodynamic compromise.

## Acute Coronary Syndrome Patients with Cardiogenic Shock

- The deleterious effects of hypotension in patients with acute ischemic hemodynamic compromise have been emphasized. Therefore, it is essential to emergently rectify hypotension in patients suffering coronary ischemia, first with pharmacologic support (vasopressors and inotropes), while preparing for definitive mechanical support. Although IABP does restore or at least improve mean arterial pressure in most patients, it does not create the direct mechanical power and CO provided by PVADs, such as the Impella. In most cases, such direct power generating PVADs are preferable if technically feasible.

- Studies of the IABP in patients with acute MI and CS undergoing reperfusion intervention suggest no mortality benefit.[6] Hemodynamic improvements have been demonstrated in small studies of the Impella 2.5 system in CS.[7] A recent exploratory randomized trial, however, involving mechanically ventilated CS patients did not show reduced 30-day mortality versus IABP.[8] In aggregate, these studies demonstrate the apparent ceiling that has limited progress in salvage of CS patients. Clearly better treatments are needed for CS in acute myocardial ischemia. Regardless, it is unthinkable not to use some type of mechanical support in STEMI patients with CS undergoing primary PCI.[9]

- Mechanical complications of MI, such as ischemic MR and postinfarct ventricular septal rupture, are increasingly uncommon in the primary reperfusion era. Regardless, they are critical to identify (clinical, echocardiographic, and hemodynamic investigation is usually definitive) and may benefit from mechanical support devices because the hemodynamic disturbance is usually acute and substantial

*Case illustration: acute anterior ST segment elevation myocardial infarction, cardiac arrest, and cardiogenic shock*

A 49-year-old man presented to the emergency department with chest pain and anterior ST elevation on ECG and then developed ventricular tachycardia. He was quickly defibrillated but was in profound CS with pulmonary edema and hypotension and evidence of hypoperfusion by cool, clammy, mottled vasoconstricted extremities.

- Initial emergency department therapy: he was intubated, started on vasopressors, and emergently brought to the cardiac catheterization laboratory, with initial BP = 84/71 mm Hg and LV end-diastolic pressure = 30 mm Hg. Fick CO/cardiac index showed 2.8 L/min, 1.3 L/min/m$^2$.

- Escalated hemodynamic support: Impella 3.0 was placed, dopamine was started, phenylephrine was discontinued, and norepinephrine down-titrated. Lasix was given IV. BP rose to 135/97 mm Hg, CO/cardiac index = 8.0 L/min, 3.6 L/min/m$^2$, and PCWP decreased to 22 mm Hg.

- Supported high-risk PCI: coronary angiography documented a thrombotically occluded proximal LAD, which, under Impella support, was successfully recanalized and stented with an excellent angiographic result with restoration of Thrombosis in Myocardial Infarction grade 3 flow (Fig. 2). The patient was admitted to the coronary care unit (CCU) and initial echocardiogram revealed a dilated diffusely hypokinetic LV with an EF of 30% (Fig. 3).

- Post-PCI CCU course: the patient improved dramatically over 48 hours and repeat echocardiogram revealed complete return of LV function (see Fig. 3), after which the Impella was weaned off and the patient extubated without hemodynamic compromise, then was rapidly up and ambulating.

- Staged nonculprit PCI: prior to discharge, he underwent staged stenting of a severely stenosed right coronary artery; he left the hospital the following day, functional class I asymptomatic.

Pre-PCI          Post-PCI

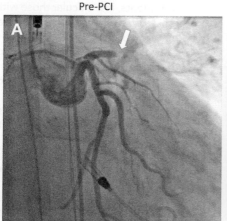 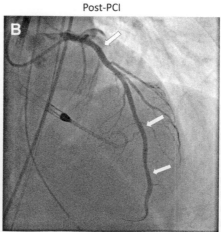

**Fig. 2.** Patient with acute anterior MI and cardiac arrest with CS. (*A*) Proximal LAD occlusion (*arrow*), with Impella in place. (*B*) Following primary PCI with stent, there is successful LAD reperfusion (*arrows*).

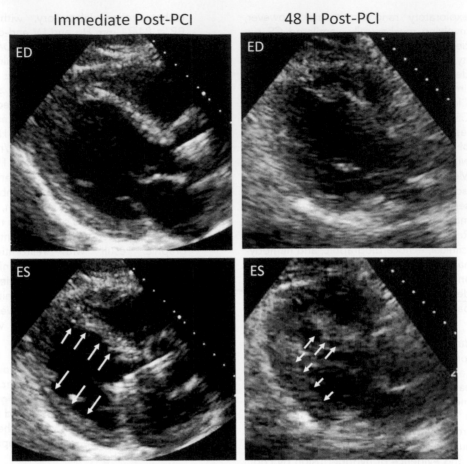

Immediate Post-PCI          48 H Post-PCI

Fig. 3. Echocardiograms in patient illustrated in **Fig. 2**. Immediately post-PCI with Impella in place, the LV is severely dilated at end diastole (ED) and there is global depression of systolic function at end systole (ES), with diffuse impairment of wall motion (*arrows*) and EF less than 30%. At 48 hours, the Impella has been removed and LV size markedly reduced at ED, with complete return of wall motion (*arrows*) and normalization of EF at ES.

### Case illustration: escalation of support in anterior ST segment elevation myocardial infarction with cardiogenic shock

- Clinical presentation and emergency department course: a 62-year-old man with type 2 diabetes mellitus, peripheral arterial disease with bilateral femoral to peroneal bypass, prior nonreperfused lateral infarct, and recent LAD stenting presents with severe chest pain and dyspnea. The patient was in respiratory distress, the BP = 59/41 mm Hg, heart rate 81, and the extremities were cool and mottled. ECG revealed new left bundle branch block. Norepinephrine was initiated and the patient was intubated urgently and taken to cardiac catheterization. Bedside echocardiogram was performed, which excluded mechanical complications of acute MI.

- Access: pelvic angiography was performed (**Fig. 4**A) to determine optimal site for Impella CP insertion. This is important for all patients, in particular those with peripheral arterial disease. Impella CP was placed prior to coronary angiography.
- Coronary angiography: chronic occlusion of the circumflex and subacute stent thrombosis of the mid-LAD coronary artery (see **Fig. 4**B)
- PCI: balloon angioplasty, intravascular ultrasound, and stenting of distal stent edge dissection (see **Fig. 4**C)
- Escalation of hemodynamic support: despite successful coronary intervention the cardiac power output was only 0.5 W and the pH remained 7.1. Therefore, via the right axillary artery, hemodynamic support was escalated from Impella CP to Impella 5.0 (see **Fig. 4**D). Cardiac power output increased to 0.8 W, pH improved

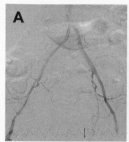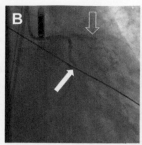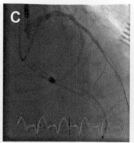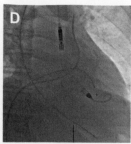

Fig. 4. Impella-supported PCI in patient with anterior MI and CS. (A) Peripheral angiogram provides map for safe insertion of Impella support. (B) Chronic occlusion of the proximal circumflex (*closed arrow*) and acute occlusion of the LAD (*open arrow*), with Impella CP in place. (C) Successful stenting of the LAD. Despite successful LAD recanalization, the patient remained hemodynamically unstable; therefore, hemodynamic support was upgraded to Impella 5.0 via axillary access (D).

to 7.36, and norepinephrine was weaned off. Patient was transferred for surgical LV assist device. This illustrates that after PCI hemodynamics must be reassessed to determine whether initial support strategies are sufficient or whether support must be escalated.

## Valvular Heart Disease and Complex Heart Failure Syndromes

Given the growing numbers of patients with compromised cardiac function undergoing percutaneous coronary and valve therapies and given the potential benefit of supporting LV function and systemic hemodynamics with a minimally invasive device, new applications for this technology are emerging. Among these, patients with severe, nonoperable valve disease represent a rapidly emerging population that may benefit from cardiac support during percutaneous aortic valvuloplasty or aortic valve replacement. Although in hemodynamically stable patients with severe symptomatic AS and CAD, PCI can be performed without significant increased risk, those with LVEF less than or equal to 30% and Society of Thoracic Surgeons score greater than or equal to 10% are at a higher risk of 30-day mortality. Such patients may benefit from percutaneous ventricular assist support during both the coronary and valvular intervention.[10] Significant CAD is present in half of patients undergoing TAVR. Although not all patients require revascularization before TAVR, PCI should be considered for severely stenotic lesions in proximal coronaries that subtend a large area of jeopardized myocardium. Special consideration should be given to patients with depressed LVEF and low-gradient severe AS. TAVR improves survival compared with medical therapy, but CAD severity and

incomplete revascularization predict worse outcomes.[11]

### Case illustration: impella-supported aortic valvuloplasty and high-risk percutaneous coronary intervention
Valvular heart disease

- Clinical presentation: an 86-year-old woman with hypertension and atrial fibrillation presented with New York Heart Association (NYHA) class III congestive HF. Echocardiogram revealed severe LV systolic dysfunction with EF = 20% and severe AS with mean gradient of 26 mm Hg and aortic valve area of 0.5 cm². Cardiac catheterization revealed 80% distal left main and 70% proximal LAD stenoses. PCWP was 28 mm Hg and pulmonary artery pressure was 64/33 mm Hg.
- Heart team discussion: the case was discussed at valve conference and it was decided to proceed with Impella-supported balloon aortic valvuloplasty and mechanical rotational atherectomy and stenting of the left main and LAD coronary arteries. Goal of care was to perform bicuspid aortic valvuloplasty (BAV) and PCI as bridge to TAVR.
- Angiography: severe calcified distal left main and proximal LAD stenoses (**Fig. 5**A)
- Impella-supported balloon aortic valvuloplasty: Impella 2.5 was inserted and BAV was performed with a 21-mm V8 (InterValve Inc, Plymouth, MN) (see **Fig. 5**B).
- Impella-supported PCI: mechanical rotational atherectomy (1.75-mm bur) and stenting (4.0-mm × 32-mm Promus stent (Boston Scientific, Boston, MA), postdilated 5.0-mm noncompliant balloon in left main) (see **Fig. 5**C, D).

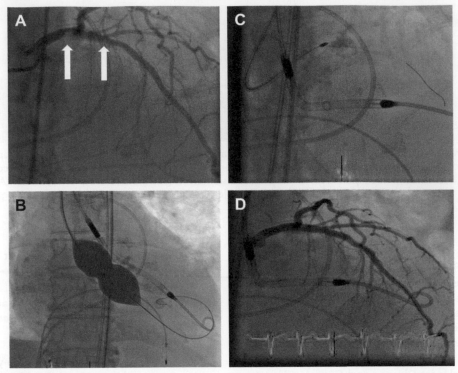

Fig. 5. (*A*) An 86-year-old woman with severe left main and LAD stenoses (*arrows*), severe AS, and severe LV systolic dysfunction. (*B*) Impella-supported balloon aortic valvuloplasty. (*C*) Impella-supported mechanical rotational atherectomy and stenting of LM-LAD. (*D*) Final angiography showing widely patent vessels.

## Case illustration: severe mitral regurgitation and aortic stenosis

- Clinical presentation: an 86-year-old woman with hypertension, type 2 diabetes mellitus, and prior coronary artery bypass graft surgery presented with acute decompensated NYHA class IV congestive HF. Echocardiogram revealed normal LV systolic function, moderate to severe AS, and severe MR due to flail A2 segment of the mitral valve (Fig. 6A, B). Invasive assessment revealed a mean aortic valve gradient of 30 mm Hg and an aortic valve area of 0.8 cm$^2$ (see Fig. 2)
- MitraClip (Abbott Vascular Inc, Santa Clara, CA) implantation: although TAVR is usually performed first in patients with combined aortic stenosis (AS) and MR (because MR is reduced by 1 grade in approximately 50% of patients), the MitraClip was implanted (see Fig. 6C) in this patient because it was thought that her sudden decompensation was secondary to chordal rupture. MR grade was reduced to mild (see Fig. 6D). The transaortic gradient increased to 65 mm Hg

with an aortic valve area of 0.5 cm$^2$ (Fig. 7B), presumably due to increased forward CO after reduction of MR.
- TAVR was performed 2 months later with a 26-mm Sapien 3 (Edwards Lifesciences, Irvine, CA) valve (see Fig. 7A) with resolution of aortic valve gradient (see Fig. 7C) and complete resolution of exertional dyspnea.

**Decompensated left ventricular pump failure.** HF is a major cause of global morbidity and mortality and is the most common admitting diagnosis in the United States. Underlying causes range from hypertensive and ischemic heart disease to valvular heart disease and primary cardiomyopathies. Nonischemic indications for use include acute exacerbation of chronic systolic failure as well as acute reversible cardiomyopathies, such as myocarditis, tachycardia-induced cardiomyopathy, takotsubo, acute transplant rejection, and so forth.

Approximately 50% of such patients suffer from diastolic HF, in whom mechanical support or percutaneous interventions are generally neither necessary nor helpful (novel drugs and

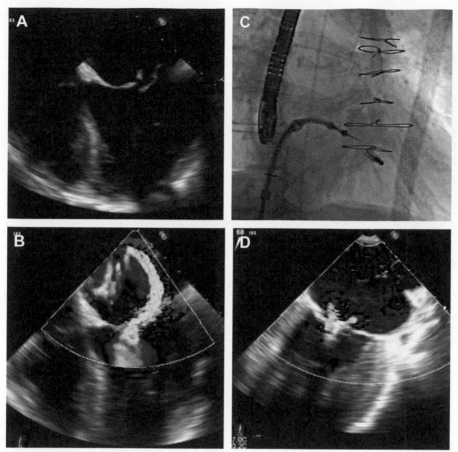

Fig. 6. An 86-year-old woman with acute decompensated NYHA class IV congestive HF, severe MR, and moderate to severe AS. (*A*) Flail A2 segment of the anterior mitral leaflet. (*B*) Severe eccentric MR. (*C*) Successful MitraClip implantation. (*D*) Mild residual MR after MitraClip.

devices are under active clinical investigation and may offer future interventions help). This section, therefore, focuses solely on decompensated HF attributable to severe LV pump failure, which may be a primary cardiomyopathy (which is often accompanied by complicating functional MR); HF may result from primary valvular lesions (AS and MR) or both primary cardiomyopathy and valve disease may coexist and complicate each other.

- Initial medical management: a majority of patients admitted with decompensated congestive HF due to LV systolic dysfunction can be successfully managed with medical therapy (IV diuretics and oral vasodilators). Unfortunately, despite appropriate initial medical measures, a significant proportion of patients suffer persistent pulmonary congestion, intractable right HF, and cardiorenal syndrome. Furthermore, it is not uncommon for

patients to dwindle along, not frankly unstable but unable to achieve progress; this frustrating cycle often occurs in which on the medical floor IV diuretics are administered with some diuresis and attempts at vasodilators are frustrated by borderline or low BP and/or elevating serum urea nibrogen and creatinine. Therefore, the patient is still decompensated or barely improved with respect to congestion and on essentially no vasodilators, thus doomed to poor functional class at best and repeated decompensation episodes at worst.

*Escalating therapies*
*Escalation step 1* Patients, as described previously with failure to thrive, should be considered for early escalation of therapy with more frequent and aggressive diuretic dosages and early initiation of inotropic support to provide augmented CO and BP, which then facilitate

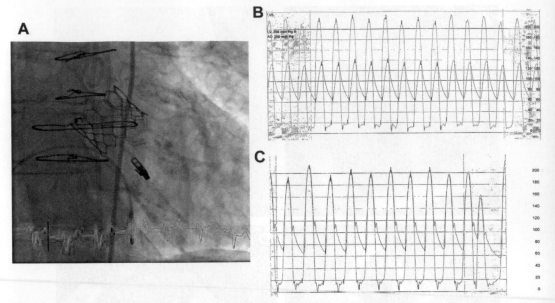

**Fig. 7.** (A) After MitraClip, the mean aortic valve gradient increased from 30 mm Hg to 65 mm Hg. (B) Staged TAVR with 26-mm Edwards Sapien 3 heart valve. (C) Resolution of aortic valve gradient after TAVR. Patient had complete relief of dyspnea.

titration of optimal vasodilator doses that are key to achieving further decongestion and optimal perfusion and restoration of organ function (including the kidneys) as well as longer-term hemodynamic compensation. These measures should in most cases be instituted in the CCU and with invasive right heart catheter monitoring.

*Escalation step 2* If these measures do not achieve adequate hemodynamic improvement, percutaneous mechanical circulatory support should be instituted. Although the IABP has been impugned in CS overall and shock associated with STEMI, in particular, and despite that direct power support devices such as Impella have been demonstrated superior in high-risk PCI, in patients with predominant decompensated HF, the IABP can be a powerful and relatively inexpensive support device to facilitate hemodynamic optimization. In this setting, the IABP accrues benefits by systolic augmentation, which augments mean aortic pressure, thereby enhancing systemic perfusion; diastolic unloading (deflation) reduces LV impedance to outflow, improving CO, and may indirectly decompress the heart by facilitating diuresis. BP stabilization then allows and aggressive titration of oral vasodilators essential for short-term and longer-term hemodynamic improvement. This device is easy to insert and inexpensive and can be performed in the CCU

without necessarily requiring the catheterization laboratory.

*Escalation step 3* In patients not responsive to steps 1 and 2, consideration of escalation of support by either surgical implantation of an LV assist device (LVAD) together with evaluation planning for transplantation as a critical strategy for appropriate candidates. In some such cases, a PVAD, such as the Impella, which provides direct cardiac support and greater cardiac power, may allow greater hemodynamic compensation and avoid the necessity of an LVAD or serve as bridge thereto. Surgically implanted LVADs as a bridge to recovery, bridge to transplant, or for use as permanent (ie, destination) therapy are now well established. Biventricular assist devices and the total artificial heart are also available as a bridge to transplant for patients with biventricular HF. These surgically definitive interventions increase the importance of PVAD devices as a treatment strategy to stabilize and advanced HF patients and render them more likely to do well with such surgical interventions. PVADs not only are attractive for the goal of stabilizing critically ill patients prior to additional therapies but also may serve to allow judicious decision regarding destination therapy and in some cases may act as a definitive intervention, allowing for myocardial recovery obviating destination therapy (eg, cases with acute HF from myocarditis).

## Right Heart Failure Syndromes

Shock due to acute RV failure is characterized by the clinical triad of hypotension–low CO, clear lungs, and disproportionately elevated jugular venous pressure. Acute RV failure may occur due to primary decreased contractility, such as in patients with acute inferior STEMI with RV involvement (RVI), post-LVAD implantation, or postcardiotomy after any cardiac surgical procedure.[12–17] Acute RV failure is also often seen as a result of acute pressure overload due to submassive or massive pulmonary emboli.

### Acute right ventricular infarction

Approximately 50% of patients with acute inferior STEMI manifest RVI by ECG or echocardiography, although fewer than half develop hemodynamic compromise. RVI is virtually always the result of proximal right coronary artery occlusion compromising RV free wall perfusion, resulting in depressed global RV performance, which diminishes transpulmonary delivery of LV preload, leading to decreased CO despite intact LV contractility. Biventricular diastolic dysfunction contributes to hemodynamic compromise.[12,13] Despite the absence of RV free wall contraction, an active albeit depressed RV systolic waveform is generated by systolic ventricular interactions mediated by primary septal contraction and through mechanical displacement of the septum into the RV cavity associated with paradoxic septal motion. Therefore, in the setting of acute RVI, global RV performance is dependent on LV contractile function. Despite LV inferior-posterior septal infarction, in most cases global LVEF is relatively preserved. When RVI develops in the setting of prior anterior myocardial infarction (MI) with impaired global LV dysfunction, however, the picture may be dominated by low output and pulmonary congestion, with right HF. These findings support the concept that under conditions of acute ischemic RV dysfunction, biventricular performance and systemic hemodynamics are critically dependent on both RV and LV contractile function, which may have clinical implications for biventricular mechanical support in some cases.

Therapeutic options for management of hemodynamically significant RVI may be categorized according to temporal format as follows.

### Prereperfusion therapies

**Rhythm.** Patients with acute RVI are at increased risk for vagal-mediated reflex induced high-grade atrioventricular (AV) block and bradycardia-hypotension without AV block, both during occlusion as well as abruptly during reperfusion. Although atropine may restore physiologic rhythm in some patients, temporary pacing is often required. Caution and expertise are required for manipulating catheters within the dilated ischemic RV may also induce ventricular arrhythmias.

**Preload.** In patients with RVI, the dilated, noncompliant right ventricle (RV) is exquisitely preload dependent, as is the LV, which is stiff but preload deprived. Therefore, any factor that reduces ventricular preload tends to be detrimental. Accordingly, vasodilators and diuretics are contraindicated. An initial volume challenge is appropriate for patients manifesting low output without pulmonary congestion, particularly if the estimated central venous pressure is less than 15 mm Hg. Caution should be exercised to avoid excessive volume administration above and beyond that documented to augment output, because the right heart chambers may operate on a descending limb of the Starling curve, resulting in further depression of RV pump performance as well as inducing severe systemic venous congestion.

**Inotropes/vasopressors.** Parenteral inotropic support is usually effective in stabilizing hemodynamically compromised patients not fully responsive to restoration of physiologic rhythm and gentle volume resuscitation. In patients with RV shock, inotropic stimulation enhances RV performance by increasing LV-septal contraction, which thereby augments septal-mediated systolic ventricular interactions.[12–15] Although an inotropic agent, such as dobutamine, which has the least deleterious effects on afterload, oxygen consumption, and arrhythmias, is the preferred initial drug of choice, patients with severe hypotension may require agents with vasopressor effects (such as dopamine) for prompt restoration of adequate coronary perfusion pressure.

### Reperfusion therapy

The term, *RV infarction*, is a misnomer, because superior oxygen supply-demand characteristics render an acutely ischemic RV relatively resistant to irreversible injury. The ischemic RV, therefore, responds favorably to successful reperfusion, even late after the onset of occlusion.[14] Successful primary mechanical right coronary artery reperfusion generally leads to rapid improvement in and later complete recovery of RV function, associated with excellent clinical outcomes. In a majority of patients who manifest initial hemodynamic compromise, successful reperfusion results in early hemodynamic improvement.

Some patients may require persistent inotropic/mechanical support, however, until RV function recovers. Also, acute reperfusion may elicit reflex bradycardia and hypotension; thus, the operator must be prepared for rapid temporary pacemaker placement.

### Persistent hemodynamic compromise in acute right ventricular infarciton

Persistent hemodynamic compromise may necessitate consideration of mechanical support and may be necessary either just prior to or during reperfusion in RVI patients with profound hypotension or in some cases with slower recovery of right heart function and. Regardless, given that ischemic RV failure is typically reversible, application of short-term percutaneous mechanical hemodynamic support may provide a bridge to recovery for refractory RV shock. First principles dictate that in the setting of acute myocardial ischemia, restoration of BP sufficient to maintain organ and coronary perfusion is essential. Recent findings in patients with acute inferior MI complicated by predominant RV shock demonstrate the hemodynamic benefits of IABP support,[16] which promptly improves aortic pressure. It is hypothesized that IABP assist likely does not directly improve RV performance but rather exerts salutary effects indirectly by improving coronary perfusion, which may augment left coronary flow and thereby benefit LV function, which imparts benefits to the failing RV via enhanced LV-septal contractile contributions. In those cases in whom balloon pump support together with reperfusion is not adequate to restore circulation, a percutaneous RV assist device with the Impella RP promptly improves hemodynamics in patients with severe RV failure complicated by refractory life-threatening low output-hypotension. The direct RV power provided by Impella RP support immediately increases cardiac index and decreases central venous pressure, thereby providing a bridge to recovery.[17]

### Right ventricular shock due to acute pulmonary embolus

Acute submassive/massive pulmonary embolus leads to hemodynamic compromise as the thrombotically occluded pulmonary bed elevates pulmonary resistance, which, similar to cases of acute RVI, diminishes effective forward RV stroke volume and thereby reduces transpulmonary blood flow, which limits LV preload delivery and CO. The RV, a volume pump by design, is ill equipped to acutely adapt to pressure overload; thus, acute RV failure may

develop, which further reduces CO. Furthermore, similar to RVI, acute RV diastolic pressure/volume overload induces septal-mediated diastolic ventricular interactions, which further impairs LV compliance and filling. The acutely dilated pressure overload RV also becomes ischemic and is at particular risk for further deterioration in pump function, particularly if mean aortic perfusion pressure is decreased; it is, therefore, critical to restore BP in this setting by pharmacologic or mechanical measures.

- Massive pulmonary embolism with RV shock: pulmonary embolism is defined as massive based not on clot burden per se but by hemodynamic criteria of severe RV failure and manifest hypotension and is now typically managed by thrombolytic therapy, either systemically or in an increasing number of institutions by direct catheter infusion in an interventional suite, in some cases In conjunction with percutaneous catheter-directed thrombus aspiration techniques.[18] In patients profoundly compromised, or with clot in transit, emergency surgical thrombectomy can be life-saving. In some cases, temporary mechanical circulatory support is needed, typically venoarterial extracorporeal membrane oxygenation. Whether direct RV mechanical support via the Impella RP may be beneficial requires clinical investigation.

- Submassive pulmonary embolism, characterized by severe RV dilation and depressed global performance but the absence of manifest hypotension, can be managed medically with traditional anticoagulation and watchful waiting. Many institutions are increasingly using thrombolytic therapy, however, in patients at reasonable risk for these drugs, such as therapy administered either systemically or in an increasing number of cases by direct catheter infusion.

### Acute right ventricular pump failure post–left ventricular assist device or cardiovascular surgery

Acute RV failure may complicate both percutaneous and implantable LVAD; its occurrence is associated with poor outcome.[17] Although the precise mechanisms leading to post-LVAD RV failure have not been fully delineated, the presence of severe RV systolic dysfunction and clinical right HF are risk factors for this potentially devastating complication. Analogous to the importance of LV-septal contraction to RV systolic performance in patients with acute RVI, when it may postulated that reduction of LV contributes to support of a chronically failing RV, may be one mechanism by which RV failure develops after surgical LVAD implantation. That is, the LV is decompressed and the interventricular septum shifts toward the LV, which may impair its contribution to RV performance. This, combined with increased RV preload in the setting of increased venous return with LVAD, creates a perfect storm of acute RV dysfunction and hemodynamic compromise. The Impella RP offers temporary active right heart support and, similar to the benefits described previously in acute RVI, its efficacy has been demonstrated in such patients suffering RV shock postcardiotomy and post-LVAD.[17]

**Chronic right ventricular failure.** In the setting of chronic left HF, RV failure is common and may be attributable to both a primary nonischemic cardiomyopathic insult to the RV as well as to the effects of postcapillary pulmonary hypertension from left HF. In the setting of chronic congestive heart failure, the magnitude of RV systolic dysfunction and clinical right HF exacerbate hemodynamic compromise for any degree of LV systolic dysfunction and increase mortality.[19] Severe RV systolic dysfunction and clinical right HF also identify patients at increased risk of hemodynamic compromise after surgical LVAD implantation or cardiac transplantation. Whether there is a therapeutic role for percutaneous RV support with the Impella RP, alone or together with LV mechanical support, requires further investigation.

# REFERENCES

1. Rihal CS, Naidu SS, Givertz MM, et al. Clinical Expert Consensus Statement on the Use of Percutaneous Mechanical Circulatory Support Devices in Cardiovascular Care From the Society for Cardiovascular Angiography and Interventions (SCAI), Heart Failure Society of America (HFSA), Society for Thoracic Surgeons (STS), American Heart Association (AHA) and American College of Cardiology Foundation (ACCF0 Co-Published in J Am Coll Cardiol 2015;65:2140–1, Catheter Cardiovasc Interv 2015;85:1112-4, and J Card Fail 2015;21:499-518.

2. Naidu SS. Novel percutaneous cardiac assist devices: The science of and indications for hemodynamic support. Circulation 2011;123: 533–43.

3. Dixon SR, Henriques JP, Mauri L, et al. A prospective feasibility trial investigating the use of the Impella 2.5 system in patients undergoing high-risk percutaneous coronary intervention (the PROTECT 1 Trial): initial US experience. J Am Coll Cardiol Cardiovasc Interv 2009;2:91–6.

4. Maini B, Naidu SS, Mulukutla S, et al. Real-world use of the Impella 2.5 circulatory support system in complex high-risk percutaneous coronary intervention: the USpella Registry. Catheter Cardiovasc Interv 2012;80(5):717–25.

5. O'Neill WW, Kleiman NS, Moses J, et al. A prospective, randomized clinical trial of hemodynamic support with Impella 2.5 versus intra-aortic balloon pump in patients undergoing high-risk percutaneous coronary intervention: the PROTECT II study. Circulation 2012;126(14):1717–27.

6. Thiele H, Zeymer U, Neumann FJ, et al. Intraaortic balloon support for myocardial infarction with cardiogenic shock. N Engl J Med 2012;367: 1287–96.

7. Seyfarth M, Sibbing D, Bauer I, et al. A randomized clinical trial to evaluate the safety and efficacy of a percutaneous left ventricular assist device versus intra-aortic balloon pumping for treatment of cardiogenic shock caused by myocardial infarction. J Am Coll Cardiol 2008 Nov 4;52(19):1584–8.

8. Ouweneel DM, Eriksen E, Sjauw KD, et al. Percutaneous mechanical circulatory support versus intra-aortic balloon pump in cardiogenic shock after acute myocardial infarction. J Am Coll Cardiol 2017;69:278–87.

9. Hochman JS, Sleeper LA, Webb JG, et al, for the SHOCK Investigators. Early revascularization in acute myocardial infarction complicated by cardiogenic shock. N Engl J Med 1999;341:625–34.

10. Goel SS, Ige M, Tuzcu EM, et al. Severe aortic stenosis and coronary artery disease—implications for management in the transcatheter aortic valve replacement era: a comprehensive review. J Am Coll Cardiol 2013;62:1–10.

11. O'Sullivan CJ, Englberger L, Hosek N, et al. Clinical outcomes and revascularization strategies in patients with low-flow, low-gradient severe aortic valve stenosis according to the assigned treatment modality. JACC Cardiovasc Interv 2015;8: 704–17.

12. Goldstein JA. State of the art review: Pathophysiology and management of right heart ischemia. J Am Coll Cardiol 2002;40:841–85.

13. Goldstein JA, Barzilai B, Rosamond TL, et al. Determinants of hemodynamic compromise with severe right ventricular infarction. Circulation 1990;82: 359–68.

14. Bowers TR, O'Neill WW, Grines C, et al. Effect of reperfusion on biventricular function and survival

after right ventricular infarction. N Engl J Med 1998;
338:933–40.

15. Goldstein JA, Kommuri N, Dixon SR. LV systolic
dysfunction is associated with adverse outcomes in
acute right ventricular infarction. Coron Artery Dis
2016;27:277–86.

16. McNamara M, Dixon SD, Goldstein JA. Impact of
intra-aortic balloon pumping on hypotension and
outcomes in acute right ventricular infarction. Coron
Artery Dis 2014;25:602.

17. Anderson M, Goldstein JA, Morris L, et al.
Benefits of a novel percutaneous ventricular

assist device for right heart failure. the prospective RECOVER RIGHT study of the impella
RP device. J Heart Lung Transplant 2015;34:
1549–60.

18. Konstantinides SV, Barco S, Lankeit M, et al.
Citation: management of pulmonary embolism:
an update. J Am Coll Cardiol 2016;67:976–90.

19. Ghio S, Gavazzi A, Campana C, et al. Independent
and additive prognostic value of right ventricular
systolic function and pulmonary artery pressure in
patients with chronic heart failure. J Am Coll Cardiol 2001;37:183–8.

# Integrating Interventional Cardiology and Heart Failure Management for Cardiogenic Shock

 CrossMark

Navin K. Kapur, MD[a],*, Carlos D. Davila, MD[a],
Marwan F. Jumean, MD[b]

## KEYWORDS

- Interventional heart failure • Mechanical circulatory support • Heart team • Cardiogenic shock

## KEY POINTS

- Cardiogenic shock remains a major clinical problem with high rates of in-hospital mortality that have not changed significantly over the past 3 decades.
- The primary objectives when managing cardiogenic shock include providing (1) circulatory support, (2) ventricular unloading, and (3) coronary perfusion.
- The use of percutaneous acute mechanical circulatory support (AMCS) has steadily grown in the last decade.
- Four primary AMCS device platforms are clinically available for hemodynamic support and include (1) the intra-aortic balloon pump (IABP), (2) TandemHeart (TandemLife, Pittsburgh, PA), (3) centrifugally driven venoarterial extracorporeal membrane oxygenation (VA-ECMO), and (4) microaxial flow catheters (Impella, Abiomed, Danvers, MA).
- Interventional heart failure (IHF) is an emerging specialty within cardiology.

## THE SPECTRUM OF ADVANCED HEART FAILURE AND CARDIOGENIC SHOCK

Cardiogenic shock remains a major clinical problem with high rates of in-hospital mortality that have not changed significantly over the past 3 decades.[1–3] One potential explanation for the lack of progress in the management of cardiogenic shock is that the profile of patients presenting with cardiogenic shock has changed. In the late 1980s, the SHOCK trial (Should We Emergently Revascularize Occluded Coronaries for Cardiogenic Shock) highlighted the beneficial impact of early revascularization on long-term outcomes among patients with acute myocardial infarction (AMI) complicated by cardiogenic shock.[4] For this reason, more patients are surviving AMI and shock, which has contributed to the growing population of patients with advanced heart failure.[5] Recent projections estimated that more than 8 million individuals in the United States alone will be diagnosed with heart failure.[6] As a result, more patients currently presenting with cardiogenic shock tend to be older, have more comorbidities, and have preexisting cardiovascular disease, including prior myocardial infarction or heart failure.[7] This new complex profile of

Disclosure Statement: N.K. Kapur receives research support, consulting fees, and speaker honoraria from Abiomed Inc, Maquet-Getinge Inc, St. Jude Inc, and Cardiac Assist Inc. He also receives NIH grant support (1R01HL133215-01). No relevant disclosures for C.D. Davila and M.F. Jumean.
a The Acute Mechanical Support Working Group, The Cardiovascular Center, Tufts Medical Center, 800 Washington Street, Boston, MA 02111, USA; b Center for Advanced Heart Failure, University of Texas Health Medical School, 6400 Fannin Street, Houston, TX 77030, USA
* Corresponding author. The Cardiovascular Center, Tufts Medical Center, 800 Washington Street, Box # 80, Boston, MA 02111.
E-mail address: Nkapur@tuftsmedicalcenter.org

http://dx.doi.org/10.1016/j.iccl.2017.03.014
2211-7458/17/© 2017 Elsevier Inc. All rights reserved.

cardiogenic shock requires a more comprehensive management approach that involves both interventional cardiologists and advanced heart failure cardiologists.

## CHANGING OBJECTIVES FOR THE MANAGEMENT OF CARDIOGENIC SHOCK

Three primary objectives when managing cardiogenic shock include providing (1) circulatory support, (2) ventricular unloading, and (3) coronary perfusion (Fig. 1). The sequence of achieving these 3 objectives must be tailored to each patient. Although early revascularization for cardiogenic shock secondary to AMI remains an important therapeutic objective, a recent analysis of patients with ST segment elevation myocardial infarction (STEMI) failed to identify any incremental reduction in in-hospital mortality with door-to-balloon reperfusion times less than 90 minutes.[8] These data suggest that timely coronary reperfusion alone may be insufficient to reduce mortality associated with cardiogenic shock and that other therapeutic objectives may take priority depending on the clinical scenario. For example, a patient with profound hypoperfusion due to low cardiac output in the setting STEMI may not benefit from immediate coronary reperfusion but instead may require stabilization of their mean arterial pressure (circulatory support) and a reduction in cardiac filling pressures before reperfusion. Typically, physicians start vasopressors and inotropes, which may partially achieve these objectives but at the cost of reducing end-organ microvascular perfusion and forcing the heart to work harder. The net result is more myocardial oxygen consumption and potentially worse myocardial ischemia. In contemporary clinical practice, the 3 objectives of shock management can be achieved using AMCS pumps.

## MECHANICAL CIRCULATORY SUPPORT: INTERVENTIONAL TOOLS FOR COMPLEX HEART FAILURE AND SHOCK

In contrast to the IABP, the rotary flow pumps that can achieve these objectives include both intracorporeal axial-flow (Impella, Abiomed) and extracorporeal centrifugal flow (Tandem-Heart, TandemLife) pumps that can directly reduce ventricular filling pressures while increasing mean arterial pressure within minutes of activation.[9] The TandemHeart left ventricular (LV) support pump requires a trans-septal puncture and diverts blood from the left atrium to the femoral artery using 2 large-bore cannulas. The Impella pump is a transvalvular pump that diverts blood from the left ventricle to the aorta. In contrast to the TandemHeart LV pump, the Impella series of pumps can be implanted via the femoral, brachial, or axillary approach. Access via the brachial or axillary approach allows for increased patient mobility, which becomes critically important when managing patients in shock awaiting myocardial recovery, a decision to advanced therapies, or palliation. Under emergent conditions, both the Impella and TandemHeart devices may be deployed quickly; however, emergent trans-septal puncture is not commonly performed in most centers. VA-ECMO is another support option that pumps

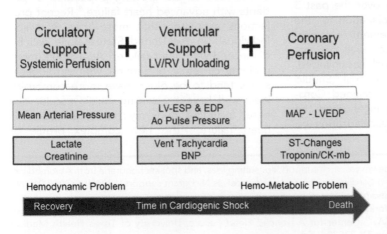

Fig. 1. Illustration of the acute hemodynamic support equation. Circulatory support is defined by an increase in mean arterial pressure. Ventricular support is defined by a reduction in LV pressure and volume, thereby reducing myocardial wall stress and oxygen demand. Coronary perfusion is defined by an increase in the transmyocardial gradient, which is determined by the difference between coronary arterial and LV end-diastolic pressure. The net effect of optimal hemodynamic support is increased urine output, reduced serum lactate, reduced pulmonary capillary wedge pressure, resolution of ischemic electrocardiographic changes, and reduced levels of myocardial injury biomarkers, such as creatine kinase–MB. An ideal mechanical circulatory support device would target all elements of the hemodynamic equation and prove safe and easy to use in the acute setting. Ao, aortic; BNP, brain natriuretic peptide; CK-MB, Creatine Kinase-MB; EDP, end-diastolic pressure; ESP, end-systolic pressure; MAP, mean arterial pressure.

and oxygenates blood from the venous to arterial circulation. In contrast to the Impella and TandemHeart devices that directly unload the left-sided circulation, VA-ECMO indirectly unloads the LV if a large enough venous drainage cannula is placed; otherwise, a concomitant use of an LV unloading device may be required.[10,11] For this use, Impella seems more beneficial than IABP. Although none of these 3 AMCS is complication-free, all can rapidly achieve the 3 primary objective of cardiogenic shock in the setting of STEMI with profound systemic hypoperfusion due to low cardiac output. Recent data support that first providing circulatory and ventricular support before coronary reperfusion reduces short-term mortality among patients with STEMI and shock.[12]

## THE HEART TEAM: AN EVOLVING MULTISPECIALTY COLLABORATION

Over the past 2 decades, growth in 3 major cardiac device domains helped to shape contemporary practice around cardiogenic shock. The REMATCH trial (Randomized Evaluation of Mechanical Assistance for the Treatment of Congestive Heart Failure) in 2001 showed a reduction of 48% in the risk of death in advanced heart failure patients receiving pulsatile left ventricular assist device (LVAD) therapy compared with optimal medical therapy.[13] A landmark study identified that the Heartmate II (Thoratec, Pleasanton, CA) rotary flow LVAD demonstrated superior clinical outcomes compared with pulsatile LVADs for patients with advanced heart failure.[14] This trial triggered immense growth in the use of LVADs. Around the same time, AMCS device use within the interventional cardiology community was growing for high-risk percutaneous coronary intervention and for cardiogenic shock.[15,16] Third, the growing use of percutaneous aortic valve replacement programs supported the ongoing cross-talk between cardiac surgery, interventional cardiology, and advanced heart failure specialists. This unique collaboration, commonly known as the heart team approach, is now applied to patients with cardiogenic shock and includes a growing role for cardiac intensive care specialists (Fig. 2).

Communication and teamwork among these 4 core groups are fundamental to optimizing clinical outcomes in cardiogenic shock. Depending on the clinical scenario, the role of each of these 4 components may change. The role of the interventional cardiologist on the heart team is to provide coronary revascularization, invasive hemodynamic assessment, and then AMCS for LV, right ventricular, or biventricular failure. This

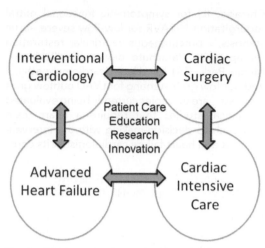

Fig. 2. Components of a cardiogenic shock team.

approach allows for reversal of underlying causes of shock and early implementation of AMCS in cardiogenic shock when necessary. The role of the cardiac surgeon on the heart team is to manage post-MI mechanical complications and surgical coronary revascularization if PCI is not an option, to assist with initiation of AMCS or VA-ECMO, and to provide input regarding candidacy for LVAD or orthotopic heart transplantation (OHTx). The advanced heart failure specialist also assists with evaluating a patient's candidacy for LVAD or OHTx, hemodynamic optimization, and management of AMCS or VA-ECMO and provides input regarding end-of-life decision making, palliation, and medical futility. Finally, the role of the cardiac intensivist is a critically important component of a successful cardiogenic shock program. In addition to assisting with hemodynamic optimization and AMCS device management, the intensivist provides key input on the management of noncardiac organ systems, including pulmonary, renal, hepatic, and hematologic abnormalities as well as prevention and management of infectious issues. Furthermore, intensivists provide input on nutrition, early mobilization, and prophylaxis against deep venous thrombosis, gastric ulcers, and cutaneous ulcers. Recent data support that incorporation of a cardiac intensivist improves short and long-term mortality for cardiogenic shock.[17]

## BEYOND SHOCK: THE EXPANDING ROLE OF INTERVENTIONAL CARDIOLOGY

Similar to the expansion in armamentarium of AMCS in acute and chronic heart failure over the past decade, a similar trend has happened in structural interventions for this increasing patient population. The use of MitraClip (Abbott,

Chicago, IL) for symptomatic functional mitral regurgitation,[18] TAVR for low-flow severe aortic stenosis,[19] percutaneous ventricular restoration therapy with Parachute device (Cardiokinetix, Menlo Park, CA) for dilated cardiomyopathy,[20] and outflow graft stenting for LVAD outflow graft stenosis[21] are therapies currently being evaluated in clinical studies that require a heart team approach to decision-making with the interventionalist and heart failure cardiologist at its core.

## INTERVENTIONAL HEART FAILURE TRAINING: IS THIS RIGHT FOR ME?

Contemporary training programs focus on developing 1 of the 4 specialists required for the heart team. As understanding of hemodynamics, metabolic failure, and the importance of early initiation of AMCS devices grows, training programs will need to adapt. Although many interventionalists may be comfortable with AMCS device implantation and invasive hemodynamic catheter placement, decision making around AMCS device management, patient candidacy, and a viable exit strategy (that is, recovery, LVAD therapy, or OHTx candidacy) or the role of pharmacologic therapy for advanced heart failure and shock is not part of the typical interventional training curriculum. Advanced heart failure fellowship offers the reciprocal training experience with no exposure to implantation of AMCS devices or advanced hemodynamics in the catheterization laboratory. Furthermore, formal training in cardiac intensive care is often lacking in most cardiology training programs. As a result, fellows in training are beginning to seek programs where they can complete combined advanced training in interventional cardiology, heart failure, or critical care.

Fellows considering training in both interventional cardiology and advanced heart failure, however, must ask themselves a fundamental question, "If you had to choose one pathway, which would it be — interventional cardiology or advanced heart failure?" If the answer is interventional cardiology, then IHF training may be the right path to pursue.[22] IHF training allows trainees to technically function as interventional operators with the ability to handle vascular, coronary, ventricular, and basic structural interventions, while at the same time acquiring the cognitive skills to understand the fundamentals of heart failure physiology and advanced heart failure decision making. This 2-year program optimally begins with advanced heart failure training for months 1 to 12 and ends with interventional training in months 13 to 24. IHF graduates should be board-eligible in both

interventional cardiology and advanced heart failure. Graduates of IHF training programs should seek interventional positions within a team-based structure for management of advanced heart failure patients.

If the answer to that fundamental question is advanced heart failure, then IHF training may not be the right path to pursue. Most fellows whose primary interest is advanced heart failure wish to pursue interventional training to gain skills for device implantation. Implanting AMCS devices is not a reason, however, to pursue interventional cardiology training. Without a strong commitment to interventional cardiology as a clinical practice, IHF training only serves to develop substandard operators who do not routinely perform cardiac interventions but rather intermittently are exposed to the catheterization laboratory. For those fellows interested primarily in advanced heart failure, new programs, such as the Training and Education in Advanced Cardiovascular Hemodynamics (TEACH) program provide an in-depth understanding of advanced hemodynamics in heart failure and shock as well as a deep understanding of mechanical support device management.

Over the next decade, understanding of acute and chronic heart failure device management will change immensely. This change will be driven by growth in the number of patients with heart failure, increasing patient complexity, and new diagnostic and therapeutic options for these patients. With appropriate training, collaboration among each of the 4 physician components of the heart team will ultimately lead to better patient outcomes.

## REFERENCES

1. Goldberg RJ, Gore JM, Thompson CA, et al. Recent magnitude of and temporal trends (1994-1997) in the incidence and hospital death rates of cardiogenic shock complicating acute myocardial infarction: the second national registry of myocardial infarction. Am Heart J 2001;141(1):65–72.

2. Goldberg RJ, Samad NA, Yarzebski J, et al. Temporal trends in cardiogenic shock complicating acute myocardial infarction. N Engl J Med 1999; 340(15):1162–8.

3. Wayangankar SA, Bangalore S, McCoy LA, et al. Temporal trends and outcomes of patients undergoing percutaneous coronary interventions for cardiogenic shock in the setting of acute myocardial infarction: a report from the CathPCI Registry. JACC Cardiovasc Interv 2016;9(4):341–51.

4. Hochman JS, Sleeper LA, Webb JG, et al. Early revascularization in acute myocardial infarction

complicated by cardiogenic shock. SHOCK Investigators. Should we emergently revascularize occluded coronaries for cardiogenic shock. N Engl J Med 1999;341(9):625–34.

5. Ezekowitz JA, Armstrong PW, Granger CB, et al. Predicting chronic left ventricular dysfunction 90 days after ST-segment elevation myocardial infarction: An Assessment of Pexelizumab in Acute Myocardial Infarction (APEX-AMI) Substudy. Am Heart J 2010;160(2):272–8.

6. Hunt SA, Abraham WT, Chin MH, et al. 2009 focused update incorporated into the ACC/AHA 2005 guidelines for the diagnosis and management of heart failure in adults: a report of the American College of Cardiology Foundation/American Heart Association Task Force on Practice Guidelines: developed in collaboration with the International Society for Heart and Lung Transplantation. Circulation 2009;119(14):e391–479.

7. Ezekowitz JA, Kaul P, Bakal JA, et al. Declining in-hospital mortality and increasing heart failure incidence in elderly patients with first myocardial infarction. J Am Coll Cardiol 2009;53(1):13–20.

8. Menees DS, Peterson ED, Wang Y, et al. Door-to-balloon time and mortality among patients undergoing primary PCI. N Engl J Med 2013;369(10):901–9.

9. Morine KJ, Kapur NK. Percutaneous mechanical circulatory support for cardiogenic shock. Curr Treat Options Cardiovasc Med 2016;18(1):6.

10. Aghili N, Kang S, Kapur NK. The fundamentals of extra-corporeal membrane oxygenation. Minerva Cardioangiol 2015;63(1):75–85.

11. Kapur NK, Zisa DC. Veno-arterial extracorporeal membrane oxygenation (VA-ECMO) fails to solve the haemodynamic support equation in cardiogenic shock. EuroIntervention 2016;11(12):1337–9.

12. O'Neill WW, Schreiber T, Wohns DH, et al. The current use of Impella 2.5 in acute myocardial infarction complicated by cardiogenic shock: results from the USpella Registry. J Interv Cardiol 2014;27(1):1–11.

13. Rose EA, Gelijns AC, Moskowitz AJ, et al. Long-term use of a left ventricular assist device for end-stage heart failure. N Engl J Med 2001;345(20):1435–43.

14. Slaughter MS, Rogers JG, Milano CA, et al. Advanced heart failure treated with continuous-flow left ventricular assist device. N Engl J Med 2009;361(23):2241–51.

15. Stretch R, Sauer CM, Yuh DD, et al. National trends in the utilization of short-term mechanical circulatory support: incidence, outcomes, and cost analysis. J Am Coll Cardiol 2014;64(14):1407–15.

16. Sandhu A, McCoy LA, Negi SI, et al. Use of mechanical circulatory support in patients undergoing percutaneous coronary intervention: insights from the National Cardiovascular Data Registry. Circulation 2015;132(13):1243–51.

17. Na SJ, Chung CR, Jeon K, et al. Association between presence of a cardiac intensivist and mortality in an adult cardiac care unit. J Am Coll Cardiol 2016;68(24):2637–48.

18. Stone G, Abraham W, Lindenfeld J, et al. TCT-627 Cardiovascular Outcomes Assessment of MitraClip Therapy in Heart Failure Patients with Functional Mitral Regurgitation (The COAPT Trial): baseline characteristics and preliminary 30-day and 1-year outcomes of the roll-in cohort. J Am Coll Cardiol 2016;68(18S):B255.

19. Martinez CA, Singh V, Heldman AW, et al. Emergent use of retrograde left ventricular support in patients after transcatheter aortic valve replacement. Catheter Cardiovasc Interv 2013;82(2):E128–32.

20. Costa MA, Mazzaferri EL Jr, Sievert H, et al. Percutaneous ventricular restoration using the parachute device in patients with ischemic heart failure: three-year outcomes of the PARACHUTE first-in-human study. Circ Heart Fail 2014;7(5):752–8.

21. Pham DT, Kapur NK, Dermody M, et al. Stenting of an outflow graft obstruction after implantation of a continuous-flow, axial-flow left ventricular assist device. J Thorac Cardiovasc Surg 2015;150(1):e11–2.

22. Kapur NK, Dimas V, Sorajja P, et al. The Interventional Heart Failure Initiative: a mission statement for the next generation of invasive cardiologists. Catheter Cardiovasc Interv 2015;86(2):353–5.

# Moving?

## Make sure your subscription moves with you!

To notify us of your new address, find your **Clinics Account Number** (located on your mailing label above your name), and contact customer service at:

**Email: journalscustomerservice-usa@elsevier.com**

**800-654-2452** (subscribers in the U.S. & Canada)
**314-447-8871** (subscribers outside of the U.S. & Canada)

**Fax number: 314-447-8029**

**Elsevier Health Sciences Division**
**Subscription Customer Service**
**3251 Riverport Lane**
**Maryland Heights, MO 63043**

*To ensure uninterrupted delivery of your subscription, please notify us at least 4 weeks in advance of move.

Printed and bound by CPI Group (UK) Ltd, Croydon, CR0 4YY

03/10/2024

01040384-0013